Konrad Maurer (Ed.)

Imaging of the Brain in Psychiatry and Related Fields

With 101 Figures, 15 in Color

Springer-Verlag
Berlin Heidelberg New York
London Paris Tokyo
Hong Kong Barcelona
Budapest

Konrad Maurer, M.D.
Professor of Psychiatry,
Neurology, Psychotherapy
Department of Psychiatry
University of Würzburg
Füchsleinstr. 15

W-8700 Würzburg, FRG

ISBN 3-540-54785-1 Springer-Verlag Berlin Heidelberg New York
ISBN 0-387-54785-1 Springer-Verlag New York Berlin Heidelberg

Library of Congress Cataloging-in-Publication Data. Imaging of the brain in psychiatry and related fields / Konrad Maurer (ed.). p. cm. Includes bibliographical references and index. ISBN 3-540-54785-1 (alk. paper). – ISBN 0-387-54785-1 (alk. paper) 1. Brain – Imaging. 2. Brain – Pathophysiology. 3. Schizophrenia – Pathophysiology. I. Maurer, Konrad, 1943– . [DNLM: 1. Brain – physiopathology. 2. Brain – radionuclide imaging. 3. Diagnostic Imaging – methods. 4. Electroencephalography. 5. Mental Disorders – diagnosis. 6. Psychiatry – methods. WM 141 131] RC386.6.D52I4 1992 616.8′04754 – dc20 DNLM/DLC

Printed in Hong Kong

Typesetting: Best-Set, Typesetter Ltd., Hong Kong
25/3130-543210-Printed on acid-free paper

Preface

In the last two decades imaging of the brain, or neuroimaging, has become an integral part of clinical and research psychiatry. This is due to recent advances in computer technology, which has made it relatively easy to generate brain images representing structure and function of the central nervous system.

Currently used clinical diagnostic imaging modalities, such as X-ray computed tomography (CT) and magnetic resonance imaging (MRI), provide predominantly anatomic information. CT images reflect X-ray attenuation distribution within the brain, whereas MRI signals depend primarily on proton sensitivity and tissue relaxivity.

The chapter "Structural Imaging Methods" reviews CT and MRI studies on schizophrenic and affective disorders and degenerative central nervous system diseases. The impact of fast three-dimensional (3-D) imaging and the automatic transfer from 3-D elements in the brain to artificial diagrams based on this information is considered.

Since the original report of the findings of Ingvar and Franzen in 1974 and the introduction of regional cerebral blood flow (rCBF) measurements, single photon emission computed tomography (SPECT) has been gaining acceptance as one of the major imaging techniques, and it is available in most nuclear medicine departments. The section "Functional Imaging Methods (Cerebral Blood Flow – CBF, Single Photon Emission Computerized Tomography – SPECT)" describes rCBF studies with the ^{133}Xe inhalation method utilizing a 254 detector system and rCBF images measured by SPECT using the tracer ^{99m}Tc-HMPAO. The authors provide a comprehensive account of this technique, including a brief summary of the basic principles, various methods of application, and recent findings in most psychiatric disorders. Analogies to its "aristocratic cousin" positron emission tomography (PET) are presented to emphasize the similarities and differences.

PET has been widely used as a research tool in the investigation of human physiology and pathology for over a decade. By labeling suitable components (i.e., glucose, amino acids, ammonia, DOPA, or drugs) with positron emitting isotopes, which are then administered in tracer amounts, blood flow, metabolism, and even cell receptor or neurotransmitter distribution can be assessed in vivo. The section "Functional Imaging Methods (Positron Emission Tomography – PET)" endeavors to explain briefly the principles of the PET technique and then outlines promising areas in which PET has become clinically useful, such as neuroreceptor and dopamine receptor imaging.

The birth of magnetoencephalography (MEG) in the 1970s and its development in the 1980s came at a time when CT and MRI were able to provide excellent structural images of the brain. The current generation of equipment with nearly 40 MEG channels has already provided a unique view in the brain, and samples from these studies are discussed in the section "Functional Imaging Methods (Magnetencephalography – MEG)."

Mapping of spontaneous and activated EEG activity and evoked potentials uses computer technology to quantify the electrophysiological data and plot out results in an understandable form. It also employs statistical tests to give significance to the data analyzed. Advantages over the other imaging methods are extremely short analysis times, in the millisecond range, and noninvasiveness, with the possibility of performing follow-up examinations as often as needed. The section "Functional Imaging Methods (Computerized Electroencephalographic Topography – CET)" describes the major findings of EEG and EP mapping in psychiatry, also including advanced methods such as dipole source estimation, neurometrics, and microstates of the brain's electrical fields.

A section has been devoted to the multimodal application of imaging measurements. Within this section imaging procedures such as CET and PET have been applied simultaneously to explore pathophysiologic and metabolic peculiarities in psychoses. The so-called biochemical imaging (BCI) describes topographic maps of biochemical data (biopsy, neurotransmitter, postmortem) and includes immunocytochemistry, autoradiography and topography of drug action. Imaging techniques can now even be used to assess neuropsychological data; this is called behavioral imaging.

The impetus for this book was provided at an international symposium entitled "Imaging of the Brain in Psychiatry and Related Fields," which took place in 1990 in Würzburg, Germany. This symposium was also the inaugural meeting of the International Society for Neuroimaging in Psychiatry (ISNIP). Participants who presented their data at the symposium were asked to prepare a contribution to this volume, discussing their recent research activities and clinical results. Altogether 54 chapters written by a total of 206 authors are presented here. These authors, who represent research laboratories and clinics in many parts of Europe, Japan,

Australia, and the United States, include original pioneers as well as current experts in the field of neuroimaging in psychiatry. Through the high quality of their scientific and clinical data, they all have made valuable contributions both to the symposium and to this volume. I wish to express my sincere thanks to all of them.

I would also like to thank Dr. Grimmel and Dr. Bergmann from Rhone-Poulenc Rorer Pharmaceuticals for their generous support and for making it possible to hold this symposium. I am also grateful to Ms. Gröbner, Ms. Möslein, Dr. Dierks, Dr. Frölich, and Dr. Ihl for their efforts in organizing the meeting and editing this volume. I am also very grateful to Dr. T. Thiekötter and Ms. B. Wehner of Springer-Verlag who made it possible to produce this book with an abundance of lavish illustrations.

As editor, it is my hope and wish that this book will help to promote research and application of neuroimaging in psychiatry and also to promote the goals of the International Society for Neuroimaging in Psychiatry (ISNIP) and its journal *Psychiatry Research – Neuroimaging*.

Konrad Maurer

Contents

Structural Imaging Methods
(Computerized Tomography/
Nuclear Magnetic Resonance Imaging)

Functional Imaging Methods (Computerized Electroencephalographic Topography)

Multimodal Application

List of Contributors

The addresses of the first authors are given at the beginning of each contribution

Structural Imaging Methods (Computerized Tomography/ Nuclear Magnetic Resonance Imaging)

Schizophrenia as an Anomaly of Cerebral Asymmetry

T.J. Crow[1]

Introduction

Science progresses by the formulation and elimination of hypotheses. This article attempts to provide an explanation for the structural changes that are present in the brain in schizophrenia and draws attention to what appears to be emerging as a consistent finding – that these changes are asymmetrical. On the basis of this finding an hypothesis is formulated that relates these changes to an evolutionary framework.

In 1879 Crichton-Browne wrote that "the cortical centres which are last organised, which are the most highly evolved and voluntary, and which are supposed to be located on the left side of the brain, might suffer first in insanity". Southard, in 1915, summarised his own studies of the neuropathology of schizophrenia as showing that "the atrophies and aplasias when focal show a tendency to occur in the left cerebral hemisphere". He endorsed Crichton-Browne's hypothesis by adding that "for this there is probably good a priori reason in the structure, late evolutionary development, and consequent relatively high lability of these regions". Radiological and post-mortem studies now support that the changes in schizophrenia are asymmetrical, and there is a case that such asymmetries are specific to psychosis. It will be argued that such findings are consistent with Southard's hypothesis, that the disease has an origin in late evolutionary developments in brain structure and that this gives us a clue to the location of the gene.

Asymmetries of Brain Structure in Schizophrenia

Air Encephalographic Studies

Ventricular enlargement in schizophrenia was first reported in air encephalographic (AEG) studies (e.g., Jakobi and Winkler 1927) (Table 1). In a number of these studies enlargement was reported to be greater on the left

[1] Division of Psychiatry, Clinical Research Centre, Watford Road, Harrow, Middlesex, HAl 3UJ, UK.

Imaging of the Brain in Psychiatry
and Related Fields
Edited by K. Maurer

Table 1. Asymmetries of brain structure in schizophrenia

Technique	Findings
Air encephalography	
Jacobi and Winkler (1927)	L > R ventricle in 9 of 19 patients R > L in one patient
Hunter et al. (1968)	Ventricular enlargement left-sided when unilateral
Haug (1982)	Temporal horn enlargement greater on the left side in patients with chronic compared to those with acute schizophrenia
Computerised tomography	
Crow et al. (1989a)	Occipital asymmetry less in patients with early onset schizophrenia
Daniel et al. (1989)	Sagittal suture more symmetrical in right-handed schizophrenic patients
Keefe et al. (1987)	Poor outcome (Kraepelinian) patients have greater ventricular enlargement on the left
Reveley et al. (1987)	Scan density decreased on the left in affected twin in discordant monozygotic pairs
Nuclear magnetic resonance imaging	
Temporal lobe size	
Johnstone et al. (1989b)	Relative reduction in temporal lobe area on the left side in schizophrenic vs affective patients and controls
Rossi et al. (1990a,b)	Left temporal lobe area reduced
Coffman et al. (1989)	Temporal lobe size reduction greater on the left side
Delisi et al. (1990)	Temporal lobe reduction in chronic patients (L > R)
Suddath et al. (1990)	Posterior temporal gray matter reduced on left side in ill as compared to well monozygotic twins
Lateral ventricular size	
Kelsoe et al. (1988)	Ventricular enlargement greater in posterior regions on the left
DeGreef et al. (1990)	Lateral ventricular enlargement in first episode patients in body, occipital and temporal horns on the left side
Schwarzkopf et al. (1990)	Left VBR and third ventricle enlargement in patients with "sporadic" disease
Superior temporal gyrus volume	
Barta et al. (1990)	Superior temporal gyrus volume reduced (L > R); L gyrus volume inversely correlated with hallucinations
Post-mortem findings	
Brown et al. (1986)	Parahippocampal gyrus width decreased on the left side in schizophrenics relative to patients with affective disorder
Crow et al. (1989b)	Temporal horn enlargement in schizophrenia but not in Alzheimer-type dementia is selective to the left side

L, left; R, right; VBR, ventricular/brain ratio.

Table 2. AEG evidence of ventricular enlargement in patients with chronic and acute schizophrenia

	Acute schizophrenia (n = 38)	Chronic schizophrenia (n = 101)	Relative increase (%)
Third ventricle	6.9	8.7	26
Cella media			
Right	12.4	14.1	13
Left	12.1	14.5	20
Temporal horn			
Right	2.8	3.6	29
Left	3.0	4.8	60

From Haug 1982.
AEG, air encephalographic.

than on the right side. For example, in their original AEG study, Jakobi and Winkler reported that the left ventricle was larger than the right in 9 of 19 patients and that the right was larger in only one patient. Hunter et al. (1968) reported that the enlargement was sometimes unilateral and usually on the left side. Haug (1962, 1982) found ventricular size to be greater in patients with chronic schizophrenia than in those with acute disease, although whether this difference relates to progression or intrinsic differences between the groups cannot be determined from assessments at a single point in time. The changes observed in patients with chronic schizophrenia in this study show a degree of selectivity to the left temporal horn (Table 2).

Computerised Tomography Studies

In our patients with chronic schizophrenia we found (Johnstone et al. 1989a) that, when other relevant variables (e.g. age and duration of illness) were controlled, age of onset predicted a number of aspects of outcome. Thus patients who were first admitted to hospital at an age below the mode for the group as a whole were more likely than those who were first admitted at a later age to show negative symptoms, intellectual impairment (e.g. age disorientation) and behavioural deterioration. It might be expected that age of onset determined whether or not structural change was present. Surprisingly, we found that the three parameters (lateral and third ventricular area and brain area) that distinguished patients with schizophrenia from other subjects did not separate those with early from those with late age of onset. However, a further structural index – the difference between the widths of the two sides of the brain in the posterior segments – did distinguish the groups. Patients with early onset had significant ($p < 0.01$)

reductions in the width of the left hemisphere in measurements taken in the occipital and temporal regions (Crow et al. 1989a) (Table 1). It seemed that early onset had arrested the development of the normal asymmetries in the posterior part of the brain.

Evidence for a loss of asymmetry in the occipital region in schizophrenia has also been reported in a computerised tomography (CT) study by Daniel et al. (1989). These authors found significant relationships between brain parenchymal and skull asymmetries: Asymmetry of occipital skull measurements was found to be less in a group of right hand and eye dominant schizophrenic patients than in controls.

There is other CT evidence for a relationship between brain asymmetry and the schizophrenic disease process. In an investigation of monozygotic twins discordant for schizophrenia, Reveley et al. (1987) demonstrated a reduction in scan density (that may indicate enlargement of CSF spaces) on the left side in the ill twin. Keefe et al. (1987), in their CT study, reported that patients with "Kraepelinian" (poor outcome) schizophrenia had significantly greater ventricular enlargement on the left than other patients with schizophrenia.

Conflicting findings with respect to cerebral asymmetry were recorded in earlier CT studies. Luchins et al. (1982) reported that "reversals" of asymmetry (i.e. brain wider on the right in the occipital region and wider on the left in the frontal region, in contrast with normal findings) were more commonly found in patients with schizophrenia than in normal controls and that this change was present in those patients in whom the ventricles were not enlarged. Although some studies (e.g. Tsai et al. 1983; Lee et al. 1985) reported similar findings, others (e.g. Andreasen et al. 1982) did not, and Luchins (1983) later concluded that "the better controlled studies have been negative". "Reversal" of asymmetry was not present in a study (Crow et al. 1989a) that showed reduced asymmetry in patients with early onset disease; here, arrest of development of the left hemisphere in the posterior (i.e., temporal and occipital) segments could account for the findings. It has to be considered that it is a failure to develop asymmetry (that is seen in changes on the later developing left side) rather than reversal that characterises the schizophrenic disease process. In assessing this possibility handedness may need to be taken into account. In two studies (Crow et al. 1989a; Daniel et al. 1989) exclusion of non-right handers revealed stronger evidence for loss of posterior cerebral asymmetry, and in two studies (Andreasen et al. 1982; Katsanis and Iacono 1989) ventricular enlargement was found to be greater in patients with schizophrenia who were left-handed. Thus the changes in left handers may be different.

Nuclear Magnetic Resonance Imaging Studies

Recent nuclear magnetic resonance imaging (NMRI) studies have reported lateralized changes in both the temporal lobe and the ventricles (Table 1).

With respect to temporal lobe area Johnstone et al. (1989b) found a relative reduction (with a diagnosis-by-side interaction) on the left in patients with schizophrenia compared to those with affective disorder and age-matched controls. Rossi et al. (1990a,b) found significant reductions in temporal lobe area on the left but not on the right side in young patients (mean age of onset 22 years) compared to normal controls. Coffman et al. (1989) observed reduction in temporal lobe size, significantly greater on the left than on the right side, in their group of schizophrenic patients. DeLisi et al. (1990) reported similar findings in a group of patients with chronic (but not those with acute) schizophrenia.

Kelsoe et al. (1988) found lateral ventricular area to be enlarged particularly in the posterior (temporal and occipital) coronal sections. In those sections in which differences were seen, their significance was greater on the left side. In a study of 25 patients with first episodes of schizophrenia Bogerts et al. (1990; see also Degreef et al. 1990) found enlargements that were significant on the left but not on the right side for the body and occipital and temporal horns, enlargement of the anterior portion of the temporal horn being present only on the left. Schwarzkopf et al. (1990) factor analyzed their assessments of ventricular size in 36 male schizophrenics and identified a factor of third ventricle and left lateral ventricular enlargement that was greater in patients without than in those with a family history.

A potentially interesting finding in a group of 15 male schizophrenic patients (Barta et al. 1990) is a reduction in the volume of the superior temporal gyrus, present on both sides but greater on the left. In this study left superior temporal gyrus volume was inversely correlated with severity of hallucinations. This possibility is supported by the study of discordant monozygotic twins by Suddath et al. (1990). Amongst the differences that these authors report between ill and well twins, a number (e.g. with respect to lateral ventricular and hippocampal areas) are present on both sides of the brain, but assessments of gray matter (Table 3) reveal an important contrast between anterior and total temporal regions. This suggests rather strongly that a structure in the posterior temporal lobe carries a change in schizophrenia that is lateralised. This structure could be the superior temporal gyrus or the planum temporale.

The nature of the brain changes and their location are further elucidated by two recent post-mortem studies. The first study (Brown et al. 1986) compared patients with schizophrenia with those with affective disorder who had died in the same institution. Brains were excluded from both groups if there was identifiable microscopic pathology (e.g., Alzheimer-type change or vascular disease). Brain structures were assessed by a photograph of a coronal section at the level of the interventricular foramina. The main findings were that, when age, sex and year of birth were controlled: (1) brain weight was reduced (by 5%–6%) in patients with schizophrenia; (2) lateral ventricular area was modestly (by 15%) but not significantly

Table 3. Monozygotic twin pairs discordant for schizophrenia

	Left	Right
Anterior temporal gray matter		
Well twin	7.86+/−1.86	8.47+/−1.27
Ill twin	7.61+/−1.36	8.57+/−1.33
	NS	NS
Total temporal gray matter		
Well twin	28.43+/−5.99	30.53+/−6.24
Ill twin	26.77+/−5.37	30.21+/−4.97
	$p < 0.002$	NS

From Suddath et al. 1990. Means +/−SD.

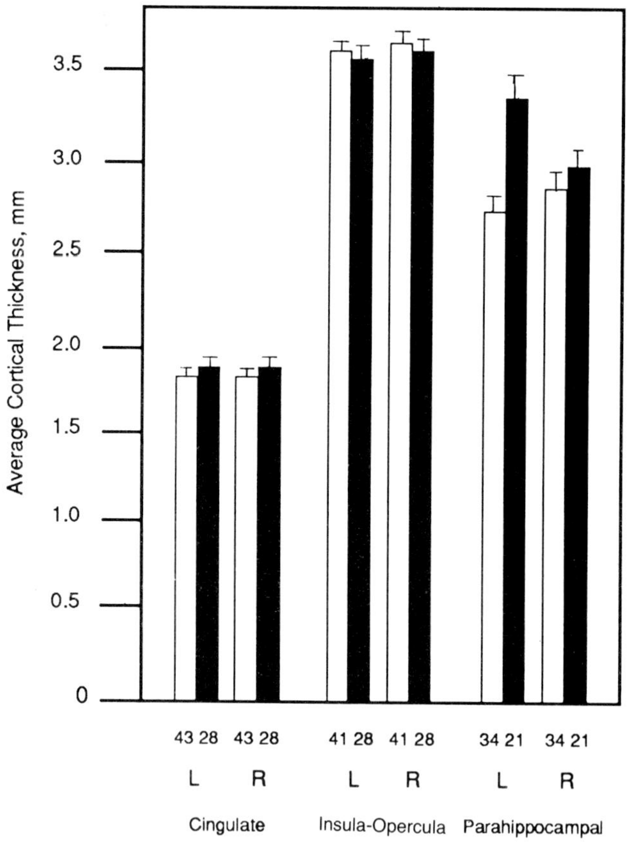

Fig. 1. Widths of various areas of cerebral cortex assessed at the level of the interventricular foramen in patients with schizophrenia and affective disorder. The width of the parahippocampal gyrus is reduced ($p < 0.01$) relative to patients with affective disorder and there is a diagnosis-by-side interaction ($p < 0.02$) by ANOVA. (Adapted from Brown et al. 1986)

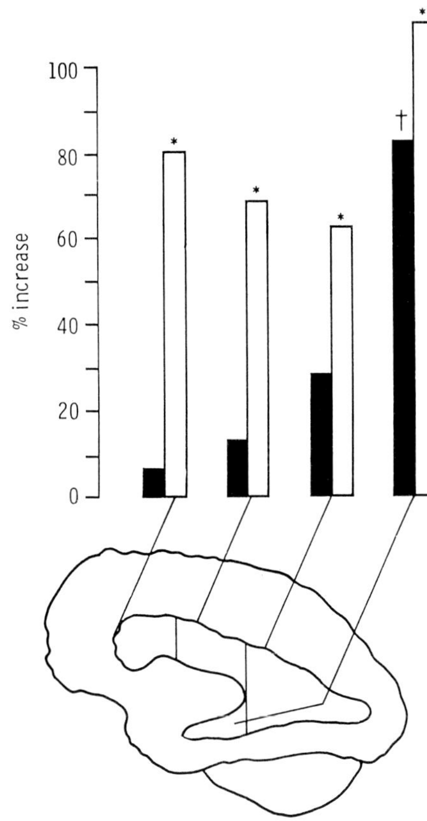

Fig. 2. Percentage increase in area of the components of the lateral ventricle as assessed from the lateral aspect in radiographs of post-mortem brain of patients with schizophrenia (*black columns*) and Alzheimer-type dementia (*open columns*) relative to age-matched controls. (Adapted from Crow et al. 1989b)

increased; (3) temporal horn area was significantly ($p < 0.01$) increased, the relative increase being over 80%; and (4) the width of the parahippocampal gyrus was reduced ($p < 0.01$). Of particular interest was a diagnosis-by-side interaction, the differences between the groups being significantly ($p < 0.02$) greater on the left side (Fig. 1). The changes in the parahippocampal gyrus are not accompanied by gliosis such as might have been expected if they had been due to an exogenous pathogen.

The second post-mortem study (Crow et al. 1989b) further emphasises the relevance of asymmetry. Brains of patients with schizophrenia were compared with those of age-matched controls. The components of the lateral ventricle were assessed on X-ray images following infusion of radio-paque medium into the ventricular spaces after formalin fixation.

The area of the posterior and particularly the temporal horn of the lateral ventricle was increased in patients with schizophrenia, in the latter site by a factor of 80% relative to the control group (Fig. 2). In patients with Alzheimer-type dementia studied at the same time, ventricular enlargement was more general, affecting the anterior horns and body and the temporal

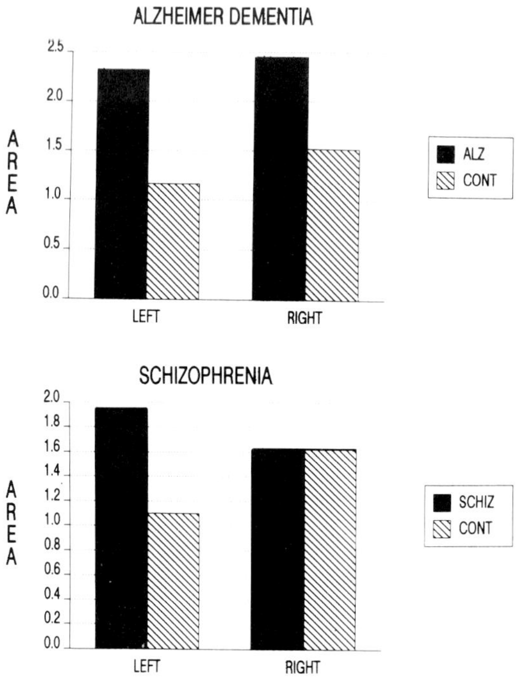

Fig. 3. Increase in temporal horn areas in patients with schizophrenia and Alzheimertype dementia on the two sides of the brain. By ANOVA there is a diagnosis-by-side interaction ($p < 0.001$). (Adapted from Crow et al. 1989b)

and posterior horns. The change in schizophrenia was selective to the left side of the brain (ANOVA $p < 0.001$), while in the Alzheimer patients there was no such lateralisation (Fig. 3). Selectivity for the left side was present in both males and females and was unaffected by inclusion or exclusion of brains in which histopathological changes could be detected.

The question raised is whether laterality of change relates to the disease process or to the normal asymmetries in the human brain, i.e. do the findings indicate that the disease process itself is lateralised or do they reflect an interaction between a bilateral process and normal anatomical and chemical asymmetries? The second post-mortem study (Crow et al. 1989b) addresses this question. Temporal horn enlargement is present in Alzheimer-type dementia but it is not lateralised; when present in schizophrenia it is selective to the left hemisphere. The findings rather strongly support the view (Crow 1984) that the disease process in schizophrenia is in some way associated with the mechanisms that determine the asymmetries in the human brain.

Anatomy of Cerebral Asymmetry

The anatomical basis of the asymmetries has been much clarified by Geschwind and colleagues. They found that, in most people, particularly

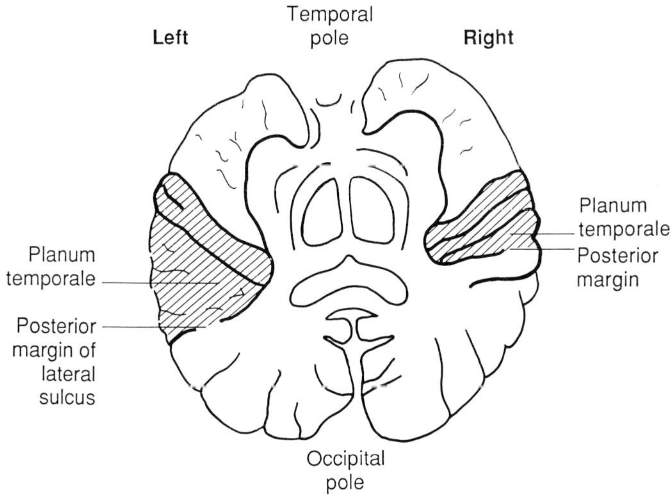

Fig. 4. The asymmetry of the human brain. (Adapted from Geschwind and Levitsky 1968)

right handers, the lateral sulcus extends back further on the left than on the right side of the brain (Geschwind and Levitsky 1968). This is because there are structures in the left temporal lobe, including the planum temporale, which forms part of the superior temporal gyrus, that are larger on the left than on the right (Fig. 4). These encompass those areas of association cortex, including Wernicke's area, that are responsible for speech and communication.

There must be a gene (or genes) that determines these developments which would be amongst those that particularly distinguish humans from other primates. The cerebral dominance gene or right shift factor is known from the studies of Annett (1985), McManus (1985) and others on handedness. Its transmission is autosomal dominant, although its location is unknown. Some 30 000 genes are said to be expressed in the brain; of these, the cerebral dominance gene seems the best candidate for the psychosis gene that we now have.

Location of the Cerebral Dominance Gene

A clue to the location of the cerebral dominance gene comes from the studies of the neuropsychology of patients with Turner's and Klinefelter's syndromes that have been conducted by Netley and Rovet (1982, 1987) (Table 4).

Turner's syndrome patients lack an X chromosome and Klinefelter's patients have an extra X. Netley and Rovet found that on IQ tests these two

Table 4. Neuropsychological impairments in sex chromosome aneuploidies

	Chromosomes	*n*	Verbal IQ	Performance IQ
Turner's syndrome	XO	35	100	88
Klinefelter's syndrome	XXY	24	83	100

In a collated sample of XXX girls, a verbal performance discrepancy similar to but of lesser magnitude than that in XXY males was seen (Netley 1986).

groups have reciprocal deficits – in Turner's there is a performance deficit (Netley and Rovet 1982) and in Klinefelter's a verbal deficit (Netley and Rovet 1987). The obvious interpretation is that in Turner's there is a right hemisphere and in Klinefelter's a left hemisphere deficit. Thus some factor located on the X chromosome is responsible for the relative development of the two hemispheres. However, because in normal females one X chromosome is inactivated, the abnormalities in Turner's syndrome are attributable to those parts of the X that are not inactivated. These include particularly the pseudoautosomal or exchange region. Therefore this suggests that the cerebral dominance gene is in the pseudoautosomal region or some other part of the X chromosome that is not inactivated (Crow 1989).

The pseudoautosomal region is that distal segment of the short arm of the X and Y chromosomes within which recombination occurs in male meiosis (Burgoyne 1986). Within this region there is strict homology of genes on the two sex chromosomes although outside it there is divergence. Since a single obligatory crossover occurs within the region in male meiosis, there is a high rate of recombination relative to other parts of the genome.

A characteristic of pseudoautosomal transmission is same sex concordance, this is, within a sibship affected individuals will more often than expected be of the same sex. This arises because when a gene within the region is passed from a father, it travels either on the X chromosome to daughters or on the Y chromosome to sons. When passed from a mother, it travels on the X chromosome without association to the sex of the children. Therefore, for a pseudoautosomal gene, concordance by sex is associated with paternal transmission. Evidence that this prediction holds for pairs of siblings with psychosis has recently been presented (Crow et al. 1989c, 1990).

There are other reasons for taking a sex chromosomal locus for psychosis seriously. Forssman (1970) discussed the excess of sex chromosome aneuploidy, particularly XXY and XXX, that has consistently been observed in populations of patients with psychosis and wrote: "Myself I am convinced that study of aberrations of the sex chromosomes will prove to have a radical effect on large sections of psychiatric thinking" and "That several

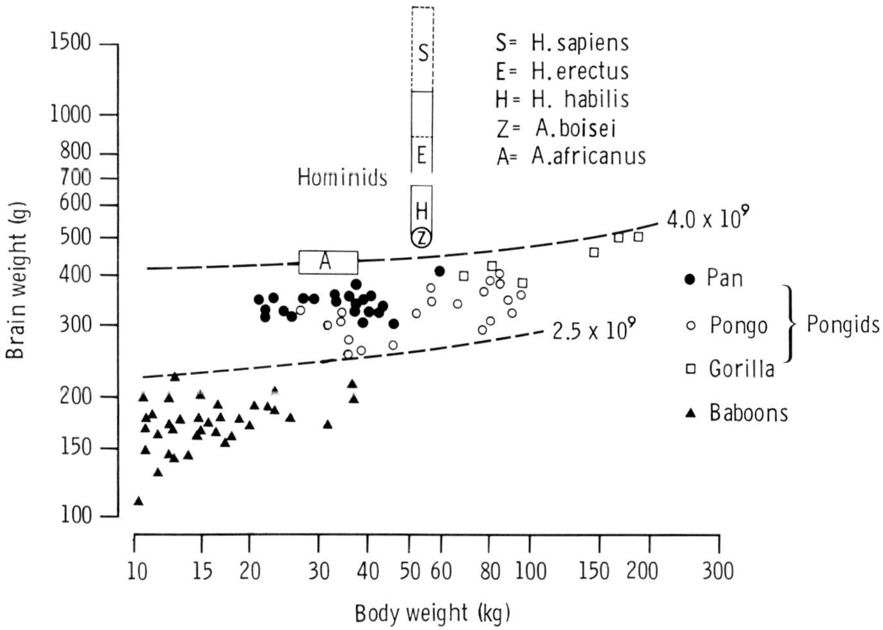

Fig. 5. Relationship between brain weight and body weight in various primate and hominid species. (Adpated from Jerison 1973)

different types of gonosomal aberration are associated with an increased risk of functional psychosis is an observation which should make us stop and think."

Evolutionary Origins

What is the evolutionary significance of this gene? In his book *Evolution of the Brain and Intelligence*, Jerison (1973) showed the relationship between brain weight and body size amongst primates (Fig. 5). The point is that in hominid species brain size has developed out of proportion to body size.

Pilbeam and Gould (1974) considered that the relationship cannot be understood in allometric terms, that is to say, the increase in size of the brain within the hominid species cannot be explained on a proportional basis (a calculation that depends upon surface area). According to these authors, if the slope of the regression line is less than 0.66, the relationship between brain weight and body size can be understood as a simple increase in body size. The relationship through *Homo habilis*, *Homo erectus* to *Homo sapiens* clearly departs from this proportionality. In the hominid species there has been a substantial and significant departure from the relationships that

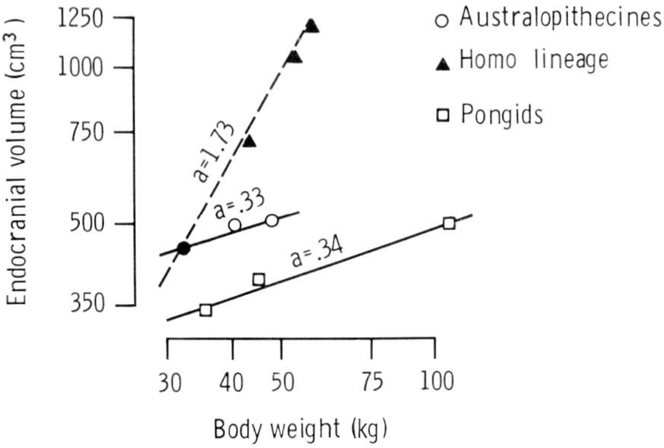

Fig. 6. Relationship between endocranial volume and body weight in homo, australopithecus and pongid species; *a*, slope of relationship. (Adapted from Pilbeam and Gould 1974)

earlier had been established. The evolution of the human brain has followed a different trajectory (Fig. 6). Jerison (1973, p. 405) spelt out what permitted these developments: "We need not look far for special selection pressures toward the major enlargements of the brain within the genus Homo. The socialized life of a predacious primate is so obviously benefited by linguistic skills, and language is so manifestly the peculiarly human development, that change in the brain to permit that advantageous supplement to perception and communication would have had obvious selective advantages throughout the period of hominid evolution."

The development of language presumably was dependent upon lateralisation of function within the brain. Levy (1977) wrote: "Bilateralization of function arose in response to specifically human pressures, occurring in a socially organized species, the members of which were mutually interdependent" and discussed the benefits of having the two hemispheres perform different functions. One such benefit is that the space available is increased, but there is also a risk associated with the consequent loss of backup capacity. Another risk may be that of developing psychosis. The significance of the cerebral dominance gene then is that it permitted new evolutionary developments; the significance of psychosis is that it reflects the disadvantageous spin-off of this essentially human evolutionary development.

Conclusions

The evolution of the human brain has been dependent upon the facility for speech and communication; this was made possible by a mutation(s) that allowed a degree of independence in the development of the two hemispheres. In psychosis an arrest or anomaly of development of cerebral asymmetry leads to structural changes which are greater on the left side of the brain and include particularly the temporal lobe and temporal horn of the ventricle. A possible locus for the cerebral dominance gene (the determinant of asymmetry) and the psychosis gene is in the pseudoautosomal (exchange) region of the X and Y chromosomes.

References

Andreasen NC, Dennert JW, Olsen SA, Damasio AR (1982) Hemispheric asymmetries and schizophrenia. Am J Psychiatry 139:427–430

Annett M (1985) Left, right, hand and brain: the right shift theory. Erlbaum, London

Barta PE, Pearlson GD, Tune LE, Powers RE, Richards SS (1990) Superior temporal gyrus volume in schizophrenia. Schizophr Res 3:22

Bogerts B, Ashtari M, DeGreef G, Alvir JMJ, Bilder RM, Lieberman JA (1990) Reduced temporal limbic structure volumes on magnetic resonance images in first episode schizophrenia. Psychiatry Res Neuroimaging 35:1–13

Brown R, Colter N, Corsellis JAN, Crow TJ, Frith CD, Jagoe R, Johnstone EC, Marsh L (1986) Post-mortem evidence of structural brain changes in schizophrenia Arch Gen Psychiatry 43:36–42

Burgoyne PS (1986) Mammalian X and Y crossover. Nature 319:258–259

Coffman JA, Schwarzkopf SB, Olson SC, Torello MW, Bornstein RA, Nasrallah HA (1989) Temporal lobe asymmetry in schizophrenics demonstrated by coronal MRI brain scans. Schizophr Res 2:117

Crichton-Browne J (1879) On the weight of the brain and its component parts in the insane. Brain 2:42–67

Crow TJ (1984) A re-evaluation of the viral hypothesis: is psychosis the result of retroviral integration at a site close to the cerebral dominance gene? Br J Psychiatry 145:243–253

Crow TJ (1989) Pseudoautosomal locus for the cerebral dominance gene. Lancet ii:339–340

Crow TJ, Colter N, Frith CD, Johnstone EC, Owens DGC (1989a) Developmental arrest of cerebral asymmetries in early onset schizophrenia. Psychiatry Res 29:247–253

Crow TJ, Ball J, Bloom SR, Brown R, Bruton CJ, Colter N, Frith CD, Johnstone EC, Owens DGC, Roberts GW (1989b) Schizophrenia as an anomaly of the development of cerebral asymmetry. Arch Gen Psychiatry 46:1145–1150

Crow TJ, DeLisi LE, Johnstone EC (1989c) Concordance by sex in sibling pairs with schizophrenia is paternally inherited: evidence for a pseudoautosomal locus. Br J Psychiatry 155:92–97

Crow TJ, DeLisi LE, Johnstone EC (1990) In reply . . . a locus closer to the telomere? Br J Psychiatry 156:416–420

Daniel DG, Myslobodsky MS, Ingraham LJ, Coppola R, Weinberger DR (1989) The relationship of occipital skull asymmetry to brain parenchymal measures in schizophrenia. Schizophr Res 2:465–472

DeGreef G, Bogerts B, Ashtari M, Lieberman J (1990) Ventricular system morphology in first episode schizophrenia: a volumetric study of ventricular subdivisions on MRI. Schizophr Res 3:18

DeLisi LE, Gupta SM, Hoff A, Shields A, Schwartz J, Halthore S, Anand A (1990) Brain morphology in first episode cases of schizophrenia. Schizophr Res 3:20

Forssman H (1970) The mental implications of sex chromosome aberrations. Br J Psychiatry 117:353–363

Geschwind N, Levitsky W (1968) Left-right asymmetry in temporal speech region. Science 161:186–187

Haug JO (1962) Pneumoencephalographic studies in mental disease. Acta Psychiatr Scand 38 [Suppl 165]
Haug JO (1982) Pneumoencephalographic evidence of brain atrophy in acute and chronic schizophrenic patients. Acta Psychiatr Scand 66:374–383
Hunter R, Jones M, Cooper F (1968) Modified lumbar air encephalography in the investigation of long stay psychiatric patients. J Neurol Sci 6:593–596
Jacobi W, Winkler H (1927) Encephalographische Studien an chronisch Schizophrenen. Arch Psychiatr Nervenkr 81:299–332
Jerison HJ (1973) Evolution of the brain and intelligence. Academic, New York
Johnstone EC, Owens DGC, Bydder GM, Colter N, Crow TJ, Frith CD (1989a) The spectrum of structural brain changes in schizophrenia: age of onset as a predictor of cognitive and clinical impairments and their cerebral correlates. Psychol Med 19:91–103
Johnstone EC, Owens DGC, Crow TJ, Frith CD, Alexandropolous K, Bydder GM, Colter N (1989b) Temporal lobe structure as determined by nuclear magnetic resonance in schizophrenia and bipolar affective disorder. J Neurol Neurosurg Psychiatry 52:736–741
Katsanis J, Iacono WG (1989) Association of left-handedness with ventricle size and neuropsychological test performance in schizophrenia. Am J Psychiatry 146: 1056–1058
Keefe RSE, Mohs RC, Losonczy MF, Davidson M, Sliverman JM, Kendler KS, Horvath HB, Nora R, Davis KL (1987) Characteristics of very poor outcome schizophrenia. Am J Psychiatry 144:889–895
Kelsoe JR, Cadet JL, Pickar D, Weinberger DR (1988) Quantitative neuroanatomy in schizophrenia: a controlled magnetic resonance imaging study. Arch Gen Psychiatry 45:533–541
Lee JH, Lee YJ, Oh SW (1985) Schizophrenia and cerebral laterality. Ann Acad Med 14:91–94
Levy J (1977) The mammalian brain and the adaptive advantage of cerebral asymmetry. Ann N Y Acad Sci 299:264–272
Luchins DJ (1983) Psychopathology and cerebral asymmetries detected by computed tomography. In: Flor-Henry P, Gruzelier J (eds) Laterality and psychopathology. Elsevier, Amsterdam, pp 625–638
Luchins DJ, Weinberger DR, Wyatt RJ (1982) Schizophrenia and cerebral asymmetry detected by computed tomography. Am J Psychiatry 139:753–757
McManus IC (1985) Handedness, language dominance and aphasia: a genetic model. Psychol Med Suppl 8:1–40
Netley CT (1986) Summary overview of behavioural development in individuals with neonatally identified X and Y aneuploidy. Birth Defects 22:293–306
Netley CT, Rovet J (1982) Atypical hemispheric lateralization in Turner syndrome subjects. Cortex 18:377–384
Netley CT, Rovet J (1987) Relations between a dermatoglyphic measure, hemispheric specialization, and intellectual abilities in 47, XXY males. Brain Cogn 6:153–160
Pilbeam D, Gould SJ (1974) Size and scaling in human evolution. Science 186:892–901
Reveley MA, Reveley AM, Baldy R (1987) Left hemisphere hypodensity in discordant schizophrenic twins: a controlled study. Arch Gen Psychiatry 44:625–632
Rossi P, Stratta P, D'Albenzio L, Tartaro A, Schiazza G, di Michele V, Bolino F, Casacchia M (1990a) Reduced temporal lobe area in schizophrenia. Biol Psychiatry 27:61–68
Rossi GF, Stratta P, D'Albenzio L, Tartaro A, Schiazza G, DiMichele V, Bolino F, Casacchia M (1990b) Reduced temporal lobe areas in schizophrenia: preliminary

evidences from a controlled multiplanar magnetic resonance study. Schizophr Res 3:1–96

Schwarzkopf SB, Nasrallah HA, Olson SC, Coffman JA (1990) A factor analytic study of ventriculomegaly in schizophrenia. Schizophr Res 3:18

Southard EE (1915) On the topographical distribution of cortex lesions and anomalies in dementia praecox, with some account of their functional significance. Am J Insanity 71:603–671

Suddath RL, Christison GW, Torrey EF, Casanova MF, Weinberger DR (1990) Anatomical abnormalities in the brains of monozygotic twins discordant for schizophrenia. N Engl J Med 322:789–794

Tsai LY, Nasrallah HA, Jacoby CG (1983) Hemispheric asymmetries on computed tomographic scans in schizophrenia and mania. Arch Gen Psychiatry 40:1286–1289

Structural Brain Changes in Schizophrenia: The Issue of Subgroups

L. Marsh[1] and D.R. Weinberger

Developments in modern neuroimaging techniques have significantly advanced our ability to examine brain structures in living subjects. As a result, replicable neuropathological changes have been demonstrated in the brains of schizophrenic patients. In schizophrenia research, though, the lack of qualitative findings and consistent clinicopathological correlations between neuroanatomical abnormalities and psychiatric symptoms leaves interpretations of the findings wide open to speculation. Some investigators (e.g., Kety 1980; Crow 1980; Jeste et al. 1982; Seidman 1983; Goetz and van Kammen 1986; Keefe et al. 1988) have argued that neuropathological changes are particular to certain clinical subgroups of patients with the syndrome of schizophrenia. The implication of this argument is that anatomical changes are markers of a distinct pathogenic and/or etiologic variety of the illness. This suggestion derives part of its appeal from the idea that schizophrenia is made up of many related diseases and is not a unitary entity. While this may turn out to be true, the neuroanatomical findings, as we will argue, do not appear to be discriminators of illness subtypes and suggest that there is a continuum of neuropathological change occurring in schizophrenia. Here, we will focus on the issue of subgroups in schizophrenia and how the current evidence from computed tomography (CT) and magnetic resonance imaging (MRI) supports the latter view.

If schizophrenia is to be regarded as a brain disorder, a comparison with other neuropsychiatric syndromes with gross structural pathology might illustrate how subtyping such illnesses according to combinations of neuropathological and clinical variables might not lead to a clearer understanding of the inherent pathological processes. In other disorders, such as Huntington's or Parkinson's disease, regardless of clinical severity and/or variability (which are great), it is generally accepted that an essential and discrete central nervous system (CNS) disease process subserves the manifestations of the illness; a quantitatively distinct neuropathological subgroup need not be assumed whenever qualitative clinical differences or

[1] Clinical Brain Disorders Branch, Intramural Research Program, National Institute of Mental Health Neuroscience Center at St. Elizabeths, Washington DC, WA 20032, USA.

Imaging of the Brain in Psychiatry
and Related Fields
Edited by K. Maurer

quantitative morphometric variation is present. A relationship between structural changes and clinical features is presumed, even when the structural changes are subtle or not grossly apparent, as in early Alzheimer's or Huntington's disease. The significant difference, though, between schizophrenia and disorders with known brain pathology is that a pathognomonic process or lesion has not been identified in schizophrenia. If the underlying pathology were known, its relationship to clinical heterogeneity could be characterized.

Progress in understanding the implications of CNS pathology in schizophrenia has thus been impeded by the heterogeneity of the clinical syndrome and the inability to demonstrate a pathognomonic lesion on MRI, CT, or at postmortem examination. A variety of clinical, biochemical, neuropsychological, and neuropathological variables have been used to define putative subgroups of schizophrenia. For example, clinical subgroups can be distinguished, in part, by phenomenology such as the predominance of positive symptoms (e.g., hallucinations, delusions, thought disorder) or negative symptoms (e.g., apathy, affective flattening, poverty of speech). Even in this realm, however, the distinctions are blurred, and few, if any, patients can be described as having only positive or only negative symptoms. The same is true of cognitive deficits, which though severe in some patients (Goldberg et al. 1988), do not clearly segregate patients into those with cognitive deficits and those without (Goldberg et al. 1990). By the same token, when examining neuroimages of the brains of patients with schizophrenia, the distinct presence or absence of neuropathogical change is also not so apparent. Yet, the attempt to subdivide populations arbitrarily based on these data has proceeded even though the reported changes are quantitatively subtle and variable, and overlap to a considerable degree with normal data.

In spite of ongoing discussions of whether neuropathological subgroups of schizophrenia exist, numerous CT and MRI studies from the last 15 years have replicated an association between structural brain pathology and schizophrenia (for review see Zigun and Weinberger 1992). Of the noted abnormalities, ventriculomegaly, sulcal widening, and temporal lobe changes are among the most replicated findings, but cerebral asymmetries and cerebellar shrinkage are also reported. Enlargement of the third and lateral ventricles is among the most consistent of reported findings. In a review of 80 CT studies of schizophrenia, Shelton and Weinberger (1986) found that the lateral ventricles and third ventricle were enlarged in schizophrenics compared to controls in 75% and 80% of the studies, respectively. MRI studies have replicated these findings of increased lateral and third ventricle size (Kelsoe et al. 1988; Suddath et al. 1989, 1990). These reports are complemented by the results of investigations using postmortem brain specimens.

Ventriculomegaly is a nonspecific indicator of brain pathology that can be found in association with almost any CNS disease. Presumably, while it reflects altered or reduced tissue in the surrounding brain regions or diffusely throughout the brain, it may represent the outcome of unique processes in different diseases. In schizophrenia, the pathological process responsible for ventriculomegaly appears in most patients to be established and static when the clinical illness is initially manifest (Weinberger et al. 1979a,b, 1982, Golden et al. 1980; Schulz et al. 1982; Ilowsky et al. 1988; Vita et al. 1988). While the basis for ventriculomegaly in schizophrenia is not known, it seems to serve as a biological marker of an abnormal brain. It is also a useful variable for testing whether neuropathological subgroups exist.

The notion that a distinct subpopulation of patients with schizophrenia has enlarged ventricles is disputed when one considers ventriculomegaly as a relative structural deviation occurring in the context of normal anatomical variability. If abnormal size is defined by values that are two standard deviations from the mean value of normal controls (a common practice in the psychiatric literature), the frequency of ventriculomegaly ranges from 6% to 40% (Seidman 1983). Thus, ventricular size in most patients with schizophrenia is well within the normal range. However, this does not necessarily mean that only a subset of patients has structural CNS abnormalities. For example, if a hypothetical CNS disease process causes ventricles in all those affected to increase by 10%–20% over what they would have been if the disease had never developed, it would follow that ventricular size in most of the affected population would still remain well within the normal range. Among the 10%–20% whose ventricles, in the absence of the disease, were near the upper limit of normal, but within the normal range, ventricular size would subsequently fall outside the upper limit of the normal range. Taking normal CNS structural variation into account, those with the largest ventricles would not, however, comprise a "neuropathological subgroup," since the same pathological process occurred in all affected individuals. This view is supported by research comparing brain images of patients with schizophrenia to those of genetically related controls.

Both CT and MRI investigations from different centers have shown that ventricular size is genetically determined to a great extent and that an additional, but unknown, process in schizophrenia accounts for greater deviations. Even when the ventricles are small in a family, the affected member demonstrates relatively enlarged ventricles. The first CT study on twin pairs, performed in England by Reveley et al. (1982), compared the ventricular/brain ratio (VBR), an expression of ventricular area as a function of brain size, in pairs of healthy monozygotic (MZ) and dizygotic (DZ) twins and MZ twins discordant for schizophrenia. Among healthy MZ twin pairs, ventricular size was highly correlated ($r = 0.98$, $p < 0.001$), but there was less correlation in VBR among the DZ or discordant MZ twins. In schizophrenic MZ twins, the mean VBR was significantly greater than that of their unaffected co-twins; this relationship was seen in six out of the seven twin pairs. Since the subtle deviations associated with schizophrenia are superimposed on normal structural variations, pathology may be present despite morphometry within the "normal" range.

The findings of Reveley et al. (1982) are strengthened and expanded upon by recent research on discordant MZ twins using MRI. Using MRI images from 15 discordant MZ twin pairs, Suddath et al. (1990) made quantitative measures of the prefrontal and temporal lobes, amygdala, anterior hippocampus, anterior and temporal horn of the lateral ventricles, and third ventricle. Compared with their unaffected sibling, the schizophrenic twin had larger lateral ventricles in 14 pairs on the left ($p < 0.003$) and in 13 pairs on the right ($p < 0.001$). Of the schizophrenic twins, 13 had a larger third ventricle than their unaffected co-twin. This relationship was seen even when the ventricles in both twins were relatively small, suggesting again that pathology may be present despite relatively "normal" size ventricles. In schizophrenic twins, there was decreased mean left temporal lobe gray matter volume and anterior hippocampal area in 14/15 twins on the left and in 13/15 on the right. None of these differences were evident in a control population of seven pairs of healthy MZ twins.

Other studies using genetically related controls have reported similar findings. In a CT study comparing ten patients with schizophrenia to their healthy siblings and a control group of 17 normal siblings from seven families, Weinberger et al. (1981) found that there was a genetic component to the size of the lateral ventricles. The mean VBR of the healthy discordant siblings was greater than that of the controls ($p < 0.001$). However, the mean VBR of the schizophrenics was even greater. In each family, the schizophrenic sibling had the largest VBR, even when the ventricles did not appear overtly abnormal. Similarly, DeLisi et al. (1986) reported enlarged lateral ventricles in schizophrenics relative to their healthy siblings.

One of the most significant aspects of the studies using control groups who are genetically related to the patients with schizophrenia is that separate subgroups of patients with neuropathology do not emerge. Relative to the healthy sibling, structural changes are present in almost every sibling with schizophrenia. While it is not clear how much anatomical variation occurs normally between MZ twins, the size of CNS structures appears to be under genetic influence. The use of MZ twins discordant for schizophrenia provides the closest approximation to comparing how the brain might have developed if additional nongenetic pathological processes were never present. The inherent pathology of schizophrenia, while presumably specific to the illness, is then colored by individual variation and genetic predisposition. Supported by the family studies, this concept can be generalized to schizophrenics who are not MZ twins. However, since the neuropathological changes are often subtle, it becomes apparent why CNS structures in many patients with schizophrenia will appear normal in size. The subtle and variable nature of these findings in the general population of schizophrenic patients also makes it unlikely that discrete subgroups could be defined.

Many groups have attempted to define a putative neuropathological subgroup by correlating clinical characteristics with the presence of ventriculomegaly (for review, see Goetz and van Kammen 1986). While positive symptoms and ventriculomegaly are generally not correlated, several groups have shown that increased VBR corresponds with higher negative symptom scores (Pearlson et al. 1984; Williams et al. 1985), poor premorbid adjustment (Weinberger et al. 1980), cognitive impairments (Johnstone et al. 1976; Donnelly et al. 1980), and poor response to neuroleptic therapy (Jeste et al. 1982). Others (Nasrallah et al. 1982, 1983; Luchins et al. 1984; Owens et al. 1985), however, have not reported such associations. These contradictory findings might be explained by relative differences in the study populations. It is possible that patients with the most severe and disabling symptoms of the illness exhibit relatively pronounced neuropathology whereas the same underlying pathological changes are not so blatant in those who are less ill.

Another approach to the question of anatomically defining subgroups of patients with schizophrenia is to look for evidence of a mixture of distributions of ventricular size data in the populations of patients with this illness. This approach was undertaken by Daniel et al. (1990) in a meta-analysis of the reported VBR values from many studies in the English literature comparing schizophrenics (n = 691) to medical controls (n = 205) or to normal controls (n = 160). VBR in each group was found to follow a normal distribution with no subgroups present in either group, suggesting that the anatomical variation occurs along a continuum. When the schizophrenic subjects were analyzed with either control population, two separate populations emerged, with the schizophrenic patients in the group with a larger VBR. While a portion of the schizophrenics had a VBR within the control range, they tended toward the range of upper normal measures. These results are consistent with the notion that there is a shift upward with respect to normals in the distribution for VBR in schizophrenia, and that this shift involves most of the ill population, not a particular subgroup.

Similar shifts in mean values occur with other CNS structures implicated as important to the pathology of schizophrenia (see Zigun and Weinberger, 1992 for review). Since the changes are often subtle and can concern relatively small structures compared to the lateral ventricles (e.g., hippocampus, parahippocampal gyrus), these relationship are not always so evident. Likewise, quantitative microstructural deviations, such as neuronal disarray (Scheibel and Kovelman 1981; Kovelman and Scheibel 1984), decreased neuronal density (Jeste and Lohr 1989; Falkai et al. 1988), or abnormal cytoarchitecture (Jakob and Beckman 1986; Falkai et al. 1988) may not always yield measureable differences on neuroimaging scans.

The issue of whether neuropathological changes occur in schizophrenia is now rarely questioned given the abundant evidence using modern research methods. Rather, the current debate focuses on whether identified neuroanatomical differences are present in all schizophrenics or if they are characteristic of a clinical and/or etiologic subgroup. Proponents of the subgroup theory generally use an arbitrary "cutoff" morphometric value or clinical criteria to define subsets and then correlate neuroanatomical features to the different groups. While this approach automatically produces clinical dichotomies even when most patients have heterogenous symptoms, it is problematic because the evidence for this practice is weak. Interpreting the neuroimages in the context of normal brain differences and genetic influences on the size of structures demonstrates how almost all schizophrenics, regardless of their symptoms, have neuroanatomical changes which appear to differ in degree, but not kind, along a continuum. It is hoped that this approach will help establish meaningful associations between the nature of the neuropathology and the clinical symptoms of schizophrenia.

References

Crow TJ (1980) Molecular pathology of schizophrenia: more than one disease process? Br Med J 280:66–68

Daniel DG, Goldberg TE, Gibbons RD, Weinberger DR (1991) Lack of a bimodal distribution of ventricular size in schizophrenia. Biol Psychiatry 30:887–903

DeLisi LE, Goldin LR, Hamovit JR, Maxwell ME, Kurtz D, Gershon ES (1986) A family study of the association of increased ventricular size with schizophrenia. Arch Gen Psychiatry 43:148–153

Donnelly EF, Weinberger DR, Waldman IN, Wyatt RJ (1980) Cognitive impairment associated with morphological brain abnormalities on computed tomography in chronic schizophrenic patients. J Nerv Ment Dis 168:305–308

Falkai P, Bogerts B, Rozumek M (1988) Limbic pathology in schizophrenia: the entorhinal region-a morphometric study. Biol Psychiatry 24:515–521

Goetz KL, van Kammen DP (1986) Computerized axial tomography scans and subtypes of schizophrenia. J Nerv Ment Dis 174:31–41

Goldberg TE, Kleinman JE, Daniel DG, Myslobodsky MS, Ragland JD, Weinberger DR (1988) Dementia praecox revisited. Age disorientation, mental status, and ventricular enlargement. Br J Psychiatry 153:187–190

Goldberg TE, Ragland JD, Torrey EF, Gold JM, Bigelow LB, Weinberger DR (1990) Neuropsychological assessment of monozygotic twins discordant for schizophrenia. Arch Gen Psychiatry 47:1066–1072

Golden CJ, Moses JA, Zelazowski R, Graber B, Zatz LM, Horvath TB, Berger PA (1980) Cerebral ventricular size and neuropsychological impairment in young chronic schizophrenics. Arch Gen Psychiatry 37:619–623

Ilowsky BP, Juliano DM, Bigelow LB, Weinberger DR (1988) Stability of CT scan findings in schizophrenia. Results of an 8 year follow-up study. J Neurol Neurosurg Psychiatry 51:209–213

Jakob H, Beckmann H (1986) Prenatal developmental disturbances in the limbic allocortex in schizophrenics. J Neural Transm 65:303–326

Jeste DJ, Kleinman JE, Potkin SG, Luchins DJ, Weinberger DR (1982) Ex uno multi: subtyping the schizophrenic syndrome. Biol Psychiatry 17:199–222

Jeste DV, Lohr JB (1989) Hippocampal pathologic findings in schizophrenia. Arch Gen Psychiatry 46:1019–1024

Johnstone EC, Crow TJ, Frith CD, Husband J, Kreel L (1976) Cerebral ventricular size and cognitive impairment in chronic schizophrenia. Lancet ii:924–926

Keefe RSE, Mohs RC, Davidson M, Losonczy MF, Silverman JM, Lesser JC, Horvath TB, Davis KL (1988) Kraeplinian schizophrenia: a subgroup of schizophrenia? Psychopharmacol Bull 24:56–61

Kelsoe JR, Cadet JL, Pickar D, Weinberger DR (1988) Quantitative neuroanatomy in schizophrenia. A controlled magnetic resonance imaging study. Arch Gen Psychiatry 45:533–541

Kety SS (1980) The syndrome of schizophrenia: unresolved questions and opportunities for research. Br J Psychiatry 136:421–436

Kovelman JA, Scheibel AB (1984) A neurohistological correlate of schizophrenia. Biol Psychiatry 19:1601–1621

Luchins DJ, Lewine RRJ, Meltzer HY (1984) Lateral ventricular size, psychopathology, and medication response in the psychoses. Biol Psychiatry 19: 29–44

Nasrallah HA, Jacoby CG, McCalley-Whitters M, Kuperman S (1982) Cerebral ventricular enlargement in subtypes of chronic schizophrenia. Arch Gen Psychiatry 39:774–777

Nasrallah HA, Kuperman S, Hamra BJ, McCalley-Whitters M (1983) Clinical differences between schizophrenic patients with and without large cerebral ventricles. J Clin Psychiatry 44:407–409

Owens DGC, Johnstone EC, Crow TJ, Frith CD, Jagoe JR, Kreel L (1985) Lateral ventricular size in schizophrenia: relationship to the disease process and its clinical manifestation. Psychol Med 15:27–41

Pearlson GD, Garbacz DJ, Breakey WR, Ahn HS, DePaulo JR (1984) Lateral ventricular enlargement associated with persistent unemployment and negative symptoms in both schizophrenia and bipolar disorder. Psychiatry 12:1–9

Reveley AM, Reveley MA, Clifford CA, Murray RM (1982) Cerebral ventricular size in twins discordant for schizophrenia. Lancet i:540–541

Scheibel AB, Kovelman JA (1981) Disorientation of the hippocampal pyramidal cell and its processes in the schizophrenic patient. Biol Psychiatry 16:101–102

Schulz SC, Koller M, Kishore PR, Hamer RM, Friedel RO (1982) Abnormal scans in young schizophrenics. Psychopharmacol Bull 18:163–164

Seidman LJ (1983) Schizophrenia and brain dysfunction: an integration of recent neurodiagnostic findings. Psychol Bull 94:195–238

Shelton RC, Weinberger DR (1986) X-ray computerized tomography studies in schizophrenia: a review and synthesis. In: Nasrallah HA, Weinberger DR (eds) The neurology of schizophrenia. Elsevier, Amsterdam, pp 207–250 (Handbook of schizophrenia, vol 1)

Suddath RL, Casanova MF, Goldberg TE, Daniel DG, Kelsoe JR, Weinberger DR (1989) Temporal lobe pathology in schizophrenia: a quantitative magnetic resonance imaging study. Am J Psychiatry 146:464–472

Suddath RL, Christison GW, Torrey EF, Casanova MF, Weinberger DR (1990) Anatomical abnormalities in the brains of monozygotic twins discordant for schizophrenia. N Engl J Med 322:789–794

Vita A, Sacchetti E, Valvassori G, Cazullo CL (1988) Brain morphology in schizophrenia: a 2- to 5-year follow-up study. Acta Psychiatr Scand 78:618–621

Weinberger DR, Torrey EF, Neophytides AN, Wyatt RJ (1979a) Lateral cerebral ventricular enlargement in chronic schizophrenia. Arch Gen Psychiatry 36:735–739

Weinberger DR, Torrey EF, Neophytides AN, Wyatt RJ (1979b) Structural abnormalities in the cerebral cortex of chronic schizophrenic patients. Arch Gen Psychiatry 36:935–939

Weinberger DR, Cannon-Spoor E, Potkin SG, Wyatt RJ (1980) Poor premorbid adjustment and CT scan abnormalities in chronic schizophrenia. Am J Psychiatry 137:1410–1413

Weinberger DR, DeLisi LE, Neophytides AN, Wyatt RJ (1981) Familial aspects of CT scan abnormalities in chronic schizophrenic patients. Psychiatry Res 4:65–71

Weinberger DR, DeLisi LE, Perman GP, Targum S, Wyatt RJ (1982) Computed tomography in schizophreniform disorder and other acute psychiatric disorders. Arch Gen Psychiatry 39:778–783

Williams AO, Reveley MA, Kolakowski T, Ardern M, Mandelbrote BM (1985) Schizophrenia with good and poor outcome, II: Cerebral ventricular size and its clinical significance. Br J Psychiatry 146:239–246

Zigun J, Weinberger DR (1992) In vivo studies of brain morphology in patients with schizophrenia. In: Lindenmayer J-P, Kay SR (eds) New biological vistas on schizophrenia. Brunner Mazel, New York

Volumetry of Limbic Structures in Schizophrenics and Controls

S. Heckers[1], H. Heinsen, and H. Beckmann

Introduction

The introduction of computerized tomography (CT) and magnetic resonance imaging (MRI) into the clinical neurosciences has renewed the interest in structural brain abnormalities in neuropsychiatric diseases. Based upon the assumption that a decrease in structural size reflects a lower or disturbed level of brain function, volumetric studies may point to an involvement of specific brain regions in the pathogenesis of neuropsychiatric diseases. Recent MRI studies have reported a volume reduction of limbic structures in the medial temporal lobes of schizophrenics (Suddath et al. 1990; Bogerts et al. 1990). These studies were interpreted as confirmation of previous postmortem studies which revealed subtle (Kovelman and Scheibel 1984; Jakob and Beckmann 1986; Jeste and Lohr 1989; Arnold et al. 1991) or even gross morphological changes (Bogerts et al. 1985; Brown et al. 1986; Falkai and Bogerts 1986) in the amygdala, hippocampus, and parahippocampal gyrus of schizophrenic patients. These structures are implicated in information processing and affective labeling of sensory input (Mesulam 1985). The aim of the present study was to revise the hypothesis of a limbic structure volume reduction in a new series of brains with a stereological study design.

Material and Methods

Material was taken from a new collection of brains established at Würzburg University beginning in 1986. There were 20 brains of schizophrenic patients (11 females, 9 males) that were closely matched according to sex and age (schizophrenics, 63.7 ± 18.9; controls, 64.4 ± 17.1) with 20 brains of control patients.

All patients were diagnosed retrospectively according to DSM III by reviewing the complete clinical records (Table 1). Morphometric analysis

[1] Present address: Department of Neurology, Harvard Medical School, Beth Israel Hospital, 330 Brookline Avenue, Boston, MA 02115, USA.

Imaging of the Brain in Psychiatry
and Related Fields
Edited by K. Maurer

Table 1. Psychiatric diagnosis according to DSM III

Predominant symptomatology	DSM III	*n*
Paranoid-hallucinatory	295.3	11
Catatonic	295.2	4
Disorganized	295.1	2
Mixed	295.9	2
Residual type	295.6	1

was performed "blind" with respect to psychiatric diagnosis. The whole hemisphere was cut in a series of coronal sections about 0.7 mm thick. Every third slice (about 70 per hemisphere) was Nissl-stained with gallocyanin. Using a stereomicroscope volumes of hippocampal formation, amygdala, and the three horns of the lateral ventricle were determined by applying the Cavalieri estimator (Gundersen et al. 1988). All volumes were corrected for tissue shrinkage during the staining procedure with an individual shrinkage factor (for further details see Heckers et al. 1991).

Results

The hippocampal formation of the schizophrenics showed a tendency to be smaller, with the left side more affected than the right (Table 2). However, this volume reduction of −6% on the left ($p = 0.187$) and −4% on the right side was not statistically significant. We found no significant side differences in either group.

Amygdala volume was slightly increased in the schizophrenic sample on both sides without showing a significant difference (Table 2). No significant side differences were found in either group.

The lateral ventricle was larger in schizophrenics on both sides (Table 2). However, these differences (left, +24%, $p = 0.359$; right , +17%, $p = 0.399$) were not statistically significant. All three horns of the lateral ventricle showed a tendency to be larger in schizophrenics. Volumes of neither the whole lateral ventricle nor the inferior horn correlated with amygdala or hippocampal volume.

Discussion

In contrast to previous postmortem findings, the results of the present study suggest that there is no marked volume reduction of limbic structures in the medial temporal lobe of schizophrenics. The hippocampal formation was the only brain region which showed a tendency to be smaller in schizophrenics.

Table 2. Mean (±SD) volumes (cm^3)

	Schizophrenics	Controls
Hippocampal formation		
L	3.58 ± 0.57	3.81 ± 0.45
R	3.81 ± 0.47	3.95 ± 0.43
Amygdala		
L	1.26 ± 0.22	1.16 ± 0.13
R	1.33 ± 0.21	1.25 ± 0.15
Lateral ventricle		
L	10.44 ± 5.46	8.39 ± 3.36
R	10.45 ± 4.72	8.90 ± 4.48
Anterior horn		
L	5.00 ± 2.60	4.18 ± 1.80
R	5.18 ± 1.95	4.56 ± 2.84
Inferior horn		
L	0.88 ± 0.40	0.74 ± 0.35
R	0.90 ± 0.22	0.88 ± 0.24
Posterior horn		
L	4.19 ± 2.47	3.53 ± 1.76
R	4.36 ± 3.13	3.46 ± 1.78

L, left; R, right.

The volumes of both the amygdala and the parahippocampal gyrus (Heckers et al. 1989) were not different in schizophrenics and controls. Furthermore, we did not find significant correlations between lateral ventricular enlargement and limbic structures volume. Thus, the most consistent finding of morphological schizophrenia research, i.e., lateral ventricular enlargement seems not to be a marker for a limbic system pathology in schizophrenia.

Postmortem studies which have revealed a cellular pathology of the limbic system in schizophrenic brains have suggested a neurodevelopmental etiology of schizophrenia (Kovelman and Scheibel 1984; Jakob and Beckmann 1986; Arnold et al. 1991). Such subtle neuropathological alterations might result in differences in cell density and volume reduction of brain regions. However, gross volumetry, as applied in the present study and in previous ones (Bogerts et al. 1985; Falkai and Bogerts 1986; Brown et al. 1986), may be misleading in the search for a morphological correlate of schizophrenia unless taking differences in cytoarchitectonics and fiber connections into account. Furthermore, volume reduction may represent cell loss, neuropil changes, or white matter reduction (Casanova and Kleinman 1990).

It is important to note that a nonsignificant mean difference between schizophrenics and controls does not rule out that a subset of schizophrenics is characterized by a marked volume reduction of limbic structures. Therefore, it is important to control for factors like sex, age, and postmortem tissue changes that raise variance not attributable to schizophrenia. We consider methodological factors as a possible reason for the failure to replicate previous findings.

The hippocampal formation was the only brain structure which showed the tendency to be smaller in schizophrenics. Further studies remain to be done to elucidate the underlying pathology of this volumetric finding.

References

Arnold SE, Hyman BT, Van Hoesen GW, Damasio AR (1991) Some cytoarchitectural abnormalities of the entorhinal cortex in schizophrenia. Arch Gen Psychiatry 48:625–632

Bogerts B, Meertz E, Schönfeldt-Bausch R (1985) Basal ganglia and limbic system pathology in schizophrenia: a morphometric study of brain volume and shrinkage. Arch Gen Psychiatry 42:784–791

Bogerts B, Ashtari M, Degreef G, Alvir JMJ, Bilder RM, Lieberman JA (1990) Reduced temporal limbic structure volumes on magnetic resonance images in first episode schizophrenia. Psychiatry Res: Neuroimaging 35:1–13

Brown R, Colter N, Corsellis JAN, Crow TJ, Frith CD, Jagoe R, Johnstone EC, Marsh L (1986) Postmortem evidence of structural brain changes in schizophrenia. Arch Gen Psychiatry 43:36–42

Casanova MF, Kleinman JE (1990) The neuropathology of schizophrenia: a critical assessement or research methodologies. Biol Psychiatry 27:353–362

Falkai P, Bogerts B (1986) Cell loss in the hippocampus of schizophrenics. Eur Arch Psychiatr Neurol Sci 236:154–161

Gundersen HJG, Bendtsen TF, Korbo L, Marcussen N, Moller A, Nielsen K, Nyengaard JR, Pakkenberg B, Sorensen FB, Vesterby A, West MJ (1988) Some new, simple and efficient stereological methods and their use in pathological research and diagnosis. Acta Pathologica, Microbiologica et Immunologica Scandinavica 96:379–394

Heckers S, Heinsen H, Heinsen YL, Beckmann H (1989) Morphometry of the parahippocampal gyrus in schizophrenics and controls. Some anatomical considerations. J Neural Transm [GenSect] 80:151–155

Heckers S, Heinsen H, Heinsen YL, Beckmann H (1991) Limbic structures and lateral ventricle in schizophrenia: a post-mortem study. Arch Gen Psychiatry 47:1016–1022

Jakob H, Beckmann H (1986) Prenatal developmental disturbances in the limbic allocortex in schizophrenics. J Neural Transm 65:303–326

Jeste DV, Lohr JB (1989) Hippocampal pathological findings in schizophrenia: a morphometric study. Arch Gen Psychiatry 46:1019–1024

Kovelman JA, Scheibel AB (1984) A neurohistological correlate of schizophrenia. Biol Psychiatry 19:1601–1621

Mesulam M-M (1985) Patterns in behavioral neuroanatomy: association areas, the limbic system, and hemispheric specialization. In: Mesulam M-M (ed) Principles of behavioral neurology. Davis, Philadelphia, pp 1–70

Suddath RL, Christison GW, Torrey EF, Casanova MF, Weinberger DR (1990) Anatomical abnormalities in the brains of monozygotic twins discordant for schizophrenia. N Engl J Med 322:789–794

Hippocampus and Basal Ganglia Pathology in Chronic Schizophrenics. A Replication Study from a New Brain Collection*

B. Bogerts[1], P. Falkai, M. Haupts, B. Greve, U. Tapernon-Franz, and U. Heinzmann

Introduction

In two previous papers (Bogerts 1984; Bogerts et al. 1985) we reported reduced volumes of limbic medial temporal lobe and basal ganglia structures in postmortem brains of schizophrenics belonging to the Vogt collection in Düsseldorf. A number of subsequent planimetric postmortem and MRI studies (Table 1) also reported anatomical anomalies in limbic structures of schizophrenics, whereas in two recent studies, which were based in part on very old cases (Heckers et al. 1989, 1990), no significant volume reductions of hippocampus, parahippocampal gyrus, and amygdala could be found.

Five years ago, we founded at the Department of Psychiatry, University of Düsseldorf, a new brain collection which contains 40 brains of schizophrenic patients and 90 brains of normal control subjects. In the present study, initial results of volume measurements of basal ganglia and hippocampus of brains from the new collection are reported.

Patients and Controls

Brains of 18 schizophrenics (9 males, 9 females; mean age/range 52.3, 39–72 years) and 21 control subjects without a history of neuropsychiatric disorders (14 males, 7 females; mean age/range 54.1, 38–76 years) were investigated. Only patients with well preserved and extensive clinical records were selected for this study. The mean disease duration (time between first hospitalization and death) was 21.3 years (range 2–30 years), all patients fulfilled both ICD-9 and DSM-III criteria, and were treated with neuroleptic drugs for most of their illness. Patients and controls died in the years 1985–1988. Details of clinical symptoms, disease duration, and cause of death of patients and controls are given elsewhere (Bogerts et al. 1990a).

* This project is supported by the Deutsche Forschungsgemeinschaft (Bo 799/1–3) and the Alfried Krupp von Bohlen und Halbach-Stiftung.

[1] Rheinische Landesklinik, Psychiatrische Klinik der Heinrich-Heine Universität Düsseldorf, Postfach 120510, Bergische Landstr. 2, W-4000 Düsseldorf 12, FRG.

Imaging of the Brain in Psychiatry and Related Fields
Edited by K. Maurer

Table 1. Planimetric postmortem and MRI studies of medial temporal lobe structures in schizophrenics

Positive results	
Bogerts et al. 1985 (Vogt collection)	Smaller volumes of left anterior hippocampus, parahippocampol gyrus, and amygdala
Brown et al. 1986 (Runwell collection)	Reduced cross-sectional area of left parahippocampal gyrus gray matter
Falkai and Bogerts 1986 (Vogt collection)	Smaller volumes of whole left hippocampus and hippocampal CA segments
Colter et al. 1987 (Runwell collection)	Reduced cross-sectional area of parahippocampal white matter
Falkai et al. 1988 (Vogt collection)	Reduced left entorhinal cortex volume
Jeste and Lohr 1989 (Yakovlev collection)	Smaller volumes of left anterior hippocampus and hippocampal CA 4 segment
Crow et al. 1989 (Runwell collection)	Left temporal horn enlargement
Bogerts et al. 1990a (new D'dorf collection)	Reduced volumes of total right and left hippocampus
DeLisi et al. 1988 (MRI)	Reduced hippocampus and parahippocampal areas
Suddath et al. 1989 (MRI)	Reduced temporal lobe gray matter at hippocampus-amygdala levels
Suddath et al. 1990 (MRI)	Smaller anterior hippocampus in discordant monozygotic schizophrenic twins
Bogerts et al. 1990b (MRI)	Reduced left hippocampus in male first episode schizophrenics
Negative results	
Heckers et al. 1990 (Würzburg collection)	No difference in parahippocampal gyrus volume
Heckers et al. 1990 (Würzburg collection)	No difference in hippocampus and amygdala volumes

Methods

Brains of patients and controls were fixed in formalin, embedded in paraplast, and cut into 20 μm thick, whole brain, coronal, serial sections. Each 50th section was then Nissl (cresylechtviolet)- and myelin (Heidenhain-Wölke or luxol fast blue)-stained. Within the basal ganglia the volumes of the following structures were blindly measured by three of the authors (P.F., M.H., B.G.): caudatum, putamen, and nucleus accumbens. Within the temporal lobe, the volume of the hippocampal formation (including subiculum and fascia dentata) from its anterior pole up to the splenium of the corpus callosum was measured. A detailed description of the histological procedures, anatomical delineation criteria, shrinkage factor determination, and planimetric methods are given in a more extended version of this report (Bogerts et al. 1990a).

phrenia. Differences in brain weight, temporal horn area and parayhippocampal gyrus compared with affective disorder. Arch Gen Psychiatry 43:36–42

Colter N, Battal S, Crow TJ, Johnstone EC, Brown R, Bruton C (1987) White matter reduction in the parahippocampal gyrus of patients with schizophrenia. Arch Gen Psychiatry 44:1023

Crow TJ, Ball J, Bloom SR, Brown R, Bruton CJ, Colter N, Frith CD, Johnstone EC, Owens DGC, Roberts GW (1989) Schizophrenia as an anomaly of development of cerebral asymmetry. Arch Gen Psychiatry 46:1145–1150

DeLisi LE, Dauphinais ID, Gershon E (1988) Perinatal complications and reduced size of brain limbic structures in familial schizophrenia. Schizophr Bull 14:185–191

Falkai P, Bogerts B (1986) Cell loss in the hippocampus of schizophrenics. Eur Arch Psychiatr Neurol Sci 236:154–161

Falkai P, Bogerts B, Rozumek M (1988) Cell loss and volume reduction in the entorhinal cortex of schizophrenics. Biol Psychiatry 24:515–521

Heckers S, Heinsen H, Heinsen Y, Beckmann H (1989) Morphometry of the parahippocampal gyrus in schizophrenics and controls. Some anatomical considerations. J Neural Transm 80:151–155

Heckers S, Heinse H, Heinsen Y, Beckmann H (1990) Limbic structures and lateral ventricle in schizophrenia. A quantitative post mortem study. Arch Gen Psychiatry 47:1016–1022

Jeste DV, Lohr JB (1989) Hippocampal pathologic findings in schizophrenia. Arch Gen Psychiatry 46:1019–1024

Stevens JR (1986) Clinicopathological correlations in schizophrenia. Arch Gen Psychiatry 43:715–716

Suddath RL, Casanova MF, Goldberg TE, Daniel DG, Delsoe J, Weinberger DR (1989) Temporal lobe pathology in schizophrenia: a quantitative magnetic resonance imaging study. Am J Psychiatry 146:464–472

Suddath RL, Christison GW, Torrey EF, Casanova MF, Weinberger DR (1990) Anatomical abnormalities in the brains of monozygotic twins discordant for schizophrenia. N Engl J Med 322(12):62–67

Torrey EF, Peterson MR (1974) Schizophrenia and the limbic system. Lancet ii:942–946

Normal Size of Temporal Areas in a Group of Schizophrenic Patients: A Magnetic Resonance Imaging Study

C. Colombo[1], G. Calabrese, S. Livian, G. Scotti, and S. Scarone

Introduction

The hypothesis of a correlation between the malfunction of temporal regions and schizophrenia was supported by neurofunctional studies of patients with temporal epilepsy associated with psychotic symptoms (Trimble and Perez 1982) and by postmortem studies (Brown et al. 1986; Reynolds et al. 1990). Using magnetic resonance imaging (MRI), it is possible to study brain structures in vivo with particular accuracy (Waddington et al. 1990), and the recent literature on the structural characteristics of temporal areas in schizophrenia has led to discordant results. In fact, whereas some studies showed a reduction in the temporal lobe size in schizophrenic patients compared to normal controls (Suddath et al. 1989; Rossi et al. 1990), other authors did not find any differences between the two groups (Kelsoe et al. 1988; Johnstone et al. 1989). This MRI study compares temporal lobe size in a sample of schizophrenic patients carefully evaluated regarding their clinical, psychopathological, and demographic characteristics with a group of normal controls matched for sex and age.

Methods

Subjects

There were 18 schizophrenics (12 males and 6 females, mean age 29.1 ± 8.4 years, mean educational level 9.8 ± 3.4 years) and 14 normal controls (9 males and 5 females, age 32.6 ± 16.5 years, mean educational level 16.9 ± 3.9 years) who underwent MRI. Whereas age was not significantly different in the two groups (F (3.8) 0.82; p 0.4, n.s), controls showed a significantly higher educational level (F (1.31) 5.47; $p < 0.001$). Nonetheless, the correlation between educational level and temporal lobe area in the two groups was not significant ($r = 0.18$ for the left side and $r = 0.18$ for the right side in the total sample; $r = 0.16$ for the left side and $r = 0.36$ for the

[1] Dipartimento di Neuroscienze HSR, Via Prinetti 29, 20127 Milano, Italy.

Imaging of the Brain in Psychiatry and Related Fields
Edited by K. Maurer

right side in the schizophrenic group; $r = 0.54$ for the left side and $r = 0.40$ for the right side in the control group). The diagnosis of schizophrenia, the clinical subtype, and the course of the illness (i.e., subchronic or chronic) were independently assessed by two senior psychiatrists according to DSM-IIIR criteria (APA 1987). Of the 18 schizophrenics, 3 were paranoid, 7 disorganized, 8 undifferentiated, 3 subchronic, and 15 chronic. All schizophrenic patients were treated with low dose neuroleptics at the time of the examination (a mean dose equivalent of approximately 4 mg of haloperidol). All normal controls had a negative history of serious medical, neurological, or psychiatric illness. None was taking medications known to affect brain size.

MRI Scans

All subjects were scanned on a Toshiba MRI unit operating at 0.5 T. The scanning sequences started with an axial pilot scan followed by sagittal and coronal scans with T1-weighted spin echo sequences (TR 500, TE 30). We obtained eight sagittal and eight coronal sections 5 mm thick with a 1.5 mm gap. The most lateral, left, parasagittal section usually readily showed the left parahippocampal gyrus and sylvian fissure; thus this section was used to obtain eight oblique coronal images perpendicular to the plane of the left parahippocampal gyrus and sylvian fissure, as recommended by Jack et al. (1988). The section that best showed amygdala and pes hippocampi was used for temporal lobe area measurement.

Anatomical Measurements

Neuroanatomical structures were identified as follows: Processing of the MR images was performed with an image analysis system (Kontron Bildanalyse, Eching/Munich, FRG). This system consists of a video camera, a light box, and an image processor (digitizer) within the computer. MRI slices were placed over the light box and stored on the computer. Measurements for each patient were calibrated with the scale determined for each MRI slice at the time of the scan.

Temporal lobe area measure ments were determined as follows: On the section showing amygdala and pes hippocampi, the temporal lobe perimeter was delineated, as defined by the subarachnoid space. Superiorly, the temporal lobe was manually disarticulated from the overlying hemisphere by tracing a line that joined (from medial to lateral) the most lateral aspect of the sylvian fissure. An automatic system was then employed to compute the temporal lobe area in square centimeters. The area was measured using a threshold method which permits automatic object boundary detection; this technique requires the establishment of a minimum gray scale value. The structural measurements were performed by two independent investigators who were blind as to the identity of the subjects. The reliability of the former was very high ($r = 0.93$ $p = 0.001$).

Statistical Analysis

Multivariate analysis of variance (MANOVA) was employed for the analysis. The areas of the left and right temporal lobes were the dependent variables; the diagnosis was the independent variable; and the side (left and right) was the intrasubject factor.

Results

Tables 1 and 2 show the mean areas for the right and the left temporal lobes according to the diagnostic group and the MANOVA results, respectively. No significant differences between schizophrenic subjects and controls regarding temporal lobe areas were noted. The effect of side and the interaction diagnosis-by-side were also not significant.

Discussion

The results of the present study did not demonstrate any significant difference in the size of temporal regions between a group of schizophrenics and a

Table 1. Temporal lobe areas: mean values (SD) by diagnosis

	Controls	Schizophrenics
Left side	12.74 (1.48)	12.99 (1.45)
Right side	12.70 (1.55)	13.11 (1.59)

Table 2. Summary of MANOVA

Source	MANOVA		
	df	*F*	*p*
Diagnosis	1.30	<1	ns
Side	1.30	<1	ns
Diagnosis × side	1.30	<1	ns

MANOVA, multivariate analysis of variance.

group of control subjects matched for sex and age. Whereas these data appear to be consistent with some of the recent literature, they are in disagreement with other recent findings in the field. The discrepancies found between different MRI studies in psychiatric populations may be due to differences in MRI data collection and its subsequent analysis. Recently, the importance of a standardized method for imaging analysis has been emphasized (Suddath et al. 1989). The geometric identification of a brain region requires correct adjustment of a number of variables, such as the background illumination conditions of the room where measurements are executed and the settings of technical instruments (light camera intensity, the distance between the camera and the plate, MRI slice density and contrast homogeneity). It is also necessary to consider the presence of magnetic field inhomogeneity, which produces a spatial distortion in the coronal and sagittal planes. We were careful to use the correct method of analysis, according to the criteria indicated by other researchers (Jack et al. 1990). Interstudy differences in clinical and psychopathological characteristics should also be taken into account. Further, our results outline the need for replicate studies which pay particular attention to the patient selection criteria and to the technical and methodological aspects of image analysis.

References

APA (American Psychiatric Association) (1987) Diagnostic and statistical manual of mental disorders, 3rd, rev edn. APA, Washington DC

Brown R, Colter N, Corsellis JAN et al. (1986) Postmortem evidence of structural brain changes in schizophrenia: differences in brain weight, temporal horn area and parahippocampal gyrus compared with affective disorder. Arch Gen Psychiatry 43:36–42

Jack CR, Gehring DG, Sharbrough FW et al. (1988) Temporal lobe volume measurement from MR images: acuracy and left-right asymmetry in normal persons. J Comput Assist Tomogr 12:21–29

Jack CR, Bentley MD, Twomey CK, Zinsmeister AR (1990) MR imaging-based volume measurements of the hippocampal formation and anterior temporal lobe: validation studies. Neuroradiology 176:205–209

Johnstone EC, Cowens DG, Crow TJ, Frith CD, Alexandropolis K, Bydder G, Colter N (1989) Temporal lobe structures as determined by nuclear magnetic resonance in schizophrenia and bipolar affective disorder. J Neurol Neurosurg Psychiatry 52:736–741

Kelsoe JR, Cadet JL, Pickar D et al. (1988) Quantitative neuroanatomy in schizophrenia a controlled magnetic resonance imaging study. Arch Gen Psychiatry 45:533–541

Reynolds GP, Czudek C, Andrews HB (1990) Deficit and hemispheric asymmetry of GABA uptake sites in the hippocampus in schizophrenia. Biol Psychiatry 27:1038–1044

Rossi A, Stratta P, D'Albenzio, Tartaro A, Schiazza G, Di Michele V, Bolino F, Casacchia M (1990) Reduced temporal lobe areas in schizophrenia: preliminary evidences from a controlled multiplanar magnetic resonance imaging study. Biol Psychiatry 27:61–68

Suddath RL, Casanova MF, Goldberg TE, Daniel DG, Kelsoe JR, Weinberger DR (1989) Temporal lobe pathology in schizophrenia: a quantitative magnetic resonance imaging study. Am J Psychiatry 146:464–472

Trimble MR, Perez MM (1982) The phenomenology of the chronic psychoses of epilepsy. In: Koella WP, Trimble MR (eds) Temporal lobe epilepsy, mania and schizophrenia and the limbic system. Karger, Basel, pp 98–105

Waddington JL, O'Callaghan E, Larkin C, Redmond O, Stack J, Ennis JT (1990) Magnetic resonance imaging and spectroscopy in schizophrenia. Br J Psychiatry 157:56–65

Ventricle Size and P300 in Elderly Depressed Patients

S. SCHLEGEL[1] and D. NIEBER

Introduction

Despite the growing body of literature on computerized tomography (CT) studies and event related potentials (ERP) in mental diseases, little attention has been paid to the relationship between brain morphology and ERP. In schizophrenia no significant relationship between P300 latencies and CT scan measurements was detected (Romani et al. 1987), but positive correlations were described between N1-P2 amplitude and ventrical size. Romani et al. (1987) referred to analogous findings for visual evoked potentials of elderly and demented patients (Cosi et al. 1982). To our knowledge, these two studies are the only ones which have examined the relationship between CT measurements and ERP. Therefore, our study was planned in order to investigate the correlation between P300 and brain atrophy in elderly depressed patients.

Methods

There were 12 patients (1 male, 11 females), with a mean age of 69.4 (SD: 5.3 years; range 63–80 years), who were included in the study. All patients met DSM-III criteria (APA 1980) for a major depressive episode. After a drug-free period of 6–10 days, dependent on premedication, the following rating scales were performed: the Brief Psychiatric Rating Scale (BPRS) (Overall and Gormann 1962), the Hamilton Depression Scale (HAMD) (Hamilton 1960), and the Bech-Rafaelsen Melancholia Scale (BRMS) (Bech and Rafaelsen 1980). The Mini-Mental State (MMS) (Folstein et al. 1975) was chosen for analysis of cognitive impairment. On the same day, P300 was measured according to the guidelines of Maurer and Dierks (1987). Auditory stimuli were presented binaurally at a level of 80 dB with randomized, infrequent, 2000 Hz target tones (duration 50 ms, rise and fall each 10 ms) and frequent nontarget stimuli of 1000 Hz; 30 target and approxi-

[1] Psychiatrische Universitätsklinik Mainz, Untere Zahlbacher Str. 8, W-6500 Mainz, FRG.

Imaging of the Brain in Psychiatry
and Related Fields
Edited by K. Maurer

Table 1. Correlations between evoked related potentials and computerized tomography measurements

	P300 latency			P3 amplitude		
	Parietal right	Parietal left	Central	Parietal right	Parietal left	Central
Third ventricle	0.79^{3}	0.85^{4}	0.70^{2}	−0.27	−0.27	−0.39
VBR	0.01	0.00	0.30	−0.25	−0.21	−0.28
SF right	0.43	0.51^{1}	0.31	0.17	−0.08	−0.15
SF left	0.57^{1}	0.56^{1}	0.42	0.21	0.24	−0.44

Pearson correlation coefficients: $^{1}p < 0.1$; $^{2}p < 0.05$; $^{3}p < 0.01$; $^{4}p < 0.001$.
VBR, ventricular brain ratio; SF, sylvian fissure.

mately 150 nontarget stimuli were presented. The stimulus rate was 0.5/s. Patients were asked to count the infrequent tones with their eyes closed. The cut-off frequencies were set at 0.05 Hz and 30 Hz (cut-off frequency). ERP were recorded on a computer (Brain Atlas, Biologic Systems Operation) which also allowed mapping of 16 electrode values (10–20 system). Here, only the values of P3, P4, and Cz are presented. The ear electrodes were used as references. CT scans were performed on a Philips scanner. Linear distances of the diameter of the third ventricle and sylvian fissures (SF) and planimetric ventricular brain ratio (VBR), as described earlier (Schlegel and Kretzschmar 1987), were measured on the viewing console.

Results

P300 latencies correlated significantly with the diameter of the third ventricle (Table 1). A positive but nonsignificant correlation was also found between the parietal P300 latencies and the diameter of the SF. No significant correlations were detected between P300 latencies and VBR or between amplitudes and CT values. P300 latencies and amplitudes did not correlate significantly with any rating scale. No significant correlations ($p <$ 0.1) were detected between age and latencies or amplitudes. Figure 1 shows that all patients will a left parietal P300 latency over 360 ms had a third ventricle diameter of at least 7 mm.

Discussion

The most important finding of this study is the highly significant correlation between P300 latencies and the diameter of the third ventricle. Less distinct correlations were found between P300 latencies and the diameter of the SF.

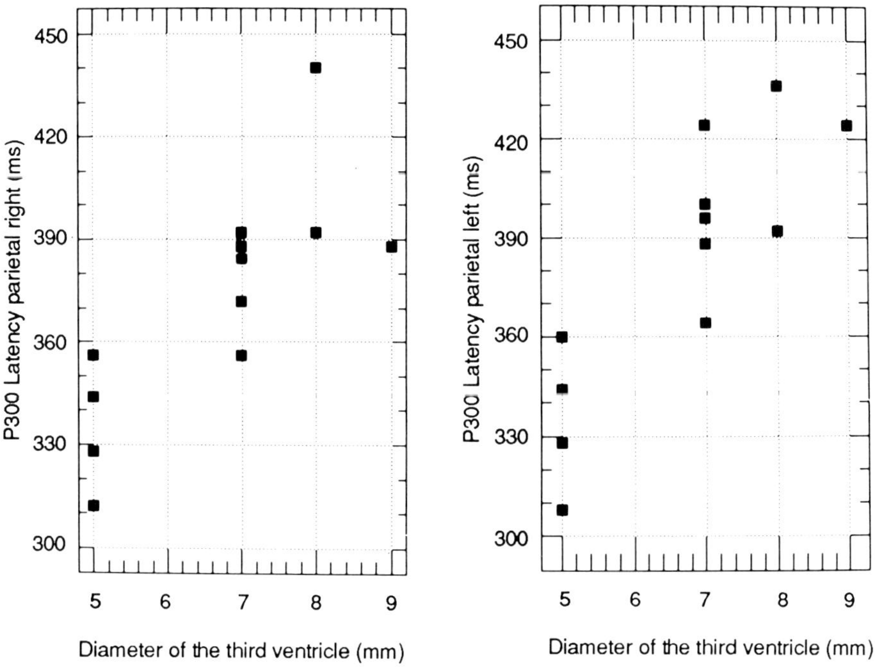

Fig. 1. P300 vs third ventricle

These findings lead to some speculations about the neural structures responsible for the generation of P300. Given the assumption that a wider third ventricle represents alterations of the thalamus, which results in a longer latency of P300, our results support the hypothesis of Yingling and Hosobuchi (1984), that P300 is generated by thalamocortical systems. These systems are thought to be involved in the regulation of selective attention processes. However, Stapleton and Halgran (1987) favored the medial temporal lobe and the hippocampus as the originating locations, suggesting that different structures could represent different types of processing.

Although the SF are not directly located near the medial temporal lobe, the correlation with P300 could indicate the involvement of the temporal area in stimulus detection. In contrast VBR, as an indicator of rather general atrophy, has no impact on P300 latencies.

The lack of a correlation between latencies and the severity of illness is in accordance with earlier studies in younger depressive patients (Roth et al. 1981; Blackwood et al. 1987). P300 did not correlate with cognitive impairment either, as measured by MMS. This discrepancy with previous studies (Brown et al. 1982; Lai et al. 1983) can be explained by the fact that the latter investigated mixed samples of depressed and demented patients.

In conclusion, our data seem to indicate that the association between P300 and the diameter of the third ventricle is independent of the severity of depression or cognitive disturbances. Further studies are in progress in order to examine these findings in various groups of patients.

References

APA (1980) Diagnostic and statistical manual of mental disorders, 3rd edn (DSM III). American Psychiatric Association, Washington DC

Bech P, Rafaelsen OJ (1980) The use of rating scales examplified by comparison of the Hamilton and the Bech-Rafaelsen melancholia scale. Acta Psychiatr Scand 62 [Suppl 285]:128–131

Blackwood DHR, Whalley LJ, Christie JE, Blackburn IM, Clair DMS, McInnes A (1987) Changes in auditory P3 event-related potential in schizophrenia and depression. Br J Psychiatry 150:154–160

Brown WS, Marsh JT, LaRue A (1982) Event-related potentials in psychiatry: differentiating depression and dementia in the elderly. Bull Los Angeles Neurol Soc 47:91–107

Cosi V, Vitelli E, Gozzoli L, Corona A, Ceroni M, Callieco R (1982) Visual evoke potentials in aging of the brain. In: Courjon J, Mauguiere F, Revol M (eds) Clinical Applications of evoked potentials in neurology. Raven, New York, (Advances in neurology, vol 32)

Folstein MF, Folstein SE, McHugh PR (1975) Mini mental state. J Psychiatr Res 12:189–198

Hamilton M (1960) A rating scale for depression. J Neurol Neurosurg Psychiatry 23:56–62

Lai J, Brown WS, Marsh JT, LaRue A (1983) Covariation of P3 latency and mini-mental-state scores in geriatric patients. Psychophysiology 20:419

Maurer K, Dierks T (1987) Topographic brain mapping of EEG and evoked potentials in psychiatry and neurology. EEG/EMG 18:1–52

Overall JE, Gormann DR (1962) The brief psychiatric rating scale. Psychol Rep 10:799–812

Pfefferbaum A, Wenegrat BG, Ford JM, Roth WT, Kopell BS (1984) Clinical application of the P3 component of event-related potentials. II. Dementia, depression and schizophrenia. Electroencephalogr Clin Neurophysiol 59:104–124

Romani A, Merello S, Gozzoli L, Zerbi F, Grassi M, Cosi V (1987) P300 and CT scan in patients with chronic schizophrenia. Br J Psychiatry 151:506–513

Roth WT, Pfefferbaum A, Kelly AF, Berger PA, Kopell BS (1981) Auditory event-related potentials in schizophrenia and depression. Psychiatry Res 4:199–212

Schlegel S, Kretzschmar K (1987) Computed tomography in affective disorders. Part I. Ventricular and sulcal measurements. Biol Psychiatry 22:4–14

Stapleton JM, Halgren E (1987) Endogenous potentials evoked in simple cognitive tasks: depth components and task correlates. Electroencephalogr Clin Neurophysiol 67:44–52

Yingling CD, Hosobuchi Y (1984) A subcortical correlate of P300 in man. Electroencephalogr Clin Neurophysiol 59:72–76

Fast Magnetic Resonance Imaging and Three Dimensional Volumetric Calculations in Degenerative Central Nervous System Diseases

G. BIRDAMER[1], S. FELBER, A. KAMPFL, F. AICHNER, F. GERSTENBRAND, and H. BENESCH

Introduction

Diagnosis of degenerative central nervous system (CNS) disorders with and without dementia is primarily based on neurological and neuropsychological examination (Gerstenbrand et al. 1990; Marsden 1985). In order to differentiate between treatable and nontreatable pathologies that cause dementia, neuroradiological examination has proven to be helpful (Le May 1986). In particular, magnetic resonance imaging (MRI), based on high tissue contrast and multiplanarity, has become a valuable tool in the detection and delineation of intracerebral pathologies (Aichner et al. 1988; Perovitch et al. 1990).

However, differentiation between senile dementia of the Alzheimer's type (SDAT) and multi-infarct dementia (MID) remains difficult, since the ischemic-like white matter lesions are detected in both types of degenerative diseases (Felber et al. 1990). To improve the capability of MRI, new gradient echo (GE) sequences have been introduced in addition to conventional spin echo (SE) sequences.

Strong, T1-weighted, GE sequences with a slice thickness of about 1 mm allow detection of even small parenchymal lesions as well as optimal differentiation between gray and white matter. Furthermore, nearly isotropic resolution allows in vivo, volumetric, computerized postprocessing.

The aim of this study was to investigate the impact of fast three-dimensional (3-D) imaging and volumetric calculation on the differentiation of degenerative disorders of various types.

Methods

All examinations were performed on a 1.5 T Magnetom using a circular polarized head coil with a field of view of 25 cm. The parameters of the 3-D

[1] Gemeinsame Institutseinrichtung für Magnetresonanztomographie und Spektroskopie, Universität Innsbruck, Anichstr. 35, 6020 Innsbruck, Austria.

Imaging of the Brain in Psychiatry and Related Fields
Edited by K. Maurer

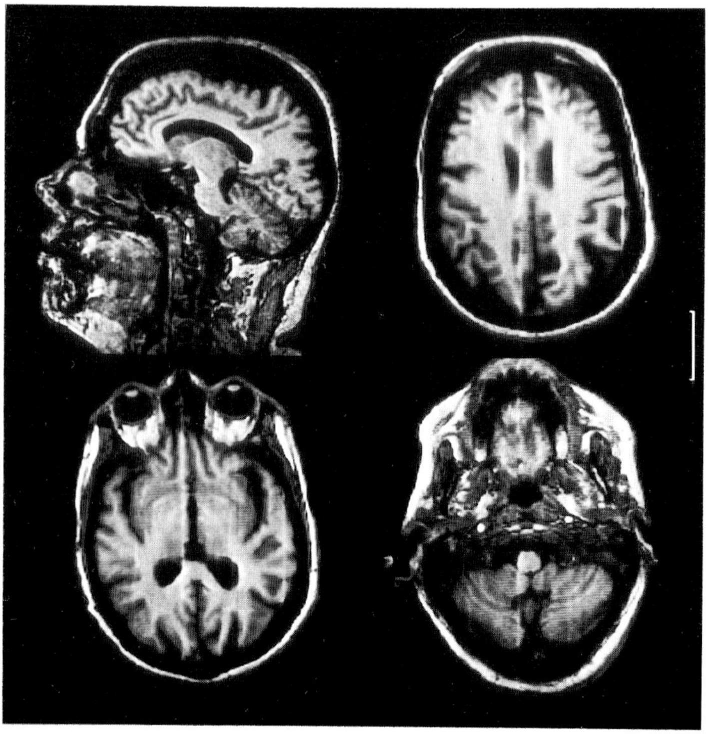

Fig. 1. A 61 year old patient with senile dementia of the Alzheimer's type. Sagittal 3-D FLASH GE sequence (see text) with axial reformations shows predominant atrophy of the temporooccipital cortex

FLASH sequence had been optimized for T1 contrast: TR, 40 ms; TE, 5–8 ms; α, 40° (Fig. 1).

Minimal pixel size and short TE times compensate for intravoxel-phased dispersion due to susceptibility effects at bony areas to soft tissue interfaces. By excitation of a 13–16 cm 3-D volume, 128 contiguous slices of the entire brain, 1–1.3 mm thick, were acquired within 21 min. The acquired data were postprocessed on a MR system computer. Brain parenchyma was isolated from the surrounding tissue using a "region-growing" segmentation algorithm. The volume of each segmentation was automatically calculated.

Patients

Between January 1989 and January 1990, 40 patients with diffuse or regional parenchymal loss were investigated. In 14 patients, additional postprocessing volumetric assessments were performed (SDAT $n = 2$, MID $n = 5$,

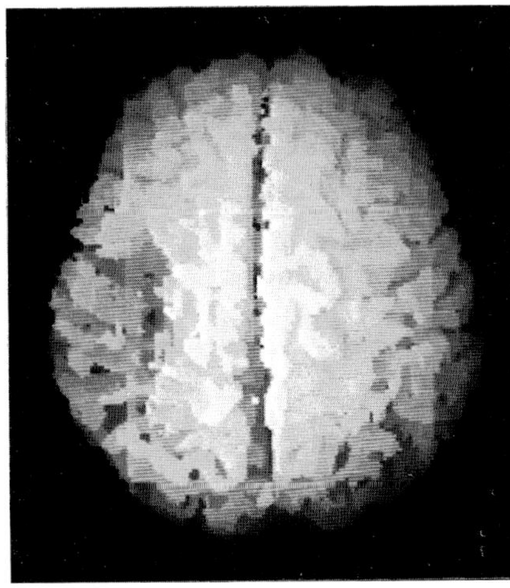

Fig. 2. A 49 year old patient with multiinfarct dementia. Surface reconstruction shows a huge postischemic defect on the right parietal lobe

spinocerebellar degeneration $n = 7$, control volunteers $n = 2$). To prove the accuracy of the volumetric values, a formalin-fixed brain was examined and the anatomical data were compared to the volumetric MR results. Surface reconstruction of the brain was done in an additional four patients (Fig. 2).

Results

A total of 14 patients, 2 volunteers, and 1 formalin-fixed specimen were scanned with a 1.5T MR system using a relatively T1-weighted GE sequence. The 3-D data were automatically segmentated and volumetrically postprocessed. In all cases the examinations were of diagnostic quality; the measurement time of 21 min for the 3D data was well tolerated by all patients. Relatively T1-weighted sequences allowed excellent delineation of gray and white matter. The contrast between cerebrospinal fluid (CSF) and cortex was sufficient for volumetric computerized postprocessing. A pixel size of $1-1.3 \times 0.9 \times 0.9$ was calculated in milliliters and was automatically processed for volumetric assessment. To evaluate the quality of this method, the anatomical volume and the 3-D volumetric data of the specimen were compared; a difference of only 4% was found (total brain volume: anatomical, 1098.1 ml; 3-D volumetric data, 1046.4 ml). The calculated brain volume of a normal female volunteer, age 45 years, was 1193.6 ml, that of a male volunteer, age 26, was 1304 ml. The two patients with SDAT, 61 and 57 years of age and both female, had a brain volume of 903.27 ml and 824 ml, respectively (Fig. 3). The five male patients with MID had a reduction of the total brain volume ranging from 1226.2 ml to 1093 ml.

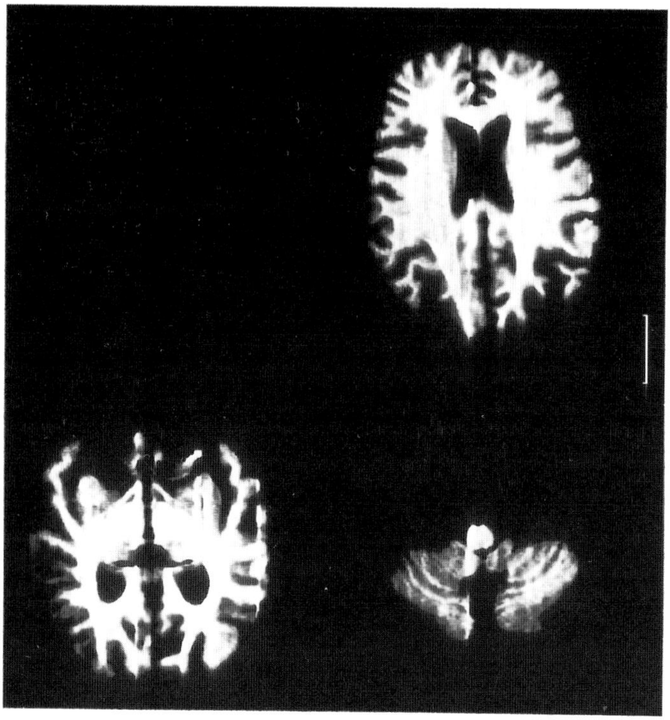

Fig. 3. Axial reformations of sagittal 3D FLASH examination in a patient with senile dementia of the Alzheimer's type postprocessed to isolate the brain from surrounding tissue. Volumetric data are: total volume, 824 ml; cortex, 705 ml; cerebellum, 118 ml

Discussion

In this preliminary study, 14 patients with different pathological conditions resulting in reduction of brain volume were volumetrically assessed. We used 1 mm thick slices and a relatively T1-weighted FLASH sequence with a nearly isotropic high resolution of less than 1 mm. With this technique, even the smallest lacunar lesions, related to vascular etiologies, can be detected. Therefore, approach may be a further step in the differentiation between MID mixed type and primary degenerative CNS disorders. In addition, this method has proven to be sufficient for volumetric postprocessing. In all patients volumetric calculation revealed a decrease in brain volume compared to nonage-matched volunteers. In SDAT and spinocerebellar atrophy, this method allows volumetric follow-up investigations which may be helpful in further understanding the course of these primary degenerative diseases.

It was found that, in patients with MID, the gray/white matter ratio in nonischemic areas was normal, whereas in patients with SDAT a thinning of the cortical gray matter was present. The excellent cortical and medullary contrast, based on the strongly T1-weighted FLASH sequences, may further allow separate volumetric calculation of gray and white matter.

In addition, surface reconstruction revealed topographic information about cortical brain structures. In order to achieve a better correlation between neurological, neuropsychological, and electrophysiological findings, this method may be helpful for future investigations of degenerative CNS diseases.

References

Aichner F, Felber S, Willeit J (1988) Magnetic resonance imaging and computed tomography in diagnosis and assessment of dementia. In: Agnoli et al. (eds) Senile dementias. 2nd International Symposium. Libbey, Paris, pp 213–217

Felber S, Birbamer G, Benesch H, Aichner F, Ehrike H (1990) Isotropic 3D-MR-imaging applied to degenerative disorders of the brain. In: Schneider GH et al. (eds) Digitale Bildgebung-Interventionelle Radiologie-Integrierte Digitale Radiologie. Blackwell/Ueberreuter, Cambridge, pp 282–285

Gerstenbrand F, Birbamer G, Rainer J (1990) Clinical aspects of dementia: a classification. In: Battistin L and Gerstenbrand F (eds) Aging brain and dementia: new trends in diagnosis and therapy. Wiley-Liss, New York, vol 54, pp 32–37

Le May M (1986) CT changes in dementing diseases: a review. AJNR 7:841–853

Marsden C (1985) Assessment of dementia. In: Frederiks J (ed) Neurobehavioural disorders. Elsevier, New York, pp 221–232 (Handbook of clinical neurology, vol 2(46))

Perovitch M, Wener L, Bryan N, Perl S, Kumar AJ (1990) Magnetic resonance imaging in the aging brain and some other pathological processes leading to dementia. In: Battistin L and Gerstenbrand F (eds) Aging brain and dementia: new trends in diagnosis and therapy. Wiley-Liss, New York, pp 465–481

Arachnoid Cysts in Psychiatric Patients: A Retrospective Computerized Tomography and Magnetic Resonance Imaging Study

T. Becker[1], M. Lanczik, E. Hofmann, T. Müller, M. Warmuth-Metz, J. Fritze, and B. Schuknecht

Introduction

The share of intracranial arachnoid cysts (ACs) in the total group of patients with intracranial space-occupying lesions is approximately 1% (Robinson 1971). ACs may be asymptomatic or give rise to a variety of neurologic symptoms. In adult patients, clinical manifestations include headache, seizures, and focal neurologic deficits. Increased head circumference and psychomotor retardation are characteristic signs in children. Some investigators have focused on psychopathologic manifestations of ACs and reported clinical improvement following cyst fenestration or shunt procedures (Colameco and DiTomasso 1983; Kuhnley et al. 1981).

In the present study the prevalence of intracranial ACs was determined in a large sample of patients examined by routine computerized tomography (CT) or magnetic resonance imaging (MRI). The psychiatric patient subgroup was compared to nonpsychiatric patients with regard to the occurrence of ACs.

Materials and Methods

During the years 1987–1988, 12088 cranial CT and 1209 cranial MRI exams were performed in the Department of Neuroradiology at Würzburg University. Clinical departments of origin (Departments of Psychiatry, Neurology, Neurosurgery, Ear, Nose, and Throat (ENT), and Pediatrics at Würzburg University) were documented for all patients; all exam reports were screened for definite diagnosis of ACs or findings suggestive of ACs. A total of 74 CT and 35 MRI exams were subjected to detailed analysis; 66 patients with inconclusive findings were excluded. Location and size of ACs, signs of brain compression, and bony changes were documented. Clinical diagnoses were derived from chart reviews. Statistical analysis was comprised of contingency tables from which expected frequencies were calculated; deviations from the latter were tested by χ^2 test.

[1] Abt. für Psychiatrie, Universitäts-Nervenklinik Würzburg, Füchsleinstr. 15, W-8700 Würzburg, FRG.

Imaging of the Brain in Psychiatry
and Related Fields
Edited by K. Maurer

Table 1. Location and size of intracranial arachnoid cysts in psychiatric and nonpsychiatric patients ($n = 43$)

	Side		Region[a]			Size[b]			Space-occupying effect present (n)
	Left	Right	Midline	Temporal	Non-temporal	1	2	3	
Psychiatric	6	2	–	7	2	3	4	1	2
Nonpsychiatric	24	9	2	24	15	5	24	6	17

[a] An arachnoid cyst can be located both temporally and nontemporally.
[b] Size 1, cross-sectional area $\leqslant 4\,cm^2$; size 2, >4 and $\leqslant 25\,cm^2$; size 3, area $>25\,cm^2$.

Results

CT showed ACs in 38 patients; MRI revealed 5 patients with cysts (prevalence rate 3.2 per 1000); left hemispheric and middle cranial fossa locations prevailed. In the psychiatric group, there was only one patient who did not have temporal lobe involvement (Table 1).

Both medium size and large ACs and space-occupying effects were more frequent in the nonpsychiatric patient group. When AC prevalence rates were compared to the expected prevalence, the only significant deviation was found in the psychiatric subgroup (all psychiatric ACs: found/expected = 8/3.3; $\chi^2 = 7.47$, $p < 0.01$; temporal lobe psychiatric ACs: found/expected: 7/2.4; $\chi^2 = 9.96$, $p < 0.01$; n.s. for nontemporal psychiatric ACs). There were no significant findings in the neurologic, neurosurgical, ENT, and pediatric patient groups. Chart reviews revealed features of psychiatric relevance in three neurologic patients (personality disorder/functional complaints, attempted suicide, depressive syndrome). The psychiatric patient group was heterogeneous regarding diagnosis (DSM III-R: hypochondriasis = 300.70; dysthymia and passive aggressive personality disorder = 300.40 and 301.84; organic delusional disorder = 293.81 ($n = 2$); dysthymia and obsessive compulsive personality disorder = 300.40 and 301.40; bipolar disorder, manic = 296.42; hysterical neurosis, conversion type = 300.11; major depression, recurrent = 296.34). In psychiatric patients nonpsychiatric diseases were not found.

Discussion

We found temporal ACs to be more frequent in psychiatric than in nonpsychiatric patients. The presence of psychopathologic features in three neurologic patients underscores the role of psychiatric manifestations of ACs.

Temporal lobe involvement has been established in a number of psychiatric disorders including amnesic syndromes, anxiety states, schizophreniform psychosis, and dementia. Temporal lobe trauma and tumors give rise to psychopathologic symptoms (Mulder and Daly 1952). Temporal lobe asymmetry and left temporal lesions may be involved in the pathogenesis of schizophrenia. The location of an AC is typically in the middle fossa (range 40%–80%); left hemispheric involvement prevails.

A literature review comprised of data on 1089 patients revealed psychopathologic symptoms in 14% (Becker et al. 1991). Temporal lobe location may be a factor contributing to psychopathologic symptoms in AC patients. Other mechanisms to be taken into consideration include increased intracranial pressure and hydrocephalus which may evolve secondary to ACs. However, in our psychiatric patients only two (out of eight) had cysts with a space-occupying effect. There were no cases of hydrocephalus.

As regards the pathogenesis of middle cranial fossa cysts the idea of temporal lobe agenesis has largely been abandoned in favor of the concept of arachnoid malformation (Robinson 1971). Pia and arachnoid mater, in the early developing embryo, most likely evolve from mesenchymal tissue surrounding the neural tube, the "perimedullary mesh" or endomeninx. The subarachnoid space is formed when, with the rupture of the rhombic roof, cerebrospinal fluid (CSF) escapes to within the layers of this mesenchymal mesh, the fluid being propelled by the pulsatile forces of the choroid plexus (Rengachary 1985). ACs may develop because of minor aberrations in CSF flow resulting in the sequestration of an enclosed chamber or diverticulum in the perimedullary mesh. These processes are dated to the first and second trimenon.

Neurodevelopmental abnormalities of neuroectodermal structures are considered by many investigators to be involved in the pathogenesis of schizophrenia (Jakob and Beckmann 1986); the same may apply to other psychiatric disorders. Our finding of an increased prevalence of ACs in psychiatric patients may indicate a common impairment of mesenchymal tissue differentiation. Noxious influences could be hypothesized to hit both neuroglia and the developing endomeninx during a sensitive period.

References

Becker T, Lanczik M, Hofmann E, Müller T, Warmuth-Metz M, Fritze J, Schuknecht B (1991) Erhöhte Prävalenz von Arachnoidalsystem bei psychiatrischen Patienten: Eine retrospektive CT- und MR-Untersuchung. Klin Neuroradiol 1:154–160

Colameco S, DiTomasso RA (1983) Arachnoid cyst associated with psychological disturbance. J Med Soc NY 79:209–210

Jakob H, Beckmann H (1986) Prenatal developmental disturbances in the limbic allocortex in schizophrenics. J Neural Transm 65:303–326

Kuhnley EJ, White DH, Granoff AL (1981) Psychiatric presentation of an arachnoid cyst. J Clin Psychiatry 42:167–168

Mulder DW, Daly D (1952) Psychiatric symptoms associated with lesions of temporal lobe. JAMA 150:173–176

Rengachary SS (1985) Intracranial arachnoid and ependymal cysts. In: Wilkins RH, Rengachary SS (eds) Neurosurgery. McGraw-Hill, New York, pp 2160–2172

Robinson RG (1971) Congenital cysts of the brain: arachnoid malformations. Prog Neurol Surg 4:133–174

Cerebral Effects of Stereotactic Subcaudate Tractotomy

A.L. MALIZIA[1], M.G. GRAVES, J.B. BINGHAM, J.R. BARTLETT, and P.K. BRIDGES

Introduction

The psychosurgical operation of stereotactic subcaudate tractotomy (SST) is performed for patients who have treatment resistant affective illness refractory to electroconvulsive therapy (ECT) and vigorous pharmacotherapy (Bartlett et al. 1981). The operation consists of placing ten yttrium-90 rods, 7 mm long by 1 mm in diameter, in the ventroposterior quadrant of the frontal lobes. They are placed stereotactically using a Macaul frame by taking repeat anteroposterior and lateral air ventriculograms and hence calculating the siting. Some 60% of patients get well either on or off medication; the response is slow, requiring 3–12 months. Some 20 patients from the whole UK are operated on every year. There are no major adverse personality changes (Goktepe et al. 1975). This pilot study was undertaken to determine the precise siting of the lesion, the effects of the operation on the brain at various postoperative times and the optimal time intervals for magnetic resonance imaging (MRI) of the patients postoperatively.

Patients and Methods

Ten consenting patients were scanned with a Philips Gyroscan operating at 1.5 T. Five patients were scanned preoperatively, at 3 months and at 1 year; the other five preoperatively and at 2 weeks postoperatively. Images were obtained in 8 mm coronal IR slices and 8 mm tranverse SE T2 slices. Psychiatric ratings included the Schedule for Affective Disorders and Schizophrenia (SADS-L), Present State Examination (PSE), Newcastle and Hamilton depression scales, and the Beck depression inventory. The mini-mental state test was also administered twice weekly in the postoperative period until discharge.

[1] Geoffrey Knight Unit, Brook General Hospital, London SE18 and Divisions of Psychiatry and Radiological Sciences, UMDS, Guy's Campus, London SE1, UK.

Imaging of the Brain in Psychiatry
and Related Fields
Edited by K. Maurer

Results

Patient Characteristics

Nine females and one male were scanned. Four patients had unipolar and six bipolar affective illness. The average Hamilton depression score was 23. The average age was 48 (range 36–62); 23 years had elapsed since the first episode of illness (range 7–35). The patients had received an average of 29 ECT treatments and maximal pharmacotherapy. They had been in the present cycle of the illness for an average of 9 years (range 1–30). Six had a family history of affective disorder.

MRI: Qualitative Analysis

Two weeks postoperatively there is prominent oedema which spreads preferentially along white matter fibres. The uncinate fasciculus, the orbital and rectus gyri, the olfactory sulcus, the middle frontal gyrus, the head of the caudate and the external and internal capsule are always involved. Extracerebrally, oedema accumulates in the sulci, especially in the lateral cerbral sulcus pressing on and widening the space between frontal and temporal lobes (Fig. 1a). Oedema can occupy between 23% and 48% of total brain size. Behavioural disturbance and auditory hallucinosis, when present postoperatively, seemed to be related to the oedema spreading posteriorly in the temporal lobe. Confusion seemed to be associated with oedema spreading to the basal and septal nuclei. However, precise local-

a 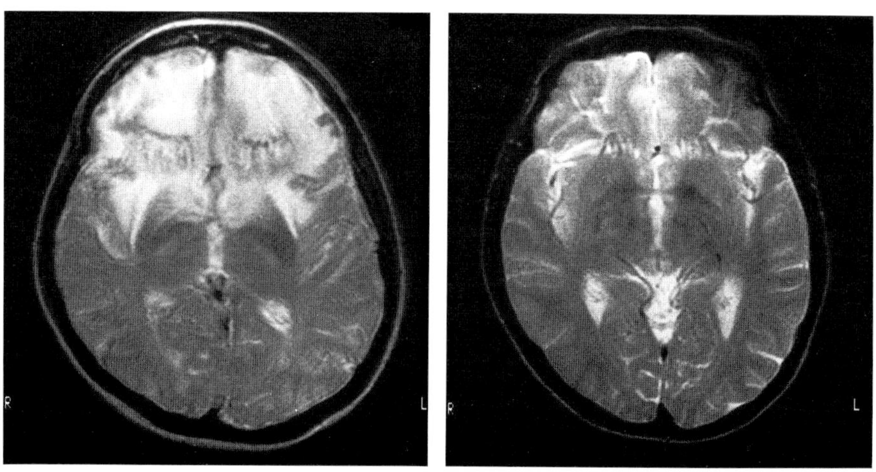 b

Fig. 1a,b. Typical appearances on T2-weighted image at 2 weeks (**a**) and at 3 months (**b**). Oedema subsides and rods are just visible

isation is difficult because of the distortion caused by the oedema. Ranking the worst postoperative mini-mental state score and correlating it to the amount of oedema failed to indicate significance (Spearman's coefficient = 0.85) but this may be due to the small number of patients involved.

At 3 months a small volume of signal change can be seen around the lesion (range 1400–4300 mm^3). The signal change extends to a minimum of 5 mm and to a maximum of 2 cm from the surface of the rods. This is limited to the posterior and inferior part of the frontal lobes. Lines of increased intensity are sometimes seen parallel to the ventricular boundary.

At 1 year only the area around the rods is visible, the whole lesion appearing in one or two slices only. The estimated volume of signal change varied between 200 mm^3 and 1300 mm^3.

MRI: Quantitative Analysis

The preoperative T2 lateral ventricle brain ratio on one slice was 8% on average (range 6.3%–11.3%). It correlated with age ($p < 0.025$) but not with number of ECTs, length of present cycle or duration of illness from first episode. It also correlated with the T1 preoperative total ventricle to brain ratio ($p < 0.005$) which had a mean of 2.1% (range 1.36%–3.34%). This latter measurement is more accurate and sensitive than single slice measurements. There was significant ventricular enlargement in all patients at 3 and 12 months when compared to preoperative findings ($p < 0.005$) but no significant difference between 3 and 12 months. The two patients with the worst outcome in terms of affective disorder had the greatest amount of enlargement. Thalamic size was unaffected by the operation.

Position of Lesion

The lesion is always in the white matter of the orbital gyri. Its posterior border on the horizontal sections was in line with the anterior border of the third ventricle in four out of five patients. In the fifth it was 5 mm in front of the third ventricle; as this patient showed very little signal change, this may represent the true lie of the rods. The head of the caudate seemed to be unaffected although up to 25% of the lesion is under it. The breadth of the lesion varied from 16 mm to 22 mm and lay 2–6 mm lateral to the medial border of the lobe.

Summary and Conclusions

Rods are placed accurately despite relying on bony and ventricular landmarks. Immediately postoperatively, oedema is the most prominent feature but it gradually subsides. It is variable in its extent and may relate to the severity of side effects and to final outcome. At 1 year the lesion is small and just the radiation necrosis is visible. The ventricles enlarge in all patients postoperatively and there is a trend for greater enlargement to be associated with poorer outcome.

Larger numbers of patients need to be scanned at 2 weeks and at least 6 months postoperatively. A change in sequence to obtain thinner slices and other orientations within the scanning time constraint are being considered at present. We are also planning to combine structural with functional and detailed neuropsychological measurements to elucidate these points further.

Acknowledgments. This work has been supported by the Guy's Hospital Special Trustees.

References

Bartlett JR, Bridges PK, Kelly D (1981) Contemporary indications for psychosurgery. Br J Psychiatry 131:249–260

Goktepe EO, Young LG, Bridges PK (1975) A further review of the results of stereotactic subcaudate tractotomy. Br J Psychiatry 126:270–280

Comparisons of Linear and Planimetric Indices as Estimators of Intraventricular Cerebrospinal Fluid Spaces (CSF) in Normal Autoptic Brains

K. Niemann[1], L. Woeckel, and J. Wasel

In cranial computerized tomography (CT), a variety of linear and planimetric indices which render estimates of the volumes of the intraventricular fluid spaces of the living brain have been suggested. The validity of these indices, however, has received little interest (Reveley 1985). We were interested in the correlation of ventricular size indices with actual cerebrospinal fluid (CSF) volumes. Measurements were achieved using digital three-dimensional (3-D) analysis of postmortem brains, transformation of the data set to a standard reference system, and computer simulated CT slicing.

The borders of the lateral ventricles of 27 formalin-fixed left hemispheres (specimens obtained from individuals age: 71.9 ± 10.4 years; 12 females, 15 males) were measured pointwise with a 3-D digitizer (von Keyserlingk DG et al. 1985). The hemispheres were free of gross pathology and distortion and there was no history of neurological or psychiatric disease. The volumes of the left lateral ventricles were calculated employing both the addition of interpolated slices (1 mm thick) and the formula proposed by Park and Lee (1977). The mean from the two procedures was considered as the real value. CT was simulated by slicing each set of points in eight horizontal standard planes parallel to the intercommissural line. The thickness of the slices was 8 mm. The section planes extended from 28 mm basal to the intercommissural plane to 35 mm dorsal. From suitable slices, the maximum spread of the anterior horn (A), the minimum spread of the anterior horn (B), the minimum width of the cella media (C), and the maximum width of the convexity of the trigone (T) were obtained. The maximum breadth of the hemisphere (D_{max}) was also determined. For the purpose of illustration, the measurement sites are drawn into analogous CT scans (Fig. 1). It should be stressed that the measurements themselves were not performed on CT scans but on each of the digitally stored point clouds representing 1 out of 27 ventricles.

From the data obtained, the cella media index (C/D_{max}; Haug 1977), Evans' ratio (A/D_{max}; 1942), the index of Hahn and Rim (B/D_{max}; 1976), and Huckman's number (A + B; Huckman et al. 1975) were determined. The calculations differ from the authors' instructions in two respects: (1) the

[1] Institut für Anatomie, Med. Fakultät der RWTH Aachen, Wendlingweg 2, W-5100 Aachen, FRG.

Imaging of the Brain in Psychiatry
and Related Fields
Edited by K. Maurer

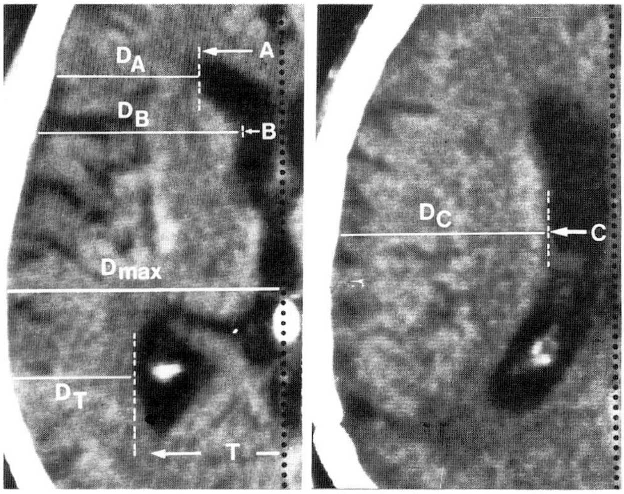

Fig. 1a,b. Measurement sites drawn into corresponding CT scans

measurements were taken only unilaterally on left hemispheres and (2) inner skull diameters were replaced by outer brain diameters. The cross-sectional areas of the lateral ventricles in each of the standard 8 mm slices were also computed.

Ventricular volumes ranged from 6.5 ml to 27.6 ml (14.5 ml ± 4.8 ml). The correlation coefficients of the linear indices with the calculated ventricular volumes were $r = 0.40$ for the cella media index, 0.50 for Evan's ratio, 0.32 for the index of Hahn and Rim, and 0.44 for Huckman's number. Age correlated with the actual ventricular volumes at $r = 0.47$.

Planimetric evaluations were performed on each of the computer sectioned ventricles. The variation between these sectioned areas in the standard plane was visualized by pseudocolors (Fig. 2). The ventricular areas 4–11 mm dorsal to the intercommissural line (Fig. 2a), which usually contain the foramen of Monro, correlated very closely ($r = 0.90$) with the actual ventricular volumes. This was not the case for the cross-sectional area 20–27 mm dorsal to the intercommissural line (Fig. 2b) which hits the cella media of the lateral ventricles ($r = 0.68$). The latter slice is often used for the calculation of the ventricle-brain ratio (VBR).

Due to the observable variation in the trigonal area (Fig. 2a), we introduced an "anterior horn-trigonum index" ($A/(A + D\mathrm{A}) + T/(T + D\mathrm{T})$) which was determined in a slice 4–11 mm dorsal to the intercommissural line. The a posteriori correlation with the actual ventricular volumes was $r = 0.82$ ($p = 0.0001$).

The brain specimens used in this study stemmed from an elderly normal population and inferences are consequently restricted. For the aging brain it may be concluded that under nonpathological conditions traditional linear

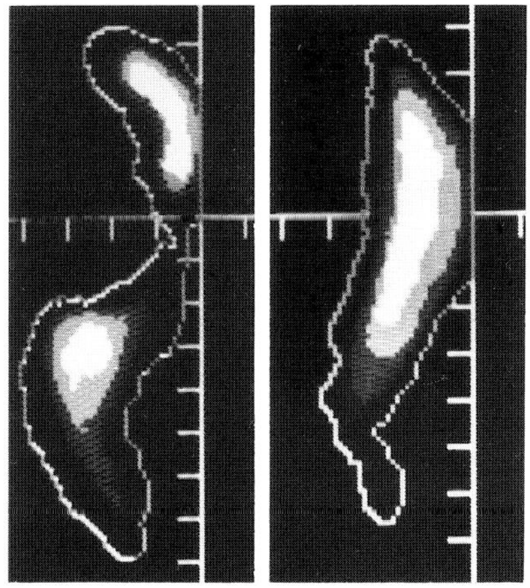

a b

Fig. 2a,b. Variability profile of 27 left lateral ventricles in a plane 4–11 mm dorsal (**a**) and 20–27 mm dorsal (**b**) to the intercommissural plane. The *white closed line* shows the total variation; the *white areas* are occupied by more than 95% of the sample; the *black areas* by less than 33% (scale = 1 cm)

indices are not valid estimators of ventricular size. However, the intuitive superiority of planimetric to linear indices cannot be taken for granted. This is demonstrated by the anterior horn-trigonum index. Here a linear index, which was defined on the basis of the known statistical variations, proved superior to the calculation of the VBR in the cella media plane. Generally, the choice of suitable estimators of ventricular size may profit from geometrical consideration and knowledge about the underlying variability profiles which should demonstrate different patterns in normal and pathological conditions.

References

Evans WA (1942) An encephalographic ratio for estimating ventricular enlargement and cerebral atrophy. Arch Neurol Psychiatry 47:931–937

Hahn FJY, Rim K (1976) Frontal ventricular dimensions on normal computed tomography. Am J Roentgenol 126:593–596

Haug G (1977) Age and sex dependence of the size of normal ventricles on computed tomography. Neuroradiology 14:201–204

Huckman MS, Fox MS, Topel J (1975) The validity of criteria for the evaluation of cerebral atrophy by computed tomography. Radiology 116:85–92

Park KS, Lee NS (1987) A three-dimensional Fourier descriptor for human body representation/reconstruction from serial cross sections. Comput Biomed Res 20:125–140

Reveley MA (1985) Ventricular enlargement in schizophrenia. The validity of computerized tomographic findings. Br J Psychiatry 147:233–240

von Keyserlingk DG, Niemann K, Wasel J, Reinold J, Poeck K (1985) A new method in computer-assisted imaging in neuroanatomy. Acta Anat 123:240–246

Automatic Transfer from Three-Dimensional Volume Elements in the Brain to Knowledge-Based Artificial Diagrams

D. Graf von Keyserlingk[1], K. Niemann, and H. Knott

Introduction

Imaging of the brain in psychiatry is usually part of a diagnostic decision process. As a computer already produces the images, it may be useful to integrate image processing and rendering into a more general knowledge-based system, e.g., a decision support system. Such systems have several basic features in common. The digital image data must be modeled; that means they must be structured in a suitable abstract arrangement so that both image data and data representing knowledge may be handled and brought into a relationship. Suitable plans for the acquisition and integration of knowledge have to be made. General rules for Conclusions must be designed such that they result in medical decisions. If the system contains different levels of symbolic representation or different kinds of knowledge, mechanisms of inference between the different parts have to be defined. In particular, the method of presentation of the procedural outcome is crucial. The results should not only be presented in a clear and concise way which is easy to grasp, but the decisions of the system must also be made transparent to the physician, who in the end accepts, corrects, or discards the proposed decisions. As any decision support system has highly ethical implications, a careful validation of the system is strongly indicated. In the following, we will refer to only some of these topics, especially the process of inference from low level data representation to higher level knowledge representation. As an example of this transition, we will describe a procedure by which lesions or other structural data from a given cranial computerized tomography (CT) scan series can be transferred to abstract documentation diagrams.

A Statistically Sound Model

As an essential part of this procedure, we established a statistically sound macroscopic brain model. It is based on anatomical measurements of 80

[1] Institut für Anatomie, RWTH Aachen, Wendlingweg 2, W-5100 Aachen, FRG.

Imaging of the Brain in Psychiatry
and Related Fields
Edited by K. Maurer

postmortem brains in standard coordinates of the anterior commissure-posterior commissure (ACPC) system (Niemann et al. 1988; von Keyserlingk et al. 1989). It is both a geometrical and a computer science model, consisting of a list of anatomical structures or terms. Each term is assigned to a set of measured reference space coordinates representing the variation in a brain structure as measured over 80 brains. These clouds of three-dimensional (3-D) points are interpreted in terms of volume density, which is equated with the presence probability of the structure in three dimensions (Weibel 1979). Presence probability is then the instrument by which structures such as sulci, gyri, or other landmarks may be identified in a given brain scan.

For this purpose the brain model must be adjusted to the CT scan series. To identify structures two things have to be brought together: (1) A segmentation procedure based on general attributes, e.g., orientation, size, form, and density, has to determine that the category of structure in question is present at that place. (2) The brain model must add a sufficient presence probability of the structure in question. This procedure is only valid for structures which can be delineated in the image, e.g., sulci, the ventricular system, or basal ganglia (Fig. 1). If segmentation is not possible, as in the case of gyri or fiber tracts, the region can only be marked when a defined (70%) presence probability exists.

Histological Extension of the Model

There are many anatomical structures which cannot be distinguished by the imaging devices available now. Nevertheless, delineation of these objects

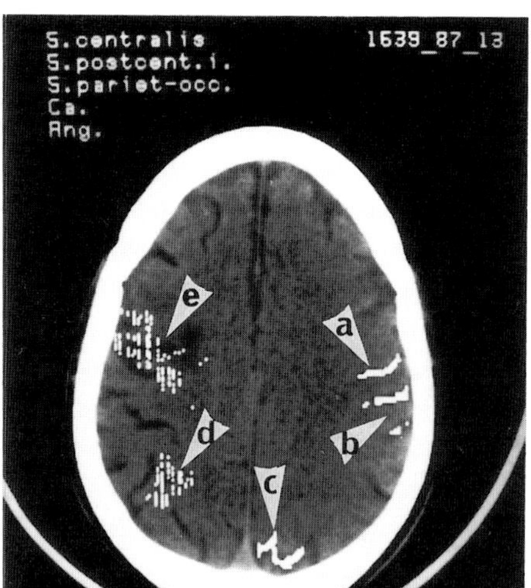

Fig. 1. Computerized tomography scan with some identified structures and regions. On the *right side*, three segmentated sulci are shown: the central sulcus (*a*), the inferior post-central sulcus (*b*), and the parietooccipital sulcus (*c*). On the *left side*, the *dotted areas* mark the angular (*d*) and precentral (*e*) gyri

may be highly desirable and can also be made possible by the statistical brain model. Besides macroscopic aspects, this morphological category includes classical histology, immunohistology, and receptor topography. There is, however, also a nonmorphological category, which can be subdivided into physiological, psychiatric, neurological, and neuropsychological data. Therefore, a procedure is necessary which links information about the topography of morphological objects and nonmorphological features to structures which can be visualized and identified in the scan. This procedure must use multiple reference structures.

Our work on the macroscopic statistical brain model was carried on with the integration of histological knowledge. The model was enriched by thorough histological examination of a selected brain specimen, which by 3-D transformations was fitted to as many of the discernible reference structures of the model as possible. The underlying assumption is that, in a brain to be examined, the invisible topography will correspond to the topography of the histologically examined and "standardized" brain (Fig. 1). This assumption may lead to a prediction uncertainty of 1–2 mm in the central regions of the brain, which may increase to 4 or 5 mm in the cortical Brodmann areas. Depending on the diagnostic question, the physician has to decide whether this uncertainty may be tolerated or not.

Functional and Clinical Extension of the Model

The transition from morphological to functional and clinical items is dominated by topographical aspects. Such relationships within the brain are excellently represented in the line drawings of von Economo and Koskinas (1925), which are a special case of "two-dimensional artificial diagrams." For a quantitative transfer from 3-D brain volumes of CT and magnetic resonance imaging (MRI) scans to such artificial diagrams, the volume which is occupied by a structure in the ACPC reference space is approxi-

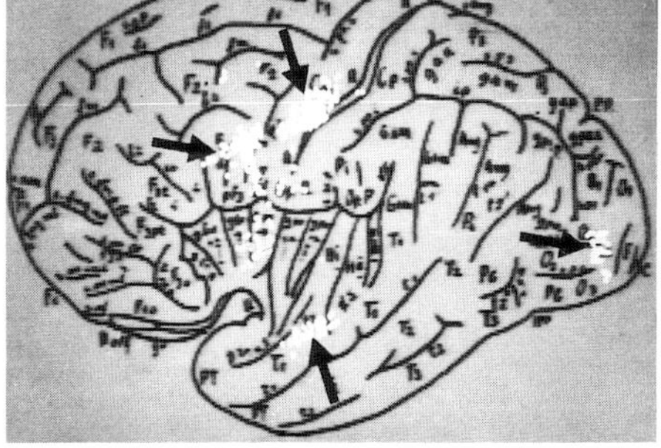

Fig. 2. Automatic 3-D/2-D transfer of the lesioned areas from a computerized tomography scan series to von Economo's artificial diagram. The *arrows* point to the lesion sites

mated by a polyhedron. The polyhedron is interactively defined by its corner points, which must be digitized both in the given scan series and in von Economo's artificial diagram. The polyhedron is then automatically subdivided into tetrahedrons by the computer and the 3-D lesion volume is mapped onto two dimensions, i.e., to von Economo's diagrams (Fig. 2).

In practice, in the scans, a structure of interest or a lesion is marked by a surrounding line. After 3-D interpolation of the structure or the lesion borders, the enclosed volume is assigned to the corresponding tetrahedrons which then, according to the principle axis transformation, are represented by points in von Economo's diagram (Fig. 2). These diagrams are pure topographical iconic representations of the human brain. They guarantee a clear layout which is easy to grasp. The actual 3-D morphology, however, is greatly distorted (Fig. 2) and may be replaced by a symbolic one (Fig. 3), which is part of a matrix giving the neighborhood relationships of all the structures of the model. The left column of abbreviations in Fig. 3 symbolizes brain structures which are lesioned. They have been digitized and brought into this artificial diagram. To their right, direct neighbors are listed in a row. The neighbors may show perifocal edema of the lesion.

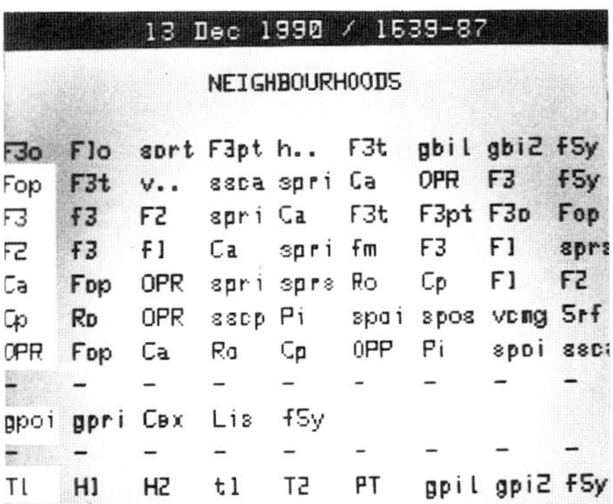

Fig. 3. The marked structures in the *left column* give a high level representation of a lesion. In the *matrix*, the rows render the mnemonic codes of the direct neighbors

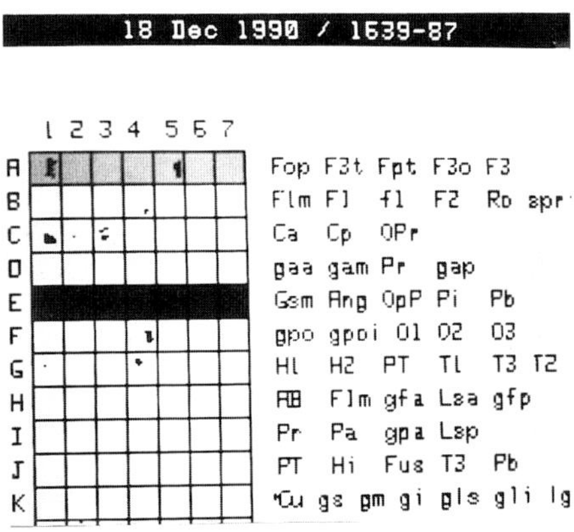

Fig. 4. In this representation of the lesion, one row of *squares* renders the structures damaged in one special syndrome. The mnemonics attached to each square can be found in the same line. Thus, row *A* gives the structures usually affected in Broca's aphasia, row *E* stands for Wernicke's aphasia. *Black* dots indicate the lesioned structures

Our standardized 3-D/2-D documentation allows for unrestricted interindividual comparison of pathological processes and morphological correlations of clinical syndromes.

Structures may also be arranged according to neurological or psychiatric syndromes. In Fig. 4, all the structures usually affected in a syndrome are arranged in a row. The first row, for example, represents structures which may be lesioned in Broca's aphasia.

High-level symbolic representation of topographical lesion data in artificial diagrams is thus advantageous in the following respects: (1) Concise documentation for both routine clinical and research purposes is facilitated. (2) The knowledge base gradually increases with every examination and an efficient strategic search for subgroups of patients is made possible. (3) It is open to changing concepts in interpretational rules, e.g., the classification of clinical syndromes. (4) Various routes of knowledge processing are opened.

References

Niemann K, von Keyserlingk DG, Wasel J (1988) Superimposition of an avaraged three-dimensional pattern of brain structures on CT scans. Acta Neurochir (Wien) 93:61–67

von Economo C, Koskinas GN (1925) Die Cytoarchitektonik der Hirnrinde des erwachsenen Menschen. Springer, Berlin Wien

von Keyserlingk DG, Niemann K, Wasel J, Maurer K (1989) Digital brain atlas for structure localization in CT combined with EEG mapping. Psychiatry Res 29:461–462

Weibel ER (1979) Stereological methods, vol 1. Practical methods for biological morphometry. Academic, London

Functional Imaging Methods
(Cerebral Blood Flow/Single Photon Emission Computerized Tomography)

Regional Cerebral Blood Flow in Schizophrenia*

S. WARKENTIN[1] and J. RISBERG

Introduction

Since the original finding of Ingvar and Franzén (1974) of a relatively reduced function in the frontal cortex of chronic schizophrenic patients, the question of its reproducibility and its significance for an understanding of schizophrenia has been a major impetus for research. Subsequent regional cerebral blood flow (rCBF) and positron emission tomography (PET) studies have in general tended to confirm a lower frontal/posterior ratio in schizophrenic patients (see Buchsbaum and Haier 1987 for a review), although it is not reported in all studies, and the findings have been variable in the extent to which the differences are manifest. The question of the specificity, or to what extent *hypofrontality* is a general phenomenon in schizophrenia, was already implicit in the original study, since not all patients showed a hypofrontal pattern. In particular, patients with shorter illness duration and with less symptoms had a normal rCBF. A similar heterogeneity is also seen in the literature of brain blood flow and metabolism, in which some studies have reported normal rCBF and metabolism (Gur et al. 1983; Mathew et al. 1982; Wiesel et al. 1987) and others have even found hyperfunction of the frontal cortex in schizophrenic patients (Cleghorn et al. 1989; Szechtman et al. 1988).

This paper is a short review of two recent studies from our laboratory addressing the question of frontal lobe dysfunction in schizophrenia:

The aim of *study 1* (Warkentin et al. 1990) was to investigate if rCBF in patients with schizophrenia varies during the course of a psychotic episode and if rCBF is correlated with the degree of psychosis.

The aim of *study 2* (Warkentin et al. 1991a) was to investigate if the frontal lobes of schizophrenic patients can be activated and if such activation is related to the clinical state of the patient at the time of investigation.

* Supported by the Swedish Medical Research Council (project number 4969), the Swedish Council for Research in the Humanities and Social Sciences, and the Söderström-Köningska Foundation.

[1] CBF Laboratory, Department of Psychogeriatrics, St. Lars Hospital, P.O. Box 638, 22009 Lund, Sweden.

Imaging of the Brain in Psychiatry
and Related Fields
Edited by K. Maurer

Study 1: rCBF in Schizophrenia During the Course of a Psychotic Episode

Patients and Methods

A total of 17 schizophrenic patients (10 men and 7 women, mean age 37.0, range 21–59 years) were recruited from intensive care units at St. Lars Hospital, Lund, Sweden. They were all in a clinically exacerbated state at admission to the hospital, displaying overt and productive symptoms. A subgroup of ten medication-free patients was studied on several occasions during the course of their psychotic episodes. The rCBF measurements were made during "rest" using the nontraumatic xenon-133 inhalation method (Obrist et al. 1975; Risberg 1980) and 32 detectors mounted in a helmet type of holder (Inhalation Cerebrograph 32 C). The first set of rCBF measurements and clinical ratings was performed as soon as possible after admission to the hospital (often within a few hours) and before neuroleptic treatment was started; the second set was performed after the first week of neuroleptic treatment; and a third set at discharge from the hospital, when the patients were clinically remitted. A control group of 17 normal healthy subjects, matched to the patients regarding age, sex, and handedness, was also studied.

Results

The mean hemispheric blood flow (CBF) was normal and not related to the clinical state of the patient or to medication. Clinically exacerbated patients showed both a normal rCBF distribution and a normal frontal-occipital (F/O) ratio. A highly significant and positive correlation ($r_s = 0.92$, $p < 0.001$) was found between clinical symptoms and the F/O ratio of the right hemisphere at admission such that the more behaviorally disturbed the patient was, the higher was the ratio. The patients improved markedly during the treatment period, as evidenced by a significant reduction in both positive and negative symptoms. The average F/O ratio *decreased* significantly during the treatment period, especially in the left hemisphere. Thus a relative hypofrontality was seen at discharge.

Discussion

A closer delineation of the specificity of frontal hypofunction in schizophrenia is of theoretical importance, as it may implicate pathophysiological evidence for dfferent subgroups of this disorder. While many researchers have attempted to explain the discrepant findings by differences in methods, technical artifacts, or effects of medication, a more intriguing possibility is that they are aspects of the disorder which pertain to the variability of the disease process. The interpretation of findings of many studies is often made difficult by the lack of information about the clinical characteristics of the patients. It is often not clear whether the patients have been examined during an actively psychotic or a more silent state. The importance of the clinical state is evident from the findings of Geraud et al. (1987), who demonstrated that hypofrontality better characterized residual types of patients, while subchronic and chronic patients with acute exacerbation did not differ from normals. They also showed that hypofrontality was a reversible phenomenon, as it disappeared with infusion of a dopamine agonist. They concluded that hypofrontality can be seen in nondeteriorated patients with several years of the illness and essentially during phases of clinical remission.

The aim of the present investigation was to test the hypothesis that the clinical state of the patient is a major determinant of frontal lobe function. To this effect, patients were examined during their most extreme clinical fluctuations during a psychotic episode, i.e., when they were in a state of acute exacerbation and when they showed a markedly reduced symptomatology. Studying patients during their most extreme fluctuations in clinical state has several advantages. It enhances the power to detect the influence of clinical state on brain blood flow, and it reduces interindividual variance. The original finding of our study was that *hypofrontality is not a stable phenomenon* but varies with the degree of psychosis during a psychotic episode. The observation was made both at the individual level and for the group as a whole. A special feature of our study was that the patients selected were responders to treatment, in that after a few weeks in the hospital they could be discharged. In this way our patients may differ from those of several other studies showing reduced frontal function (Ingvar and Franzén 1974; Weinberger et al. 1986; Berman et al. 1986). The possible differenced in responsiveness to neuroleptic drug treatment could thus be an important factor for determining frontal lobe functioning in schizophrenia and might explain some of the heterogeneity in the findings. Cohen and coworkers (1988) suggested the presence of two types of prefrontal metabolic deficits, one which was sensitive to neuroleptic treatment, and thus to a change in the presumed imbalance of regional brain dopamine, and one which was unaffected by neuroleptic treatment. Similar attempts to differentiate patients on the basis of responsivity to neuroleptic treatment have been promising but not yet conclusive. Losonczy and coworkers (1986) found that the ventricle/brain ratio (VBR) was not related to neuroleptic treatment response (haloperidol) or to symptom picture (negative-positive). This was also shown by Smith et al. (1987), who found no relationship between clinical response to neuroleptic drugs (haloperidol or thioridazine) and brain morphology as revealed by computerized tomography (CT). In addition, Wolkin and coworkers (1989) reported that the failure to respond clinically was not a function of neuroleptic uptake or binding in the central nervous system (CNS). Instead, what differed responders from nonresponders was less dopamine receptor availability in the nonresponders. This could be one possible explanation of the findings in a recent study from our group (Graae et al. submitted), in which the young patient group reported in the original study by Ingvar and Franzén (1974) was followed up with renewed investigations 18 years later. No correlation was found between rCBF or clinical symptoms and the total amount of neuroleptic drugs consumed by the patients during 18 years. Despite these findings, the feasibility of the treatment response as a subgrouping variable in schizophrenia is not yet clear, and the questions concerning the reliability of the distinction, the consistency in neuroleptic responsiveness over time, and the association between neuroleptic responsiveness and clinical features are still largely unanswered. Even if the patient complies to treatment, apparent nonresponse is difficult to assess because of possible placebo effects, pharmacokinetic differences, or inadequate or too high doses of the neuroleptic agent.

There is, to date, no convincing evidence of structural deficits in the frontal lobes of nondemented chronic and deficient schizophrenic patients. In the absence of clear-cut structural abnormalities in the frontal cortex, it is possible to view a reduced frontal function in patients with schizophrenia as a secondary phenomenon to a more primary limbic system pathology, as evidenced by the anatomical findings of enlarged ventricles and the reduced size of the amygdala, hippocampus, and other temporal cortical areas (Bogerts et al. 1985; Suddath et al. 1990; Rossi et al. 1989; Dauphinais et al. 1990). However, these structural abnormalities are largely nonspecific to the disorder of schizophrenia and seem unlikely to explain our findings in remitted patients, as they have not been related to any clinically specific subgroup of patients, despite some evidence suggesting a higher prevalence of negative symptoms and cognitive disturbances in patients with these subcortical changes (Berman et al. 1986).

Study 2: Frontal Lobe Activation by the Word Fluency Test in Different Clinical Stages of Schizophrenia

Patients and Methods

Eight schizophrenic patients (five men and three women, mean age 33.9 years, part of the series of study 1) were investigated during clinical exacerbation and during remission at discharge from the hospital. Two rCBF measurements were performed, the first during rest and the second during performance of a word fluency test (FAS; Benton 1968). This test has been found to reliably activate the prefrontal areas, especially on the left side, in normals (Warkentin et al. 1991b).

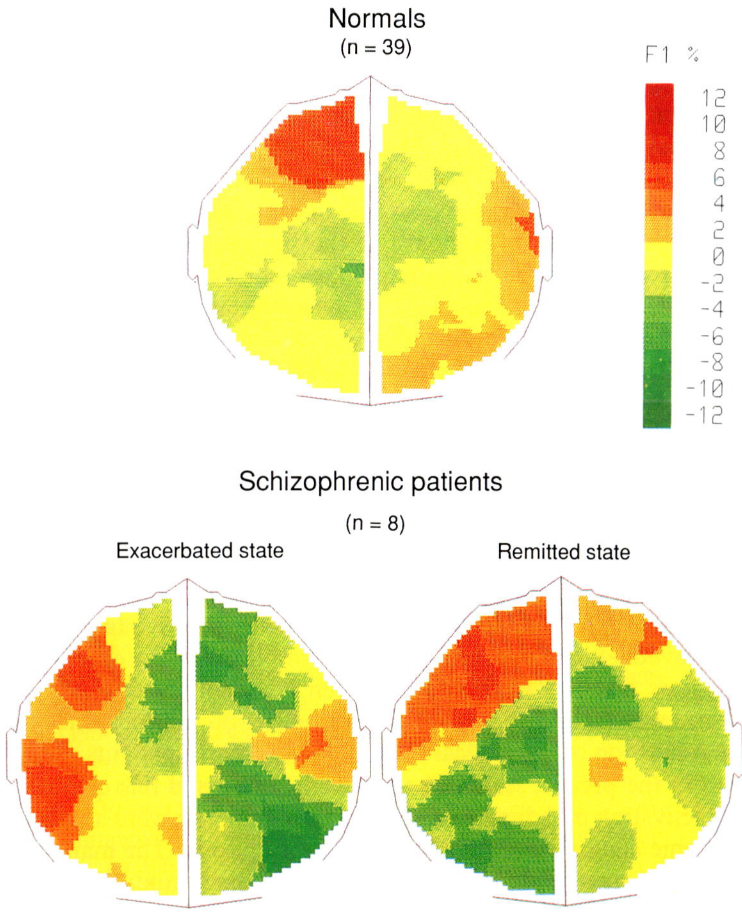

Fig. 1. Changes in cortical blood flow distribution (F_1) from rest to activation by a word fluency test in normals and in schizophrenic patients during exacerbation and clinical remission. Degree of change is defined by the color key (*upper right*). Note the left prefrontal increase in the normals, the lack of this response in the exacerbated schizophrenics, and the return of the response at remission

Results

The mean CBF did not change from rest to test and was not related to the clinical state of the patient or to medication. In the exacerbated state the patients did not activate their prefrontal cortex during performance of the word fluency test. In the remitted state the patients did activate their prefrontal cortex in a similar way as the normals did (Fig. 1).

King DJ (1990) The effect of neuroleptics on cognitive and psychomotor function. Br J Psychiatry 157:799–811

Koh SD (1978) Remembering of verbal materials by schizophrenic young adults. In: Schwartz S (ed) Language and cognition in schizophrenia. Erlbaum, Hillsdale, pp 55–99

Losonczy MF, Song, IS, Mohs RC, Small NA, Davidson M, Johns CA, Davis KL (1986) Correlates of lateral ventricular size in chronic schizophrenia. I: Behavioural and treatment response measures. Am J Psychiatry 143:976–981

Mathew RJ, Duncan GC, Weinman ML, Barr DL (1982) Regional cerebral blood flow in schizophrenia. Arch Gen Psychiatr 39:1121–1124

Obrist WD, Thompson HK, Wang HS, Wilkinson WE (1975) Regional cerebral blood flow estimated by 133-Xe inhalation. Stroke 6:245–256

Risberg J (1980) Regional cerebral blood flow measurements by 133-Xe inhalation: methodology and applications in neuropsychology and psychiatry. Brain Lang 9:9–34

Sattler JM, Nordmark T (1971) Verbal learning in schizophrenics and normals. Psychol Res 21:241–246

Smith RC, Baumgartner R, Ravichandran GK, Largen J, Calderon M, Burd A, Mauldin M (1987) Cortical atrophy and white matter density in the brains of schizophrenics and clinical response to neuroleptics. Acta Psychiatr Scand 75:11–19

Suddath RL, Christison GW, Torrey EF, Casanova MF, Weinberger DR (1990) Anatomical abnormalities in the brains of monozygotic twins discordant for schizophrenia. N Engl J Med 322:789–794

Szechtman H, Nahmias C, Garnett S, Firnau G, Brown GM, Kaplan RD, Cleghorn JM (1988) Effect of neuroleptics on altered cerebral glucose metabolism in schizophrenia. Arch Gen Psychiatry 45:523–532

Warkentin S, Nilsson A, Risberg J, Karlson S, Felkkøy K, Franzén G, Gustafson L, Rodriguez G (1990) Regional cerebral blood flow in schizophrenia: repeated studies during a psychotic episode. Psychiatr Res: Neuroimag 35:27–38

Warkentin S, Nilsson A, Risberg J, Graae E (1991a) Clinical state determinants of frontal lobe functioning in schizophrenia. In: Brain dysfunction: regional cerebral blood flow correlates of psychotic episodes in schizophrenia and cycloid psychosis. Thesis, University of Lund, Sweden

Warkentin S, Risberg, J, Nilsson A, Karlson S, Graae E (1991b) Cortical activity during speech production. A study of regional cerebral blood flow in normal subjects performing a word fluency task. Neuropsychiatr Neuropsychol Behav Neurol 4:305–316

Weinberger DR, Berman KF, Zec RF (1986) Physiologic dysfunction of dorsolateral prefrontal cortex in schizophrenia: I. Regional cerebral blood flow evidence. Arch Gen Psychiatry 43:114–124

Wiesel F-A, Wik G, Sjögren I, Blomqvist G, Greitz T (1987) Altered relationships between metabolic rates of glucose in brain regions of schizophrenic patiens. Acta Psychiatr Scand 76:642–647

Wolkin A, Barouche F, Wolf AP, Rotrosen J, Fowler JS, Shiue C-Y, Cooper TB, Brodie JD (1989) Dopamine blockade and clinical response: evidence for two biological subgroups of schizophrenia. Am J Psychiatry 146:905–908

The Regional Cerebral Blood Flow Landscape in Chronic Schizophrenia: An 18 Year Follow-up Study

E. Cantor-Graae[1], S. Warkentin, G. Franzén, D.H. Ingvar, and J. Risberg

Introduction

Ever since the first intra-arterial regional cerebral blood flow (rCBF) investigations in chronic schizophrenic patients (Ingvar and Franzén 1974; Franzén and Ingvar 1975), a number of studies using a variety of techniques have continued to reveal evidence of a subtle physiological brain dysfunction associated with this disorder. A hypofrontal pattern of rCBF has been observed in schizophrenic patients both at rest (Ariel et al. 1983; Chabrol et al. 1986) and during frontal lobe challenge (Weinberger et al. 1986; Berman 1987). However, relatively little is known about the long-term stability of the rCBF landscape in chronic schizophrenic patients. Recent follow-up studies show that for most patients a clinical plateau of deterioration is reached after 5–10 years of illness, with only a minority of patients expected to show a progressively downhill course (McGlashan 1988). Nevertheless, it is still not possible to predict the clinical course of schizophrenia for any one patient.

The variability in clinical course raises the question of whether chronic long-term schizophrenia may be accompanied by changes in cerebral metabolism, either intrinsic to the disease process itself or related to secondary aspects more associated with psychiatric treatment. The stress of repeated hospitalizations plus the unremitting administration of various forms of neuroleptic treatment are nonspecific aspects of chronic schizophrenia which hypothetically may contribute to varying levels of functional activity in the brain. Ingvar and Franzén's (1974) demonstration of abnormal patterns of rCBF in elderly patients yet relatively normal values in younger ones provided the impetus for a rCBF follow-up study of the younger subset of patients utilizing parallel neuroimaging techniques.

[1] Department of Psychiatry, University Hospital, Lund, Sweden.

Imaging of the Brain in Psychiatry and Related Fields
Edited by K. Maurer

Methods

Subjects

Of the original 11 younger patients, 7 consented to participate. The diagnosis of schizophrenia was reconfirmed according to the DSM III-R criteria (APA 1987). The patients were reevaluated clinically by G.F. with the Rockland-Pollin (RP) rating scale used in 1972 (Rockland and Pollin 1965), the Brief Psychiatric Rating Scale (BPRS) (Overall and Gorham 1962), and the Scale for Assessment of Negative Symptoms (SANS) (Andreasen and Olsen 1982) for negative symptoms. Laboratory tests were normal, and screening for substance abuse, somatic illness, and cranial injury revealed nothing of importance for cerebral functioning. The mean age for the group was 41.4 ± 5.0 years (range 35–50), age of onset 18.6 ± 2.9 years (range 14–22), and illness duration 22.9 ± 2.9 years (range 20–28). The mean number of days hospitalized since illness onset was 3104.1 ± 2010.6 (range 926–6065). Although two of the patients had recently been hospitalized for exacerbation of symptoms, none of the patients had florid illness at the time of the study. None were employed or living under self-sufficient circumstances. All but two of the patients had received electroconvulsive therapy (ECT) during the course of their illness, none, however, more recently than 2 years prior to the present study. At the time of the present investigation, the patients were taking a variety of neuroleptic medications. Transformed into chlorpromazine equivalents, the mean was 352 mg ± 340 per day (range 25–1120). The total amount of medication since contact with psychiatric services based on information provided by hospital records was 3437 grams ± 1371 per patient (range 1582–5286).

Measurement of rCBF

The rCBF was measured with the xenon-133 inhalation method, as modified by Risberg et al. (1975), utilizing a 254 detector system (Cortexplorer, Scan Detectronic, Hadsund, Denmark). For the purposes of comparison with the 1972 study, the f_1 index, representing the fast-flowing compartment of the gray matter, was chosen as the index most closely approximating the originally used Fg blood flow parameter, calculated off-line from the fast component.

Results are based on flow distributions in percent of hemispheric mean. As the original study utilized 32 detectors placed on the dominant hemisphere, detector placement was not replicable using the 254 detector system. Instead, detectors were collapsed into regions approximately comparable with those used by Ingvar and Franzén to calculate an anterior/posterior ratio based on mean regional distribution values. Thus, an index of frontality was obtained for each hemisphere.

rCBF measurements were performed during rest and during activation procedures which normally challenge the frontal lobes (the Chicago Word Fluency Test and the Wisconsin Card Sort, WCST). A baseline procedure controlled for the motoric and attentional aspects of the WCST.

Results

Paired and unpaired *t* tests were performed to examine within group and between group differences. The Wilcoxon signed ranks test was used to examine changes in RP clinical rating scores from 1972 to 1990.

No significant change in mean hemispheric flow at rest was observed from 1972 to 1990 (left hemisphere 1972: 74.6 ± 19.2; left hemisphere 1990: 70.1 ± 5.3; right hemisphere 1990: 70.3 ± 5.9). The inhalation technique would have tended, if anything, to underestimate the gray matter flow due to sensitivity differences between the two methods. Allowing for the decreases caused by normal aging, the differences from 1972 to 1990 became even less. The regional distribution for the group as a whole looked normal, or hyperfrontal (Fig. 1). No significant change was observed in the anterior/posterior index calculated during rest (Fig. 2). Although two subtrends were observed, the patients who had increased or decreased frontality indexes did not differ in any of the following measures: clinical symptoms (current or change), total medication since illness onset, current medication, self-reported anxiety, pCo_2, pulse, respiration, or demographic clinical variables. Furthermore, no significant group differences were observed between 1972 and 1990 on any RP scale dimension. The mean BPRS global symptom score for the group was 28.3 ± 10.7 (range 17–46), and the mean total SANS scale score was 58.3 ± 24.5 (range 34–104). Analyses of regression revealed no obvious relationship between clinical ratings and any blood flow measurements. Activation procedures revealed an absence of significant activation in the frontal lobes during both tests for the group as a whole.

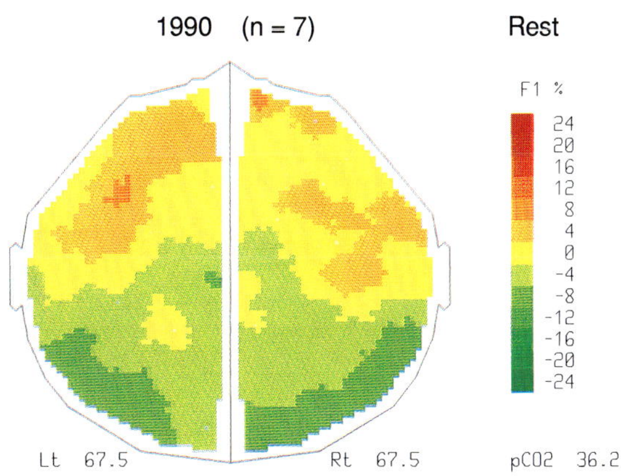

Fig. 1. Vertex view showing superficial areas of the cerebral cortex. *Yellow*, values close to hemispheric mean; *red* and *green* show higher and lower values, respectively, in per cent of hemispheric mean

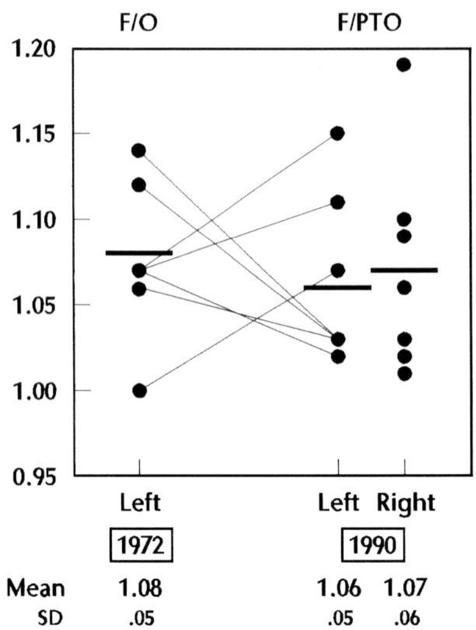

Fig. 2. Anterior-posterior ratio, or index of frontality, in an 18 year schizophrenia follow-up study

Discussion

At present, the stability of the rCBF landscape and the lack of change in clinical symptoms from 1972 to 1990 would tend to confirm the notion of schizophrenia as a nonprogressive disease process in these patients. Moreover, the absence of a significant activation response confirms indications shown by previous studies (Weinberger et al. 1986) of a subtle physiological dysfunction in the brain, a manifestation of which may be decreased response to frontal challenge. Although the consequences of long-term neuroleptic treatment are unknown, the net effect did not appear deleteriously toxic for rCBF, as measured in terms of absence of change both in hemisphere flow and frontality index. Whether or not the rCBF will continue to remain stable in these patients at a future point in time remains to be seen.

References

Andreasen NC, Olsen SA (1982) Negative vs. positive schizophrenia: definition and validation. Arch Gen Psychiatry 39:781–794

APA (1987) Diagnostic and Statistical Manual of Mental Disorders, DSM-III-R, 3rd rev edn. American Psychiatric Association, Washington, DC

Ariel RN, Golden CJ, Berg RA, Quaife MA, Dirksen JW, Forsell T, Wilson J, Graber B (1983) Regional cerebral blood flow in schizophrenics: test using the Xe 133 inhalation method. Arch Gen Psychiatry 40:258–263

Berman KF (1987) Cortical "stress tests" in schizophrenia: regional cerebral blood flow studies. Biol Psychiatry 22:1304–1326

Chabrol H, Guell A, Bes A, Moron, P (1986) Cerebral blood flow in schizophrenic adolescents. Am J Psychiatry 143:126–135
Franzén G, Ingvar DH (1975) Absence of activation in frontal structures during psychological testing of chronic schizophrenics. J Neurol Neurosurg Psychiatry 38:1027–1032
Ingvar DH, Franzén G (1974) Abnormalities of cerebral blood flow distribution in patients with chronic schizophrenia. Acta Psychiatr Scand 50:425–462
McGlashan TH (1988) A selective review of recent North American long-term followup studies of schizophrenia. Schizophr Bull 14:4:515–542
Overall J, Gorham D (1962) The brief psychiatric rating scale. Psychol Rep 10:799–812
Risberg J, Ali Z, Wilson EM, Wills EL, Halsey JH (1975) Regional cerebral blood flow by 133-xenon inhalation. Stroke 6:142–148
Rockland LH, Pollin W (1965) Quantification of psychiatric mental status. Arch Gen Psychiatry 12:23–28
Weinberger DR, Berman KF, Zec RF (1986) Physiological dysfunction of dorsolateral prefrontal cortex in schizophrenia: I. Regional cerebral blood flow evidence. Arch Gen Psychiatry 43:114–124

Cortical and Subcortical Brain Function in Schizophrenia

P. RUBIN[1], L. FRIBERG, S. HOLM, P. VIDEBECH, H.S. ANDERSEN, B.B. BENDSEN, N. STRØMSØ, J.K. LARSEN, N.A. LASSEN, and R. HEMMINGSEN

Introduction

During the last two decades there has been an increasing number of studies of regional brain function in psychoses of unknown etiology, especially schizophrenia. The applied techniques have included regional cerebral blood flow (rCBF) and regional metabolism measurements with two- or three-dimensional techniques and structural analysis by means of computerized tomography (CT) and magnetic resonance imaging (MRI) (Weinberger 1987; Pfefferbaum et al. 1990; Rubin et al. 1991).

In order to understand the mechanism behind regional brain dysfunction in psychosis it is necessary to investigate untreated and medically treated patients. It is also important to analyze changes in all relevant brain regions both during a resting state and during cognitive activation of relevant brain regions. Furthermore, it is necessary to reexamine the same patient at several occasions during the course of disease.

The majority of neurobiological studies in schizophrenia have been cross-sectional and have comprised heterogeneous patient populations. With the cross-sectional design it is difficult or impossible to establish whether a measured dysfunction represents a state marker or whether it is a trait marker, i.e., a disorder of brain function throughout the course of disease. Furthermore, cross-sectional studies make it highly difficult to establish possible correlations between specific psychopathology and specific regional brain function.

Which brain regions are relevant when trying to disentangle the neurobiology of schizophrenia? The dopamine theory suggests an increased dopaminergic activity in schizophrenia, mainly in the striaturm. Anatomical and physiological studies have tried to disclose defects of the prefrontal and temporal cortical regions in schizophrenic patients. These cortical regions are involved in structured thinking, interpretation of perception, and memory and are essential to anticipation, including planning of verbal expression and of action, all functions which might be affected in schizophrenia.

[1]Department of Psychiatry E, Bispebjerg Hospital, Bispebjerg Bakke 23, 2400 Copenhagen NV, Denmark.

Imaging of the Brain in Psychiatry and Related Fields
Edited by K. Maurer

In order to meet some of the methodological demands outlined above, we have initiated a prospective study of patients with schizophrenia and schizophreniform disorder admitted to the hospital for the first time. In order to map out regional brain activity we have applied the three-dimensional single photon emission CT (SPECT) technique to visualize cerebral blood flow distribution during rest and during activation of the prefrontal cortex.

Subjects and Methods

The initial part of the study comprised 19 patients (mean age 27 years, range 21–42 years) admitted to a psychiatric hospital in Copenhagen for the first time and meeting the DSM III-R criteria for schizophrenia or schizophreniform disorder. Patients with organic brain disorders, alcohol or drug abuse, or pregnancy and forensic patients were excluded from the study. Seven healthy volunteers (mean age 26 years, range 21–35 years) were recruited as controls and subjected to exactly the same investigational program as were the patients. rCBF distribution was measured by SPECT using the retained type of tracer technetium 99m hexamethylpropilene-amino-oxime (Tc 99m-HMPAO) (Ceretec). Within an interval of less than 1 h, two separate SPECT studies (rest and activation) were performed in each patient and volunteer. This design served to minimize irrelevant intraindividual variation. Some 10 min after each injection of Tc 99m-HMPAO the regional tracer distribution was depicted in eight transverse slices assessed over 20 min. The slice levels were parallel to the orbitomeatal plane with a slice separation of 10 mm. At rest the subjects were lying quietly, with their eyes closed and without moving. Activation of the prefrontal cerebral cortex was established by the Wisconcin Card Sorting Test. This is a problem solving, abstract reasoning test that has been adopted in a number of studies of frontal brain lesions and other types of cerebral dysfunction (Weinberger et al. 1986). For each slice a set of relevant regions of interest (ROIs; see Fig. 1) was outlined on the basis of anatomical reference (Aquilonius and Eckemäs 1980). The images were transformed by simple linear operations to a standard size and position allowing subsequent individual comparisons. Furthermore, the regional tracer distribution during the first CBF measurement (rest) was subtracted from the activation picture. A correction restoring CBF in relatively highly perfused areas was applied (Lassen et al. 1988). The relative flow distribution was normalized with reference to the mean tracer uptake in cerebellum, and flow distribution was calculated for each ROI as a value relative to the global mean value in that specific subject. The Mann-Whitney test for unpaired data and the Wilcoxon test for paired data were used for statistical analysis.

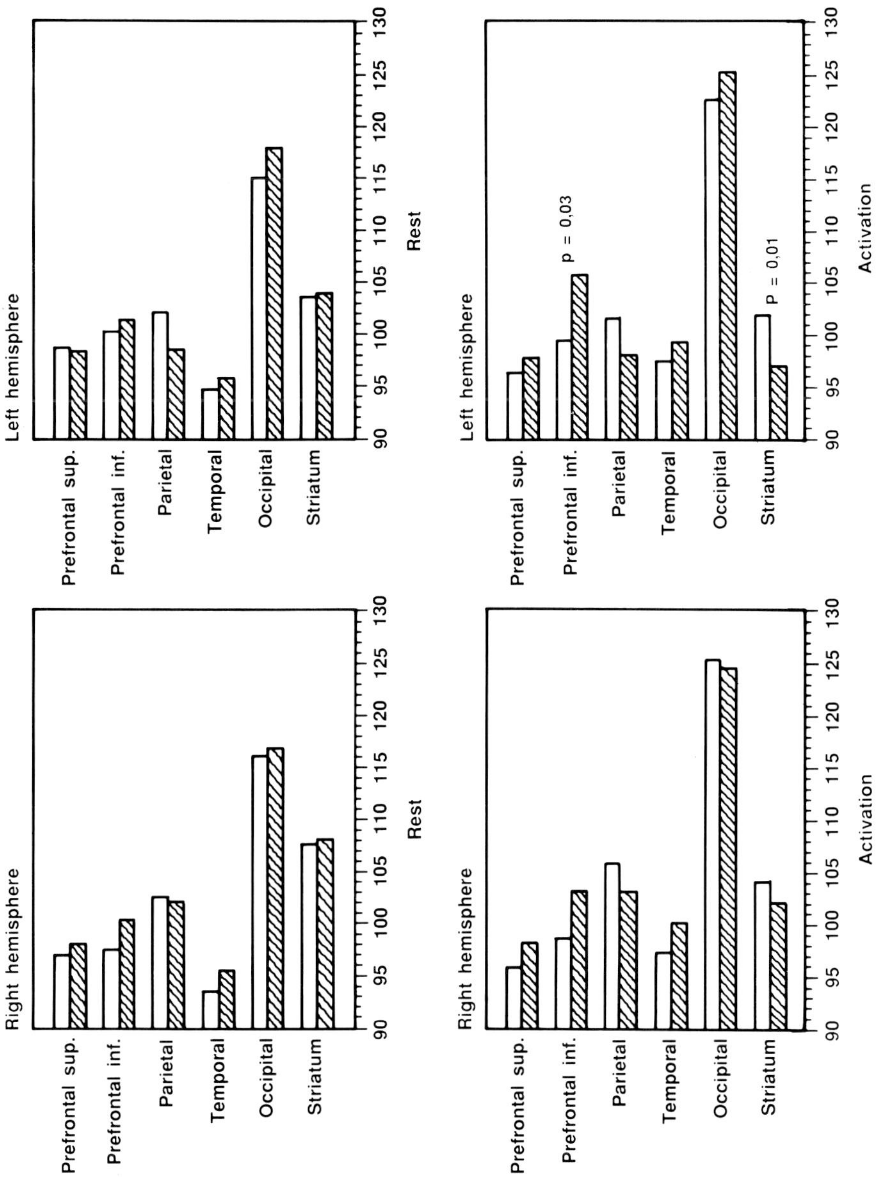

Fig. 1. Regional cerebral blood flow distribution. Values in percent (brain mean = 100). ▧, Healthy volunteers (n = 7); □, schizophrenic patients and patients with schizophretiform psychosis (n = 19)

Results

Among the 19 patients, 7 were completely unmedicated prior to the CBF study. The remaining 12 patients received short-lasting treatment with neuroleptics, the maximum period of treatment being 3 weeks. The rCBF distribution is shown in Fig. 1. During rest there were no differences between patients and normal healthy volunteers in any of the brain regions investigated. During activation with the Wisconsin Card Sorting Test the schizophrenic patients were unable to increase activity in the prefrontal inferior region compared to normal healthy volunteers. This difference was most pronounced on the left side ($p < 0.03$). Furthermore, the schizophrenic patients were unable to reduce striatal activity on the same side ($p < 0.01$). Both normal healthy volunteers and patients had increased regional activity in the temporal and occipital regions due to the auditory and visual component of the activation paradigm.

Discussion

Theoretically the prefrontal cortex and striatum may be considered as parts of a feedback circuit in which cortex pertains to negative symptoms of schizophrenia and striatum to positive symptoms (Weinberger 1987).

The normal cortical flow distribution at rest in newly diagnosed patients is in concert with the findings from one study made on a comparable series (Early et al. 1987). Our findings of cortical prefrontal dysfunction during activation are also compatible with the very subtle abnormalities seen with a stationary detector system and xenon-133 inhalation by Weinberger and collaborators (Berman et al. 1986; Weinberger et al. 1986). In their positron emission tomography (PET) study Sheppard et al. (1983) found normal regional activity except for a possible change of laterality.

Hypothetically, the organization of semantically adequate and potentially relevant verbal consciousness may be related to the development of language and hence to the dominant hemisphere. In this context it is noticeable that results from empirical pathoanatomical studies and MRI and CT studies recently put forward indicate a relationship between schizophrenia and development of brain lateralization (Reveley et al. 1987; Kelsoe et al. 1988; Crow et al. 1989). Such lateralizaton may offer an explanation as to our findings of defective left hemisphere modulation.

Histologically the prefrontal cortex communicates both with a large number of cortical regions and with subcortical regions including the striatum. Thus the defect may not necessarily or exclusively be localized prefrontally. Either the function of this region is actually defective or it does not receive an adequate input stimulus for the performance of sequential, environment-related, verbalized ideation. The schizophrenic patients' relative inability to establish relevant motivational linearity of thought may invalidate the propagation of concepts to be acted upon. Such a primary defect of anticipatory consciousness may affect the patients ability to convey affect, motivation, spontaneity, and social engagement. Hence the integrational defect in the dominant prefrontal cortex may well be an upstream defect relative to the observed negative symptoms of affect, energy, volition, and social spontaneity, which might be processed through the prefrontal cortex in normals. At any rate, the prefrontal cortex seems to represent an "output gate" disorder in schizophrenia and this pertains to both communication and relevant action. The relationship between prefrontal cortex and subcortical dopaminergic regions is very complex (Clark and White 1987). The present finding of a combined cortical activation deficit and indication of a striatal suppression deficit does not enable us to localize the primary "lesion" within the neuronal circuit connecting the two sections of the brain. The lack of abnormal flow distribution during rest, the asymmetry during activation, and the clinical fact that defect symptoms may prevail with few positive symptoms – also during neuroleptic treatment – may, however, indirectly point to a (mainly left) neocortical deficit as the primary "lesion." Weinberger (1987) suggested a relative striatal (dopaminergic) hyperactivity during cognitive awareness in schizophrenia which may be due to a deficient feedback inhibition from mesocortical dopamine neurones to mesolimbic dopamine modulation (see also Pycock et al. 1980). It should be noted that cognitive awareness is the state that normally prevails in awake humans. Thus the relative subcortical dopaminergic hyperactivity may prevail most of the time in patients.

References

Aquilonius SM, Eckernäs SV (1980) A colour atlas of the human brain. Esselte, Herzogs, Nacka

Berman KF, Zec RF, Weinberger DR (1986) Physiologic dysfunction of dorsolateral prefrontal cortex in schizophrenia: II. Role of neuroleptic treatment, attention, and mental effort. Arch Gen Psychiatry 43:126–135

Clark D, White FJ (1987) Review: D1 Dopamine receptor – the search for a function: a criterial evaluation of the D1/D2 Dopamine receptor classification and its functional implications. Synapse 1:347–388

Crow TJ, Ball J, Bloom SR, Brown R, Bruton CJ, Colter N, Frith CD, Johnstone EC, Owens DGC, Roberts GW (1989) Schizophrenia as an anomaly of development of cerebral assymmetry. A postmorten study and a proposal concerning the genetic basis of the disease. Arch Gen Psychiatry 46:1145–1150

Early TS, Reiman EM, Raichle ME, Spitznagel L (1987) Left globus pallidus abnormality in never-medicated patients with schizophrenia: (cerebral blood flow/positron emission tomography). Proc Natl Acad Sci USA 84:561–583

Kelsoe JR, Cadet JR, Pickar D, Weinberger DR (1988) Quantitative neuroanatomy in schizophrenia: A controlled magnetic resonance imaging study. Arch Gen Psychiatry 45:533–541

Lassen NA, Andersen AR, Friberg L, Paulson OB (1988) The retention of ^{99m}Tc-d, 1-HM-PAO in the human brain after intracarotid bolus injection: a kinetic analysis. J Cereb Blood Flow Metab 8:13–22

Pfefferbaum A, Kelvin OL, Rosenbloom M, Zipursky RB (1990) Brain magnetic resonance imaging: approaches for investigating schizophrenia. Schizophr Bull 16:453–476

Pycock CJ, Kerwin RW, Carter CJ (1980) Effect of lesion of cortical dopamine terminals on subcortical dopamine in rats. Nature 286:74–77

Reveley MA, Reveley AM, Baldy R (1987) Left hemisphere hypodensity in discordant schizophrenic twins: a controlled study. Arch Gen Psychiatry 44:625–632

Rubin P, Holm S, Friberg L, Videbech P, Andersen HS, Bjerg Bendsen B, Strømsø N, Larsen JK, Lassen NA, Hemmingsen R (1991) Altered modulation of prefrontal and subcortical brain activity in novel diagnozed schizophrenia and schizophreniform disorder: a regional cerebral blood flow study. Arch Gen Psychiatry 48:987–995

Sheppard G, Manchanda R, Gruzelier J, Hirsch SR, Wise R, Frackowiak R, Jones T (1983) $^{15}0$ positron emission tomographic scanning in predominantly never-treated acute schizophrenic patients. Lancet 31:1448–1452

Weinberger DR (1987) Implications of normal brain development for the pathogenesis of schizophrenia. Arch Gen Psychiatry 44:660–669

Weinberger DR, Berman KF, Zec RF (1986) Physiologic dysfunction of dorsolateral prefrontal cortex in schizophrenia: I. Arch Gen Psychiatry 43:114–124

Technetium-99m Hexamethylpropilene-amino-oxime Cerebral Single Photon Emission Computerized Tomography in Drug-Free Schizophrenic Patients

A. VITA[1], G. INVERNIZZI, M. GARBARINI, G.M. GIOBBIO, M. DIECI, C. MORGANTI, G. POGGI LONGOSTREVI, E. SACCHETTI, and C.L. CAZZULLO

Introduction

The interest in the study of regional cerebral blood flow (rCBF) in schizophrenia was stimulated by the initial work of Ingvar and Franzen (1974), who were the first to observe, through intracarotid injection of xenon-133, a decrease of frontal CBF in schizophrenic patients as compared to controls.

This finding has since been replicated by studies performed with positron emission tomography (PET) and single photon emission computerized tomography (SPECT) (Andreasen 1988). However, the majority of the studies were undertaken with chronic patients treated with psychotropic drugs. These may induce substantial modifications of both CBF and images of regional cerebral metabolism. Our SPECT study was conducted on young, drug-free, schizophrenic patients. The newly introduced Tc-99m-HMPAO (technetium-99m hexamethylpropilene-amino-oxime) (Ell et al. 1985) was used as a tracer.

Subjects and Methods

Subjects

A total of 17 consenting patients (mean age 22 ± 8 years) with a diagnosis of schizophrenia according to DSM III-R criteria (APA 1987) were selected for the study. None of the patients subjected to SPECT had medical or neurological illnesses or a history of alcohol, substance abuse, or electroconvulsive therapy; for at least 2 months, they had not been in treatment with neuroleptics or other psychotropic drugs or with drugs capable of interfering with blood flow.

The control group was comprised of 14 subjects of the same age as the patients who had been examined for minor functional disturbances. All the subjects were right-handed.

[1] Institute of Psychiatry and Schizophrenia Research Center Milan University, School of Medicine, Policlinico – Pad. Guardia II, Via F. Sforza 35, 20122 Milan, Italy.

Imaging of the Brain in Psychiatry
and Related Fields
Edited by K. Maurer

Methods

SPECT was performed with a SELO rotating γ-camera. The tracer used in this investigation was Tc-99m HMPAO (Ceretec, Amersham Int.) This tracer distributes in the brain proportional to local blood flow, has a cellular uptake, minimal redistribution, and provides therefore a quite accurate estimate of rCBF and an indirect representation of regional metabolism (Ell et al. 1985).

The patients were examined under resting conditions, with eyes and ears open, in a silent dimly lit room 30 min after injection of 15 mCi of the tracer.

Six slices, parallel to the orbitomeatal line, were obtained and two were considered for quantitative analysis. One was more superficial, immediately above the lateral ventricles and involving the cortex and centrum semiovale (level A). The other was deeper, passing just below the third ventricle and involving most of the temporal lobe (level B).

Each hemisphere was divided into three areas: (1) anterior or frontal; (2) intermediate, coinciding with the parietal lobe (level A) or temporal lobe (level B); (3) posterior or occipital. The regions of interest included both cortical and subcortical areas, with the exclusion, however, of ventricular spaces. The boundaries of cerebral areas and the ventricular system were traced manually on the SPECT computer video.

Analysis of the images was semiquantitative, based on calculation of the amount of radioactivity emitted by each region normalized for dimension. In order to control for calibration errors, these values were divided by those observed in a reference region represented by the cerebellum (analogously normalized for dimension). The ratio obtained was a corrected index of tracer uptake and of rCBF.

All measurements were completed by the same rater, who was unaware of the diagnosis of the subject and nature of the study. The intrarater reliability was measured and turned out to be high (Pearson $r = 0.90$).

Results

Comparison of the photon emission values of the individual areas demonstrated diffuse cerebral hypoemission (hypoperfusion) in schizophrenic patients compared with controls. This difference reached statistical significance in both levels of the left frontal area (Table 1). Analysis of interhemispheric differences of tracer uptake revealed that schizophrenic patients showed a relative hypoemission from the left hemisphere in the frontal region at both levels examined (Table 1).

There were no statistically significant correlations between uptake values in each region under examination and the patients' age, age at onset, and duration of illness.

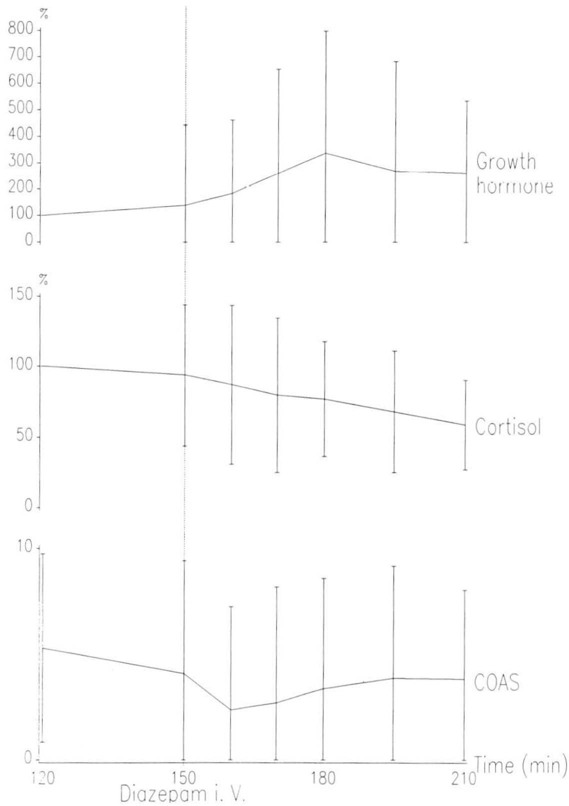

Fig. 3. Clinical effects of diazepam over time. Anxiolysis/sedation is given by the *Coas* (Covi Anxiety Scale); growth hormone and cortisol are displayed as relative values (value at t_{120} = 100%)

(Fig. 3). Thus, the clinical effects of diazepam and the displacement of iomazenil were temporarily related.

Discussion

The distribution of iomazenil in our study was found to be similar to the known distribution of benzodiazepine receptors, as visualized with flumazenil PET (Persson et al. 1985; Savic et al. 1988) and with iomazenil SPET (see Schubiger and Hasler 1990), with a predominantly cortical benzodiazepine receptor uptake. The iomazenil activity in the white matter was found to be very low. As benzodiazepines hardly exist in this area, this finding, as well as the displacement of iomazenil by diazepam confirm a specific binding of iomazenil.

Benzodiazepine receptor uptake of diazepam – corresponding to iomazenil displacement – was shown by two independent methods, i.e., digital substraction of SPET images and the time course of iomazenil plasma concentration. Since the clinical diazepam effects and the time course of iomazenil appeared to be temporarily related, the assumption that iomazenil was indeed displaced from the benzodiazepine receptor was further strengthened.

In the patient whose images were digitally substracted, a relatively reduced diazepam receptor uptake was found in the left prefrontal and parietotemporal cortices, although the iomazenil distribution and thus the senzodiazepine receptor distribution appeared to be symmetrical. This finding warrants further investigations and statistical confirmation. Should it be confirmed, it may be due to the fact that benzodiazepine receptors of different brain regions vary in their affinity towards diazepam. In biochemical studies (Seeburg 1990; Sieghart 1989), evidence for the heterogeneity of benzodiazepine receptors has been obtained. Yet, the asymmetrical diazepam uptake may also be related to a relatively reduced left prefrontal cerebral blood flow, as suggested in some studies on schizophrenics (Rubin et al. 1990; Schröder et al. 1989).

These findings can only be considered tentative, as a statistical analysis has, as yet, not been carried out. Nevertheless, our findings indicate that iomazenil SPET is a suitable technique to assess the distribution of benzodiazepine receptors in schizophrenia and that the receptor uptake of benzodiazepines can be evaluated indirectly in a diazepam displacement study.

Acknowledgments. We are grateful to Mrs. S. Demisch, Dr. U. Grethe, and Dr. K. Grupp, for their skilled assistance.

References

Bartenstein P, Ludolph A, Schober O et al. (1989) Vergleich von Blutfluß und Benzodiazepin-Rezeptor-Verteilung bei fokaler Epilepsie: Vorläufige Ergebnisse einer SPECT-Studie. Nucl Med 28:181–186

Beckmann H, Haas S (1980) High dose diazepam in schizophrenia. Psychopharmacology 71:79–82

Beer H-F, Bläuenstein PA, Hasler PA et al. (1990) In vitro and in vivo evaluation of iodine-123-Ro 16-0154: a new imaging agent for SPECT investigations of benzodiazepine receptors. J Nucl Med 31:1007–1014

Dauth J, Höll K, Deisenhammer E (1990) Time curves of radioactivity in plasma after injection of iomazenil Ro 16-0154. In: Schubiger PA, Hasler PH (eds) Iomazenil and other brain receptor tracers for SPECT. Roche, Basel

Goldberg HL, Finnerty R (1982) Comparison of buspirone in two separate studies. J Clin Psychiatry 43:87–91

Hommer DW, Matsuo V, Wolkowitz O et al. (1986) Benzodiazepine sensitivity in normal human subjects. Arch Gen Psychiatry 43:542–551

Hunkeler W, Mohler H, Pieri L et al. (1981) Selective antagonists of benzodiazepines. Nature 280:514–516

Mazière M, Hantraye P, Prenant C et al. (1984) Synthesis of ethyl 8-fluoro-5,6-dihydro-5-[C-11]methyl-t-oxo-4H-imidazo[1,5-a][1,4]benzodiazepine-3-carboxylate (Ro 15-1788-C-11): a specific radioligand for the in vivo study of central benzodiazepine receptors by positron emission tomography. Int J Appl Radiat Isot 35:973–976

Overall JE, Gorham DR (1962) The Brief Psychiatric Rating Scale. Psychol Rep 10:799–812

Persson A, Ehrin E, Eriksson L et al. (1985) Imaging of 11-C-labelled Ro 15-1788 binding to benzodiazepine receptors in the human brain by positron emission tomography. J Psychiatr Res 19:609–622

Rubin P, Friberg L, Madesen SM et al. (1990) Impaired modulation of prefrontal and striatal regions during first episode schizophrenia and schizophreniform psychosis studied by rCBF tomography (SPECT). Paper read on the 2nd international congress on imaging of the brain in psychiatry and related fields

Savic I, Persson A, Roland P et al. (1988) In-vivo demonstration of reduced benzodiazepine receptor binding in human epileptic foci. Lancet 8616 ii:863–866

Schröder J, Sauer H, Wilhelm K-R et al. (1989) Regional cerebral blood flow in endogenous psychoses: A Tc 99m HMPAO-SPECT pilot study. Psychiatry Res 29:331–333

Schubiger PA, Hasler PH (eds) (1990) Iomazenil and other brain receptor tracers for SPECT. Roche, Basel

Seeburg PH (1990) Elucidating $GABA_A$ receptor heterogeneity: an integrated molecular approach. In: Biggio G, Costa E (eds) GABA and benzodiazepine receptor subtypes. Raven, New York

Sieghart W (1989) Benzodiazepine receptor subtypes and their possible clinical significance. In: Dahl SG, Gram LF (eds) Clinical pharmacology in psychiatry. Springer, Berlin Heidelberg New York, pp 131–140

van Kammen DP, Gelernter J (1987) Biochemical instability in schizophrenia II: the serotonin and γ-aminobutyric acid systems. In: Meltzer HY (ed) Psychopharmacology: the third generation of progress. Raven, New York

Parietal Lobe Effects of Somatosensory Stimulation in Single Photon Emission Computerized Tomography: A Study on Mood Disorders and Schizophrenia

D. EBERT[1], H. FEISTEL, A. BAROCKA, T. MOKRUSCH, and W. KASCHKA

Introduction

The parietal lobes have only infrequently been implicated as being important in schizophrenia or affective disorders. However, in recent years, there has been some evidence that they might be considered as a possible site of damage or dysfunction, especially in schizophrenia but also in affective disorders. First, some positron emission tomography (PET) studies showed abnormalities in the parietal lobes in schizophrenia, especially a hypoparietal pattern on the right (Kishimoto et al. 1987; Cleghorn et al. 1989; Buchsbaum et al. 1990). Second, the right inferior parietal lobe may play an important role in the mediation of selective attention, which is thought to be impaired in schizophrenia (Buchsbaum et al. 1990). Third, the inferior parietal lobe has direct and reciprocal connections to most regions which have been found to play a role in schizophrenia, for example, the dorsolateral prefrontal cortex.

In this study, we investigated the effects of somatosensory stimulation (SSS) on the parietal lobes with technetium 99m-hexamethylpropileneamine-oxime (TC 99m-HMPAO) single photon emission computerized tomography (SPECT), since SSS can be expected to affect the parietal lobes by stimulating somatosensory pathways and selective attention.

Methods

Five inpatients with bipolar disorder, depressed, and six inpatients with schizophrenia, residual type, participated in the study. Diagnoses were made according to DSM III-R. All patients were right-handed. Demographic and clinical characteristics are shown in Table 1.

All subjects were investigated twice; the second scan was performed 48 h later, at approximately the same time of day (between 9 and 10 a.m.).

[1] Abt. für Psychiatrie, Universität Erlangen-Nürnberg, Schwabachanlage 6-10, W-8520 Erlangen, FRG.

Imaging of the Brain in Psychiatry
and Related Fields
Edited by K. Maurer

Table 1. Demographic and clinical characteristics of the two patient groups

	Patient number	Sex	Age	Age of onset (years)	Hospitalization (days)	HRSD	Medication
	1	F	38	25	2	29	Sulpiride
Bipolar disorder	2	F	18	16	12	26	Sulpiride
296.5	3	F	42	30	5	20	Sulpiride + amitryptiline
	4	F	66	28	11	21	Sulpiride + amitryptiline
	5	F	47	20	8	20	Sulpiride
Mean			42.2	23.8	7.6	23.2	
	1	F	65	23	2	29	Sulpiride + amitryptiline
Schizophrenia	2	M	39	25	12	25	Sulpiride
295.6	3	M	25	20	11	20	Sulpiride
	4	F	61	22	2	19	Sulpiride
	5	F	21	19	5	18	Sulpiride
	6	F	24	19	8	23	Sulpiride + amitryptiline
Mean			39.2	21.3	6.7	24	

HRSD, Hamilton rating scale.

Table 2. Change of regional perfusion indices during somatosensory stimulation (testretest differences compared by t-test, paired, two-tailed)

	Right		Left	
	295.6	296.5	296.5	296.5
SP	−3.6 + 1.5 ($p < 0.05$)	−0.2 + 1.3 (n.s.)	−1.3 + 1.6 (n.s.)	+0.2 + 1.9 (n.s.)
IP	−1.3 + 1.0 (n.s.)	+3.0 + 1.1 ($p < 0.05$)	−0.5 + 1.0 (n.s.)	+0.8 + 1.5 (n.s.)

SP, superior parietal lobe; IP, inferior parietal lobe.

SPECT 1 was performed under resting conditions, SPECT 2 with SSS. Medication and psychopathological ratings remained unchanged.

Somatosensory stimuli consisted of electrical impulses of 0.2 ms duration and 0.5 c/s frequency delivered to the right median never at the wrist and achieving a painless but clear motor response of the thumb. Stimulation was performed for 1 min before and 10 min after the injection of HMPAO. For semiquantitative evaluation 18 anatomically significant areas were depicted as regions of interest and a regional perfusion index (RPI) was calculated. The RPI is the ratio between counts per voxel of one region and mean counts per voxel of all brain regions. For statistical data evaluation in this study, the RPIs for the superior and inferior parietal lobes were calculated.

Results

Statistical analysis (*t* test) showed no significant differences in the parietal lobes between the two groups under resting conditions. However, the pattern of response to SSS was different in the two groups, as shown in Table 2 where one can see the differences in RPI between resting and stimulated conditions. These test-retest differences were significantly different in the two groups only in the right inferior parietal lobe (Fig. 1).

Discussion

The bipolar and the schizophrenic group showed a different pattern of response to SSS in the parietal lobes. The first group had an average

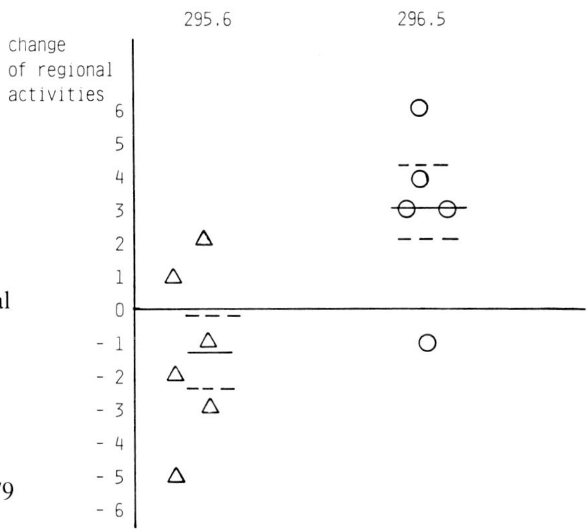

Fig. 1. Differences in regional perfusion index between rest and stimulation in the right inferior parietal lobe. Comparison between schizophrenic and affective groups (student's *t* test, unpaired, two-tailed); $t = 2.79$ ($p < 0.021$)

increase of relative regional activity, the second a relative decrease. The effects were significantly different between the two groups in the right inferior parietal lobe and are probably not due to medication or depressive affect since these did not differ in the two groups. As all schizophrenics were residual type (295.6) with predominantly negative symptoms, including attentional deficits, and as it has been shown that healthy subjects showed an increase of activity in (right) parietal regions unter attentional activating tasks (Buchsbaum et al. 1990), it is assumed that the missing positive response in the schizophrenic group in this study is connected to negative symptomatology, as also seen in type-II schizophrenia. For future research, the right inferior parietal lobe should be examined more closely in larger samples of type-II schizophrenia patients using tasks that can be expected to activate attention and the parietal lobes more specifically.

References

Buchsbaum MS, Nuechterlein KH, Haier RJ, Wu J, Sicotte N, Hazlett E, Ascarnow R, Potkin S, Guichi S (1990) Glucose metabolic rate in normals and schizophrenics during the continous performance test assessed by positron emission tomography. Br J Psychiatry 156:216–227

Cleghorn J, Kaplan R, Nahmias C, Garnett E, Szechtman H, Szechtman B (1989) Inferior parietal region implicated in neurocognitive impairment in schizophrenia. Arch Gen Psychiatry 46:758–759

Kishimoto H, Kuwahara H, Ohno S, Takazu O, Nomnra Y, Yokio S, Jio M (1987) Three subtypes of chronic schizophrenia identified using ^{11}C-Glucose positron emission tomography. Psychiatry Res 21:285–292

Changes in the Regional Activation Pattern in the Normal Human Brain During Dreaming and Rapid Eye Movement Sleep as Measured with Single Photon Emission Computerized Tomography

P.L. MADSEN[1], L. FRIBERG, S. HOLM, S. VORSTRUP, N.A. LASSEN, and G. WILDSCHIØDTZ

Introduction

In the sleep-wake, cycle, rapid eye movement (REM) sleep represents a distinct mental condition, as it is closely correlated to the dream experience (Dement and Kleitman 1957). The present understanding of the dream phenomenon is very limited. We do not know the functional significance of dreams and the physiological state of the dreaming brain is largely unknown.

In the normal brain there is a close coupling between cerebral blood flow (CBF) and neuronal activity (Sokoloff 1981). This coupling also exists on the regional level allowing an interpretation of regional CBF (rCBF) in terms of regional neural activity (Olesen 1971). While the functional landscape of the wakeful brain has been assessed by the measurement of rCBF in a large variety of conditions (Lassen and Ingvar 1978), only very few measurements of rCBF during the different sleep stages have been performed so far (Sakai et al. 1980; Reivich et al. 1968). The explanation for this is undoubtedly the elusive character of sleep, imposing severe restrictions on examination methodology. To study rCBF during sleep, the examination technique should allow sleep in a segregated room without causing interference. Furthermore, the examination methodology should not impose major restrictions on body movements during sleep.

Single photon emmision computerized tomography (SPECT) and the new tracer Tc 99m-d, 1-hexamethylpropylene-amine-oxime (Tc 99m-HMPAO) meet these criteria. The aim of the present investigation was, through use of this new technique, to measure rCBF during well-defined REM sleep.

Material and Methods

A total of 11 healthy young volunteers (5 women, 6 men) were studied. None of the subjects used medication on a regular basis, and all had a

[1] Department of Clinical Physiology, Bispebjerg Hospital, 23, Bispebjerg Bakke, 2400 Copenhagen NV, Denmark.

Imaging of the Brain in Psychiatry and Related Fields
Edited by K. Maurer

normal stable sleep-wake cycle. All volunteers gave informed consent, and the study was approved by the local ethics committee.

rCBF was measured by SPECT with a retainable tracer, Tc 99m-HMPAO (Ceretec). The tracer is administered as a bolus in a peripheral vein. While sufficiently stable in vitro, Tc 99m-HMPAO undergoes rapid conversion when in contact with blood cells and tissue. The injected lipophilic form is transported over the blood-brain barrier. Intracellulary, the compound is enzymatically converted into a hydrophilic substance that is trapped. Therefore, the distribution of Tc 99m-HMPAO in brain tissue reflects the regional tracer supply, i.e., rCBF at the time of injection. Measurements were performed using a rotating multidetector SPECT instrument (Tomomatic 232). In the present study, the regional tracer distribution was depicted in eight transverse slices.

The sleep stages were assessed by standard sleep laboratory polysomnography, including EEG, submental electromyography (EMG), and electrooculography (EOG). The sleep stages were scored according to the criteria of Rechtschaffen and Kales (1968).

rCBF was measured on separate nights during REM sleep and during EEG-verified wakefulness, with a randomized order of measurements. Before measurements were undertaken, the subject spent a night in the sleep laboratory during mimicked test procedures to secure acquaintance with the test conditions. To assure pleasant and undisturbed surroundings facilitating sleep, the subject was left alone in a comfortable bed in a quiet dark room. A long catheter and a cable carrying the polysomnographic data were led through a hole in the door to a neighboring observation room. From the observation room the state of sleep was monitored and the infusion of Tc 99m-HMPAO controlled. When the subject had spent 7 min in the second REM phase of the night, as verified by polysomnographic readings, 250 MBq of Tc 99m-HMPAO were administered from the observation room Exactly 5 min after the Tc 99m-HMPAO injection, with the subject still in uninterrupted REM sleep, the subject was awakened and questioned about the occurrence of dreams and dream content. Measurements during wakefulness were performed on separate days between 10 and 12 p.m. in the same surroundings as described above.

On the two sets of rCBF distribution images the following procedures were applied:

1. For each slice a set of relevant regions of interest (ROI) was demarcated on the basis of anatomical reference.
2. The two sets of distribution images were normalized relative to the mean count rate in their respective cerebellar regions.
3. The mean value of each ROI was calculated and taken as a percentage of the mean value of the upper six slices (orbitomeatal plane (OM) + 30 mm–OM + 80 mm).

A four-way analysis of variance (ANOVA) was performed using the mean of the linearized count rate in each ROI.

Results

In all subjects, verified REM sleep was maintained during injection of Tc 99m-HMPAO and throughout the following 5 min period. On awakening all subjects reported the occurrence of dreams.

Statistical analysis revealed no statistically significant difference in regional side-to-side blood flow distribution between measurements obtained during wakefulness and REM sleep.

During REM sleep there was a statistically significant increase by 4% ($p < 0.01$) in relative rCBF in the associative visual area. In contrast, a significant decrease in relative rCBF in the lower frontal cortical areas, including the inferior frontal cortex (−9.2%, $p < 0.01$), the inferior mesial frontal cortex (−5.4%, $p < 0.02$), and the lateral frontal cortex (−5.7%, $p < 0.03$), was observed during REM sleep (Madsen et al. 1991a). During REM sleep, no other significant changes vere found in relative rCBF in any other cortical or subcortical region (Madsen et al. 1991a).

Discussion

The Tc 99m-HMPAO compound allows, for the first time, tomo-graphic measurements of rCBF during unrestrained well-defined REM sleep. However, due to major difficulties in obtaining a valid arterial input curve, only relative rCBF values are measured. Furthermore, it has been shown that the tracer is not retained in a linear proportion to flow (Lassen et al. 1988). This problem has been partly solved by introducing an algorithm linearizing blood flow values (Lassen et al. 1988). The relative rCBF values from the present study have been linearized according to this algorithm, but the method probably still underestimates high flow values and overestimates low flow values. Thus the flow changes observed in the present study are primarily a measure of the direction of change, and it is not possible from our data to obtain more than an impression of the magnitude of change.

Quantitative results from experimental animal studies have all shown an increased CBF during REM sleep (Reivich et al. 1968; Santiago et al. 1984; Lenzi et al. 1987). In humans, an unchanged or increased CBF have been found during REM sleep (Townsend et al. 1973; Sakai et al. 1980; Madsen et al. 1991b). The REM sleep-associated relative rCBF increase in the associative visual area found in the present study may therefore be considered an absolute flow increase. The regional distribution of this flow increase compares to the regional increase in cerebral metabolism found during complex visual stimulation in the studies of Phelps et al. (1981a,b).

Hence our results suggest that visual dream experiences are accompanied by activation of cerebral structures processing complex visual material.

In the present study we observed a decrease in relative rCBF in the inferior frontal cortex during dreaming. In this context it is interesting that awake patients with schizophrenia, in recent investigations, have been shown to display an impaired activation response in the dorsolateral prefrontal cortex during the performance of certain frontal activation tasks (Berman et al. 1986; Weinberger et al. 1986). The idea that psychosis and dreaming may share many of the same psychological features has been brought forward by many authors (e.g., Hartmann 1976; Jacobs and Trulson 1979). A REM sleep-induced decrease in relative rCBF, in the same part of the brain in which a hypofunction has been demonstrated in the schizophrenic patient, could therefore suggest that there is some kind of functional correlation between the often odd and distorted events experienced during dreams in normal humans and the altered sense of reality that might be so prominent in the awake schizophrenic patient.

References

Berman KF, Zec RF, Weinberger DR (1986) Physiologic dysfunction of dorsolateral prefrontal cortex in schizophrenia: II. Role of neuroleptic treatment, attention, and mental effort. Arch Gen Psychiatry 43:126–135

Dement W, Kleitman N (1957) The relation of eye movements during sleep to dream activity: an objective method for the study of dreaming. J Exp Psychol 53:339–346

Hartmann E (1976) Schizophrenia: a theory Pschopharmacology (Berlin) 49:1–15

Jacobs BL, Trulson ME (1979) Dreams, hallucinations and psychosis – the serotonin connection. Trends Neurosci 2:277–280

Lassen NA, Ingvar DH (1978) Brain function and blood flow. Sci Am 239:62–72

Lassen NA, Andersen AR, Friberg L, Paulson OB (1988) The retention of [99m-Tc]-d, l-HM-PAO in the human brain after intracarotid bolus injection: kinetic analysis. J Cereb Blood Flow Metab 8:S13–S22

Lenzi P, Cianci T, Guidalotti PL, Leonardi GS, Franzini C (1987) Brain circulation during sleep and its relation to extracerebral hemodynamics. Brain Res 415: 14–20

Madsen PL, Holm S, Vorstrup, Friberg L, Lassen NA, Wildschiødtz G (1991a) Regional cerebral blood flow in man during rapid eye movement sleep. J Cereb Blood Flow Metab 11:502–507

Madsen PL, Schmidt JS, Wilschiødtz G, Friberg L, Holm S, Vorstrup S, Lassen NA (1991b) Cerebral O_2 Metabolism and cerebral blood flow in humans during deep and rapid-eye-movement sleep. J Appl Physiology 70:2597–2607

Olesen J (1971) Contralateral focal increase of cerebral blood flow in man during arm work. Brain 94:635–646

Phelps ME, Kuhl DE, Mazziotta JC (1981a) Metabolic mapping of the brain's response to visual stimulation: studies in humans. Science 211:1445–1448

Phelps ME, Mazziotta JC, Kuhl DE, Nuwer M, Packwood J, Metter J, Engel J Jr (1981b) Tomographic mapping of human cerebral metabolism: visual stimulation and deprivation. Neurology 31:517–529

Rechtschaffen A, Kales A (1968) A manual of standardized terminology, techniques and scoring system for sleep stages of human subjects. UCLA Brain Information Service/Brain Research Institute, Los Angeles

Reivich M, Isaacs G, Evarts E, Kety SS (1968) The effect of slow wave sleep and REM sleep on regional cerebral blood flow in cats. J Neurochem 15:301–306

Sakai F, Meyer JS, Karacan I, Derman S, Yamamoto M (1980) Normal human sleep: regional cerebral hemodynamics. Ann Neurol 7:471–478

Santiago TV, Guerra E, Neubauer JA, Edelman NH (1984) Correlation between ventilation and brain blood flow during sleep. J Clin Invest 73:497–506

Sokoloff L (1981) The relationship between function and energy metabolism: its use in the localization of functional activity in the nervous system. Neurosci Res Prog Bull 19:159–210

Townsend RE, Prinz PN, Obrist WD (1973) Human cerebral blood flow during sleep and waking. J Appl Physiol 35:620–625

Weinberger DR, Berman KF, Zec RF (1986) Physiologic dysfunction of dorsolateral prefrontal cortex in schizophrenia: I. Arch Gen Psychiatry 43:114–124

Evaluation of Total Sleep Deprivation by Single Photon Emission Computerized Tomography

S.H. Kaendler,[1] S. Volk, F.D. Maul, R. Weber, K. Georgi, A. Hertel, B. Pflug, and G. Hör

Introduction

Total sleep deprivation (TSD) has a clear-cut positive effect on mood in depressed patients. Pflug and Tölle (1971) demonstrated that TSD can produce a dramatic effect on depressive symptoms within 24 h. Wu and Bunney (1990) pointed out that an average of 59% of patients respond to TSD as a treatment.

Two studies on the effects of TSD using positron emission tomography (PET) have been published. Wu et al. (1988) reported on normal controls: they found a decrease in metabolic rates in the caudate nucleus. Gillin et al. (1990) demonstrated that responders to TSD have a higher metabolic activity in the cingulate nucleus than nonresponders prior to TSD. The higher activity was followed by a significant decrease the day after TSD.

Up to now, to our knowledge, no study has been performed using single photon emission computerized tomography (SPECT) for analyzing the effects of TSD on regional cerebral perfusion in depressed patients. In the present study, we used SPECT to investigate depressed patients prior to and after TSD in order to find reproducible individual patterns or certain changes in the perfusion rate that would be predictive with respect to response to TSD.

Methods

The 20 studied patients (12 females and 8 males; mean age 48.5 years, range 27–65 years) all suffered from major depression (DSM III-R, APA 1987). All were treated with anti-depressant medication, in most cases with trimipramine. Medication was not changed during the week of the study. No patient suffered from organic brain disorders, occlusive cerebral disease, hypertension, kidney diseases, or other serious diseases.

[1] Abteilung Klinische Psychiatrie II, Johann Wolfgang Goethe-Universität Frankfurt/M., Heinrich Hoffmann Str. 10, W-6000 Frankfurt/M. 71, FRG.

Imaging of the Brain in Psychiatry
and Related Fields
Edited by K. Maurer

DAY / TIME	0	1	2
8.00 a.m.	Hamilton Rating Scale for Depression	Hamilton Rating Scale for Depression	Hamilton Rating Scale for Depression
8.30 a.m.	SPECT 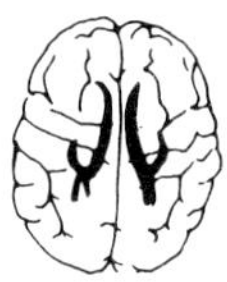	SPECT 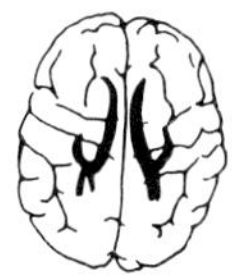	
	Total Sleep Deprivation		

Fig. 1. Design of the study

The morning prior to and after TSD, brain SPECT studies, using the perfusion marker technetium 99m-hexamethylpropilene-amino-oxime Tc 99m-HMPAO (550 MBq of Tc 99m), were carried out. The patients were sitting with eyes open while the radiopharmaceutical was administered. Within 30min the SPECT examination was performed. Before the examination the patients were not allowed to eat or take their medication (Fig. 1). For the examination a γ-camera fitted for emission computerized tomography (ECT) with a high resolution collimator was used. Within a rotation of 360°, 64 frames were taken. For the evaluation, reconstructions were made. Filtered backprojections were utilized using a Hamming-Hann filter. Standard slices of 14mm were defined; the reference was the orbitalmeatal line. Count rates were quantified in various brain regions, based on the assumption that count rates were equivalent to cerebral blood flow (CBF). Four slices were analyzed, and in defined areas symmetrical regions of interest (ROI) were drawn manually as shown in Fig. 2. In a first evaluation the cerebellum served as a reference ROI in order to compare the changes

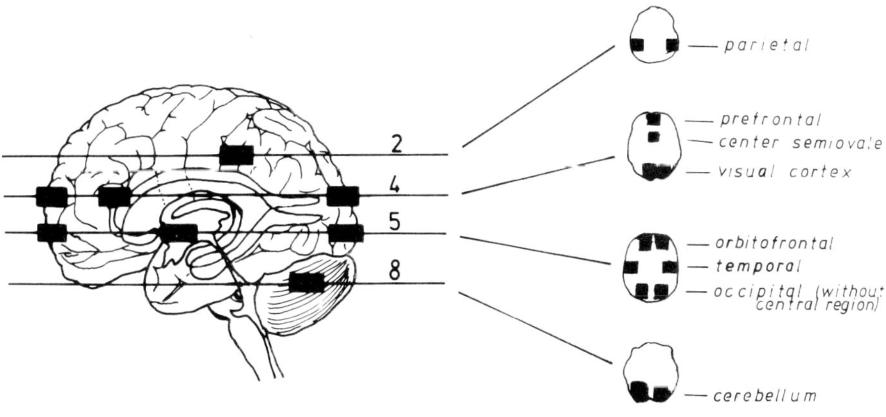

Fig. 2. Placement of the regions of interest (ROIs)

in CBF with those of other brain regions both intra- and interindividually. However, the CBF in the cerebellum, usually preferred as a referral region, showed differences between the right and left sides. Therefore the optical cortex was chosen as the reference region. It had the highest regional contrast due to the fact that the patients had their eyes open during administration of the radiopharmaceutical.

To assess the severity of the depression, the Hamilton Rating Scale of Depression (HRDS) was used. Sleep items were excluded for analysis. The mean HRDS score with sleep items on day 1 was 23.1 ± 6.3. Responders and nonresponders did not differ in HRDS scores. A response to TSD was assumed if the Hamilton index improved more than 30%. Day 2 responders were not computed separately because of the small size of the group ($n = 2$).

The SPECT variables of interest were parametrically evaluated. All distributions were tested against a normal distribution with the Kolomogorow – Smirnow goodness of fit test. No significant differences were found. To test differences between the response types to TSD and hemispheric differences, one-way analysis of variance (ANOVA) with a repeated measurement design for dependent samples and *t* tests were performed. Two-tailed probability was also determined. Significance was postulated for a probability of $p < 0.05$. Since numerous *t* tests were performed and the nature of the study was exploratory, *p* values have to be regarded as descriptive.

Results

In the examined group, 11 patients responded to TSD, 2 of them on the second day; 9 patients were nonresponders to TSD.

Table 1. Mean ratios and standard deviation in the regions showing significant differences before and after total sleep deprivation

Region	Responder			Nonresponder		
	Mean	SD	p	Mean	SD	p
Before TSD						
Temporal						
Right	0.87	0.08	NS	0.96	0.29	0.05
Left	0.88	0.07		0.99	0.28	
Cerebellar						
Right	1.81	0.45	0.008	1.83	0.41	NS
Left	1.90	0.45		1.88	0.41	
After TSD						
Temporal						
Right	0.94	0.08	NS	0.91	0.06	NS
Left	0.93	0.07		0.93	0.05	
Cerebellar						
Right	1.00	0.08	0.013	1.75	0.33	NS
Left	1.06	0.09		1.81	0.36	

TSD, total sleep deprivation; NS, not significant; SD, standard deviation; p value, two-tailed.

Table 2. Mean ratios and standard deviation in the regions showing significant differences before and after total sleep deprivation

Region	Before TSD		After TSD		
	Mean	SD	Mean	SD	p
Responder					
Parietal					
Right	0.81	0.05	0.86	0.05	0.040
Left	0.82	0.04	0.86	0.05	0.047
Temporal					
Right	0.88	0.08	0.94	0.08	NS
Left	0.89	0.07	0.93	0.07	0.008
Nonresponder					
Parietal					
Right	0.89	0.26	0.81	0.05	NS
Left	0.88	0.22	0.82	0.05	NS
Temporal					
Right	0.96	0.29	0.91	0.07	NS
Left	0.99	0.28	0.94	0.09	NS

TSD, total sleep deprivation; SD, standard deviation; NS, not significant; p value, two-tailed.

Responders and nonresponders significantly differed from each other before and after TSD. Nonresponders had significantly lower CBF in their right temporal area than in the left before TSD. After TSD this difference was equalized. In contrast, temporal differences were not observed in the responders. However perfusion in the right cerebellar region was lower than in the left before and after TSD (Table 1).

No significant differences concerning the perfusion ratio in the evaluated regions before and after TSD were found when responders and nonresponders were compared. The ratios of each side were compared separately with and without regard to the type of response to TSD.

All responders had a significant increase in the perfusion ratio within the left temporal area and in both parietal regions. The ratio decreased in both parietal and temporal areas after TSD in the nonresponders but not significantly (Table 2).

The statistical analysis of these 20 patients does not support our first results in 15 patients (Kaendler et al. 1990) of a frontal-occipital redistribution in responders.

Discussion

Measurements of CBF in depressed patients have shown controversial results (Hedde and Reischies 1986; Schlegel et al. 1989). A reduced perfusion of the left hemisphere was described by Gustafson et al. (1981). Uytdenhoef et al. (1983) found an increased perfusion within the left frontal region and reduced rates in the right posterior region. By a dynamic SPECT study in depressive patients Hedde and Reischies (1986) demonstrated a global perfusion rate not differing from that of normal subjects.

Due to the design of our study we cannot compare our findings with those from normal subjects. We could not demonstrate a common pattern of change in CBF after TSD treatment in depressed patients. However, in distinguishing responders and non-responders by the HRDS scores, differential effects of TSD on cerebral perfusion were found. The perfusion patterns of the temporal and parietal lobe have not yet been reported.

In conclusion our data suggest that state-dependent changes of perfusion involve temporal and parietal brain regions. The interpretation must remain speculative until further studies confirm the reported results.

References

APA (American Psychiatric Association) (1987) diagnostic and statistical manual of mental disorders, DSM III-R, 3rd rev edn. APA, Washington DC

Gillin JC, Buchsbaum MS, Dupont R, Wu J (1990) Localized cerebral metabolism in man: effects of sleep and sleep deprivation. In: Abstracts Book 10th Congress of the European Sleep Research Society, p 40

Gustafson L, Risberg J, Silversskiöld P (1981) Cerebral blood flow in dementia and depression. Lancet 275

Hedde JP, Reischies FM (1986) Bildgebende Diagnostik in der Psychiatrie. Nervenarzt 57:65–79

Kaendler SH, Weber R, Volk S, Maul FD, Hertel A, Pflug B, Hör G (1990) Evaluation of total sleep deprivation by SPECT. In: Abstract Book 2nd International Symposium Imaging of the brain in Psychiatry and related fields p 110

Pflug B, Tölle R (1971) Therapie endogener Depressionen durch Schlafentzug. Nervenarzt 42:117–124

Schlegel S, Aldenhoff JB, Eissner D, Lindner P, Nickel O (1989) Regional cerebral blood flow in depression: associations with psychopathology. J Affective Disord: 211–218

Uytdenhoef P, Protelange P, Jacquy J, Charles G, Linkowski P, Mendlewicz J (1983) Regional cerebral blood flow and lateralized hemispheric dysfunction in depression. Br J Psychiatry 143:128–132

Wu J, Bunney WE (1990) The biological basis of an antide-pressant response to sleep deprivation and relapse: review and hypothesis. Am J Psychiatry 147:14–21

Wu J, Buchsbaum MS, Gillin JC (1988) Positron emission tomography study of sleep deprivation. Sleep Res 16:796

Correlation of ^{99m}Tc-Labeled HMPAO-SPECT with Spectral EEG Activity in Dementia of Alzheimer Type

L. Frölich[1], C. Eilles, R. Ihl, T. Dierks, and K. Maurer

Introduction

Since the introduction of ^{99m}Tc-labeled hexamethylpropyleneamineoxime (HMPAO) as a tracer for studying regional cerebral blood flow (rCBF; Nowotnik et al. 1985), a number of studies have been conducted to investigate its relevance as a diagnostic tool in dementia of Alzheimer type (DAT). A typical pattern of temporoparietal flow deficits could be observed in DAT, as could stage-dependent reductions of the regional cerebral blood flow extending from temporoparietal to frontal areas (Frölich et al. 1989). Computed electroencephalographic topography (CET) is another functional imaging technique which has some relevance in the diagnosis of DAT (Maurer and Dierks 1987). A slowing and an anterioritzation of the peak mean frequency has been described depending on the severity of the disease (Dierks et al. 1991). Thus, both functional neuroimaging methods demonstrate changes which can be correlated with the severity of clinical symptoms of dementia. However, there have been only few studies which tried to correlate results from both imaging methods with each other. Stigsby et al. (1981) found no clear correlation between rCBF and EEG parameters. None of these earlier studies used a mapping system for EEG analysis and single photon emission computed tomography (SPECT) for measuring regional cerebral perfusion.

In the present investigation in clinically diagnosed DAT patients the EEG recorded by a BIO-LOGIC Brain Atlas III Plus was related to tracer ratios reflecting regional cerebral perfusion obtained from HMPAO-SPECT. Numeric correlations were calculated between the regional cerebral blood flow ratios, the amplitude of conventional frequency bands and the frequency, amplitude and location of the peak mean frequency of the EEG.

[1] Abt. für Psychiatrie, Universitäts-Nervenklinik Würzburg, Füchsleinstr. 15, W-8700 Würzburg, FRG.

Imaging of the Brain in Psychiatry
and Related Fields
Edited by K. Maurer

Methods

From a group of 47 DAT patients (DSM-III-R diagnosis of dementia, NINCDS/ADRDA criteria for DAT), 23 patients were selected because both EEG and HMPAO-SPECT had been recorded. Mean age was 67 ± 11 years (age range 45 to 84 years). All patients were right handed. All neuroimaging studies were carried out at rest, i.e., with the patients awake and conscious, but as far as possible undisturbed by sensory stimulation. Each patient received a battery of neuropsychological tests of which the

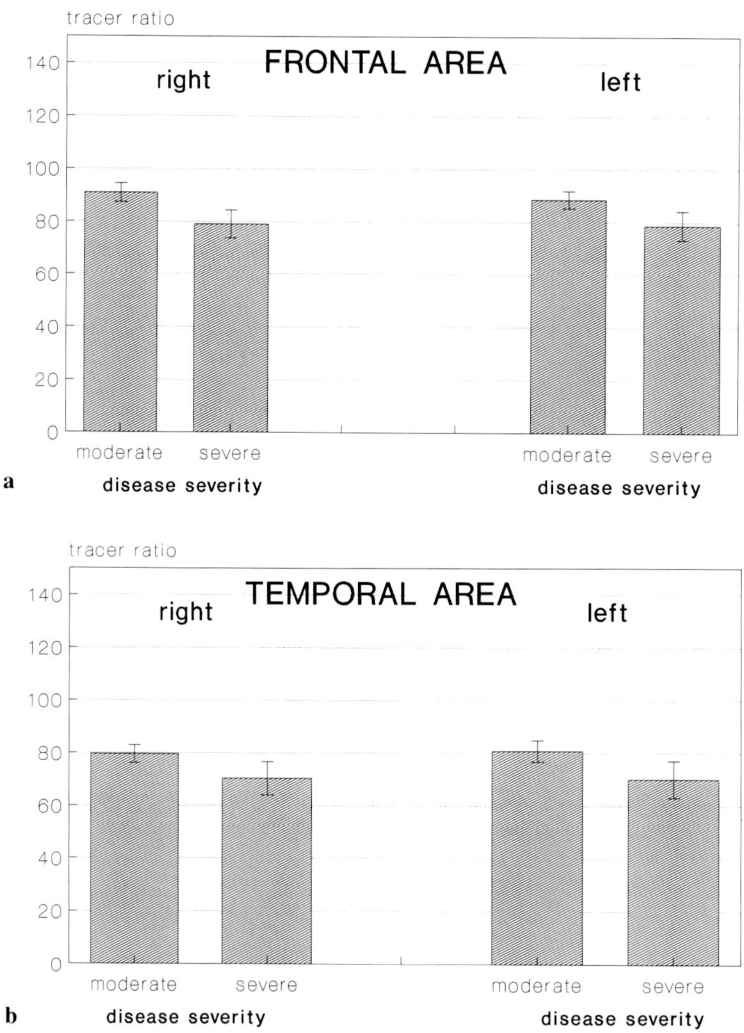

Fig. 1a–d. HMPAO-SPECT in dementia of Alzheimer type. Tracer ratios vs. disease severity according to the Short Syndrom Test in **a** the frontal, **b** temporal

Short Syndrome Test (SKT) (Erzickeit 1977) was selected to grade the patients into mildly-moderately (17 patients) and severely demented (six patients).

EEG was recorded using a 19-channel BIO-LOGIC Brain Atlas III Plus. The electrodes were placed according to the international 10–20 System. For quantification of the EEG data, spectral analysis was performed using a fast Fourier transformation (FFT); however, the EEG was visually inspected to avoid artifacts. The following frequency bands were studied: delta (1.0–3.5 Hz), theta (4.0–7.5 Hz), alpha (8.0–11.5 Hz), betal (12.0–

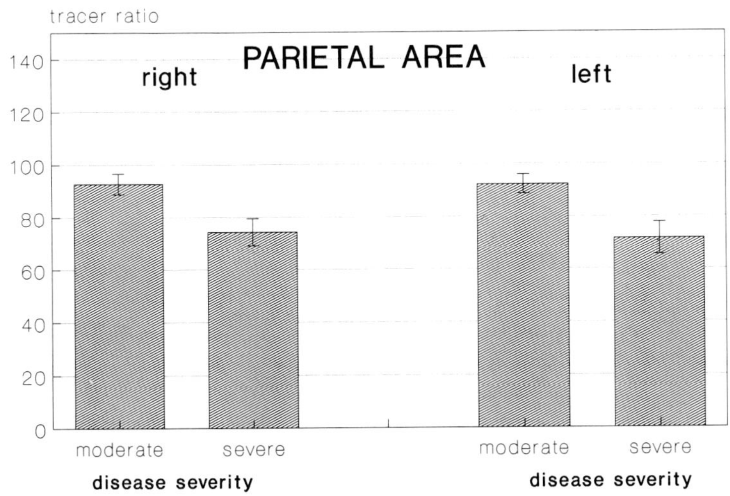

c

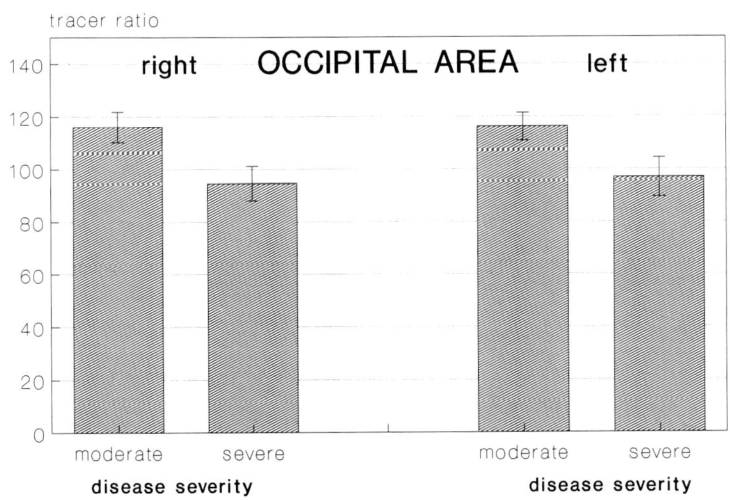

d

Fig. 1c. Parietal, and **d** occipital areas

15.5 Hz), beta2 (16.0–19.5 Hz), beta3 (20.0–23.5 Hz). The data in the frequency bands were logarithmically transformed for better Gaussian distribution. Further analysis involved calculation of the mean peak frequency, mean amplitude of the peak frequency and the localization of the maximal amplitude of the peak frequency.

HMPAO-SPECT was performed as described earlier (Frölich et al. 1989). Briefly, ca. 740 MBq HMPAO were injected into an antecubital vein. SPECT was performed 45–60 min later using a rotating gamma camera with a high resolution collimator. Transversal planes were reconstructed from the data and regions of interest (ROI) of 8 cm^3 minimal size were placed over frontal, temporal, parietal and occipital areas of both hemispheres and the cerebellum. For calculating tracer ratios, cortical tracer uptake was related to the mean cerebellar uptake. Interhemispheric asymmetries were estimated by the standard deviation between the right and left side values. For correlation of EEG and HMPAO-SPECT parameters, four regions of interest reflecting the four cortical lobes were formed using parameters from both methods, respectively: mean EEG amplitudes under electrodes F3 + F4 (= frontal activity), T3 + T4 (= temporal activity), P3 + P4 (parietal activity), and O1 + O2 (= occipital activity) were used. Mean tracer ratios of both hemispheres for frontal, temporal, parietal and occipital ROI's were used in HMPAO-SPECT. By this procedure, ROI's of comparable size and location were formed from both imaging methods and used for correlation.

Statistical comparisons were performed by calculating Pearson's correlation coefficients between 50 EEG parameters (eight selected electrodes in six frequency bands plus peak frequency and its amplitude) and eight values reflecting blood flow in the cerebral lobes. Because of the high number of correlations, the results are only meant to have descriptive significance. Results are only presented for p values below 0.05.

Results

1. Tracer ratios were calculated for four cortical regions. For the group of 23 DAT patients as a whole rCBF was lowest in the temporal area, followed by the parietal and frontal areas. The flow in the occipital area was approximately equal to cerebellar flow. Data are presented as mean ±SD.

Temporal:	76.1 ± 13.6 right side, 77.4 ± 13.4 left side
	Interhemispheric asymmetry: 3.76 ± 3.10
Parietal:	85.7 ± 15.4 right side, 85.4 ± 15.0 left side
	Interhemispheric asymmetry: 3.05 ± 3.07
Frontal:	87.2 ± 14.4 right side, 85.2 ± 13.3 left side
	Interhemispheric asymmetry: 2.20 ± 2.31
Occipital:	106.8 ± 18.9 right side, 108.8 ± 18.1 left side
	Interhemispheric asymmetry: 3.19 ± 3.21

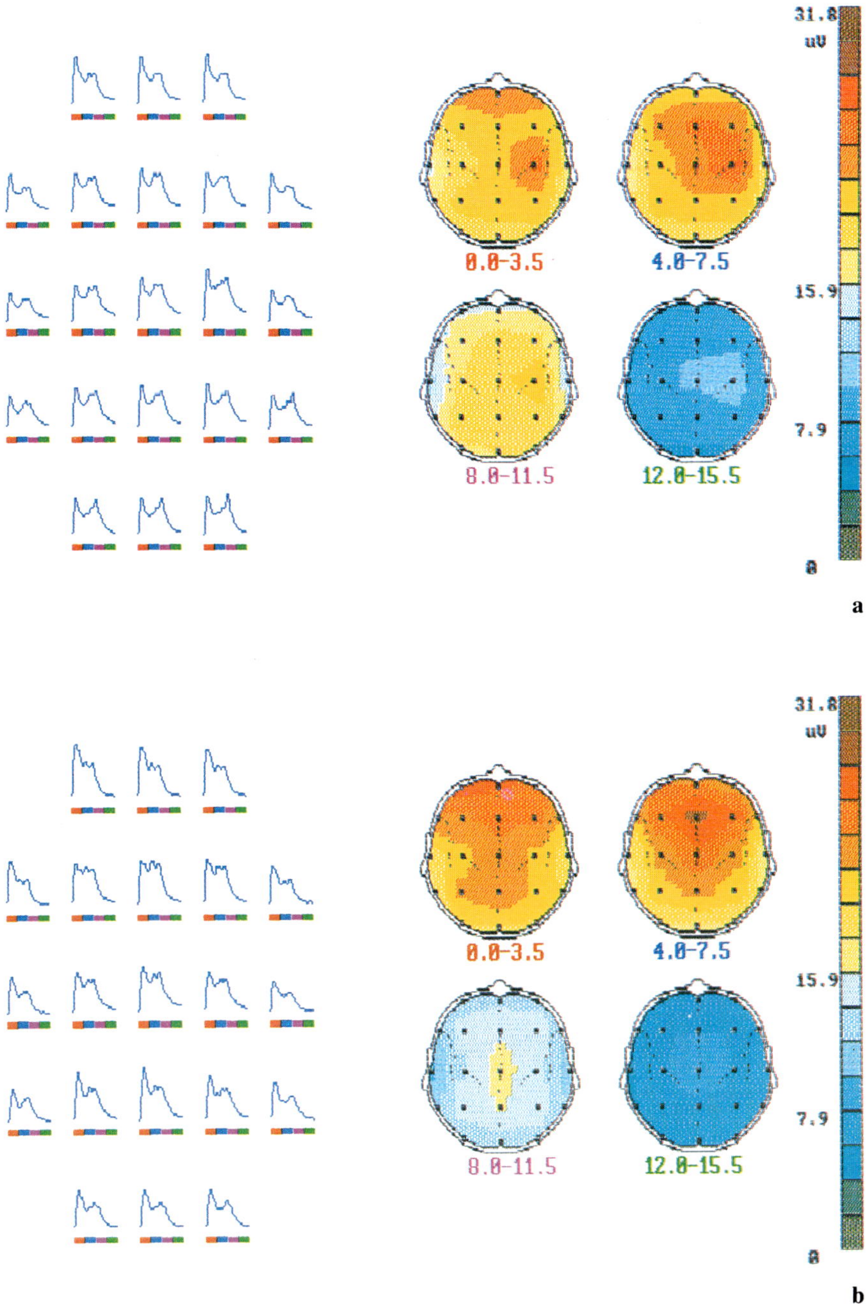

Fig. 2a,b. Spectral EEG activity in the **a** mildly–moderately and **b** severely demented group

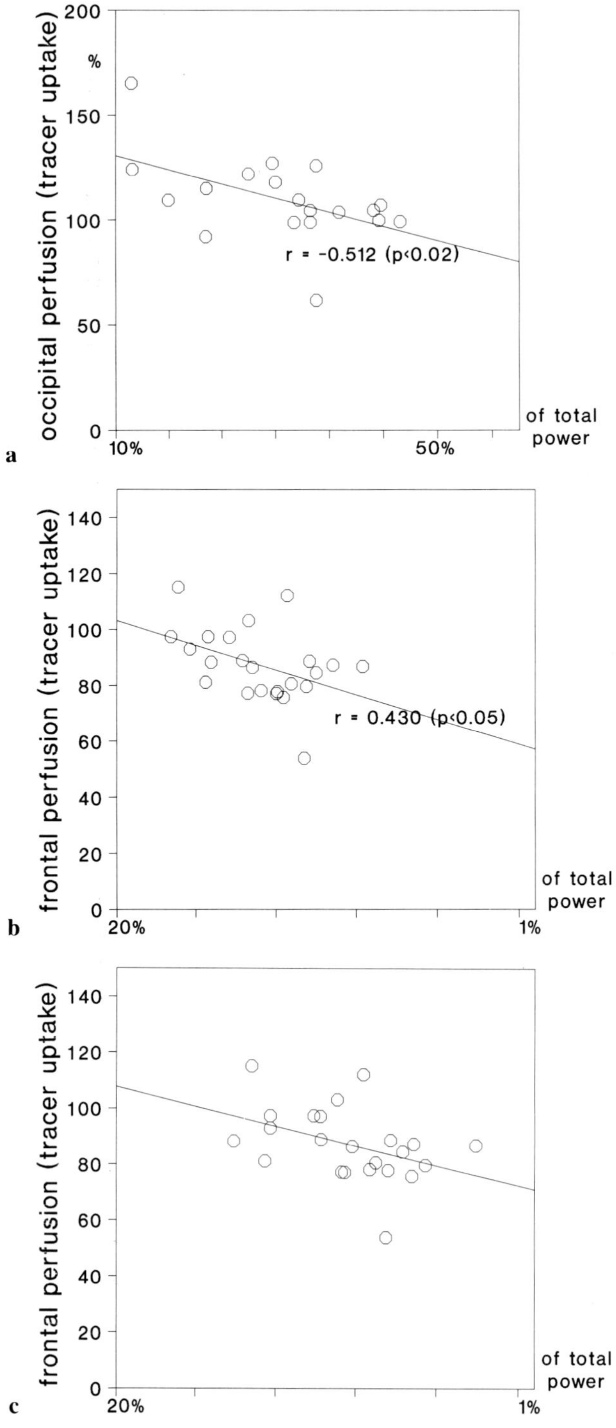
occipital perfusion (tracer uptake)
%
r = -0.512 (p<0.02)
of total power
10%
50%
a
frontal perfusion (tracer uptake)
r = 0.430 (p<0.05)
of total power
20%
1%
b
frontal perfusion (tracer uptake)
of total power
20%
1%
c

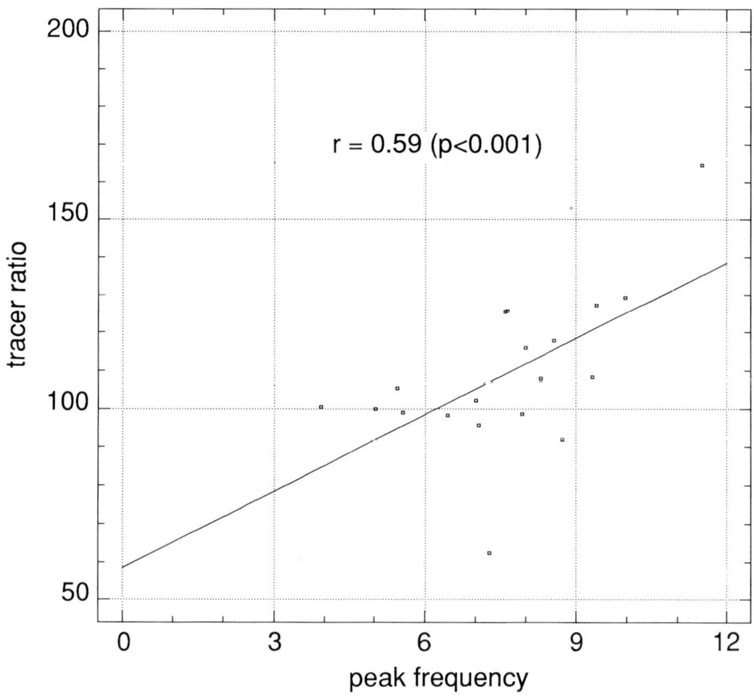

d

Fig. 3a–d. Correlation of **a** occipital theta activity, **b** frontal beta2 activity, **c** frontal beta3 activity with cerebral perfusion in the corresponding brain areas, and **d** peak frequency with occipital flow in dementia of Alzheimer type

2. When the patients were subdivided into two groups according to the neuropsychological deficits in the SKT, the perfusion ratios in all areas declined according to the severity of the disease. Interestingly, also in the occipital areas a reduction of the perfusion ratios according to the severity of the disease could be found.

3. Delta activity in DAT patients increased with the severity of the cognitive impairment, and a similar but clearer increase could be seen for the theta band. In the slightly demented patients, alpha activity was high but decreased with increasing severity of dementia. Decreased beta activity has been found for all three beta bands, most pronounced for beta2 and beta3 band. It appears that the theta and beta 2/3 bands show the earliest changes in DAT. The spectral EEG showed a slowing of the mean peak frequency and an anteriorization of the peak location dependent on the severity of the disease.

4. Correlation of regional perfusion ratios with spectral EEG values showed that theta activity under occipital electrodes (O1 + O2) correlated inversely with occipital perfusion ratio (correlation coefficient −0.512). For

beta2 and beta3 activity over frontal regions (electrode location F3) there was a correlation with frontal perfusion ratios (correlation coefficients 0.430 and 0.451). Occipital blood perfusion ratio correlated with the peak frequency (correlation coefficient 0.59). Although both EEG and HMPAO-SPECT parameters showed a clear dependence on the severity of the clinical symptomes of dementia, no further numeric correlations between results from the two imaging methods were found.

Discussion

Theta, beta2 and beta3 activity were the only frequency bands of the EEG, which correlated with HMPAO-SPECT tracer ratios reflecting cerebral perfusion in DAT. Topographic analysis showed for theta activity that this held true only for occipital brain regions, where beta activity and cerebral blood flow correlated over frontal brain areas. A correlation between the mean peak frequency and regional cerebral perfusion could also be demonstrated in occipital areas. Both beta activity and peak frequency may be regarded as positive indicators of a physiological functioning of the brain, while slow wave activity, i.e. theta activity, may be regarded as a negative indicator, that is an indirect indicator of cellular degeneration, which is the molecular basis for organic brain dysfunction. Occipital brain areas are known to be least involved in the cellular degeneration in DAT (Brun and Englund 1983). A coupling between EEG frequency, cerebral perfusion and oxidative metabolism has been demonstrated under normal conditions. Since in the present investigation this coupling could only be demonstrated in the presumably most undisturbed brain areas, it may be speculated that specific pathophysiological alterations due to the disease might have led to the dissociation of EEG and regional cerebral perfusion in more affected areas. Such pathopysiological alteration might involve a primary abnormality in glucose metabolism in DAT (Hoyer et al. 1988), which leads to imbalance between of oxidative metabolism and cerebral perfusion in early DAT. EEG activity depends more directly on an umimpaired glucose metabolism as the basis of neuronal activity than on the cerebral perfusion. Other alterations which might explain the present results include the degeneration of the cholinergic neurotransmitter system, which might influence the EEG frequency more than the cerebral perfusion. The cerebral perfusion might be influenced more by the degree of neuronal degeneration, which is most pronounced in the tertiary association areas.

In summary, the present results show that significant correlations between EEG parameters and indices of cerebral perfusion may be obtained in corresponding brain areas in DAT, leading to speculations on an uncoupling of physiological brain functions due to the disease process.

References

Brun A, Englund E (1983) Regional pattern of degeneration in Alzheimer's disease: neuronal loss and histopathological grading. Histopathology 5:549–555

Dierks T, Perisic I, Frölich L, Ihl R, Maurer K (1991) Topography of the quantitative EEG in dementia of Alzheimer type: relation to severity of dementia. Psychiatry Res (Neuroimaging) 40:181–194

Erzigkeit H (1977) Manual zum Syndrom Kurztest. Vless, Vaterstetten, München

Frölich L, Eilles C, Ihl R, Maurer K, Lanczik M (1989) Stage-dependent reductions of regional cerebral blood flow measured by HMPAO-SPECT in dementia of Alzheimer type. Psychiatry Res 29:347–350

Hoyer S, Österreich K, Wagner O (1988) Glucose metabolism as the site of the primary abnormality in early-onset dementia of the Alzheimer type? J Neurol 235:143–148

Maurer K, Dierks T (1987) Topographic brain mapping of EEG and evoked potentials in psychiatry and neurology. Z. EEG EMG 18:4–10

Nowotnik DP, Canning LR, Cumming SA et al. (1985) Development of a Tc-99m-labelled radiopharmaceutical for cerebral blood flow imaging. Nuclear Med Commun 6:499–503

Stigsby B, Johannesson G, Ingvar DH (1981) Regional EEG analysis and regional cerebral blood flow in Alzheimer's and Pisk's disease. Electroencephalogr Clin Neurophysiol 51:537–547

The Dynamic Investigation of Brain Function with Split-Dose Tc 99m-Exametazime Single Photon Emission Computerized Tomography

G.M. Goodwin[1], K.J. Shedlack, R. Hunter, and D. Wyper

Introduction

There has been a widely felt desire to extend the use of single photon emission computerized tomography (SPECT) with Tc 99m-exametazime to the investigation of dynamic change in brain function. The present study illustrates the application of a methodological innovation, split-dose Tc 99m-exametazime SPECT. Advantage has been taken of two important properties of Tc 99m-exametazime. The first is the relatively short window of time over which activity is likely to be sampled by a single injection of the tracer. The second is the stability of its distribution over time following its trapping in brain (Neirinckx et al. 1987). This allows the superposition of an activated state upon a stable basal distribution in a single examination of an individual subject.

Split-Dose Exametazime SPECT Scanning

Subjects were injected at rest with eyes patched and ears unplugged using 25% of the usual dose of Tc 99m (125 MBq). Exametazime (Ceretec, Amersham International) was constituted as recommended by its data sheet; a separate vial was used for each injection of radionuclide. The head was aligned with reference to the orbitomeatal line (OML) and scanned with a tomographic section scanner (Novo 810). Scan duration was increased (900 s per slice) and slice number decreased (to two) to compensate for reduced counts at the low dose. Without moving the subject, but again with eyes patched, subjects were then injected with a further tracer dose (375 MBq) during an activation task. The subject was rescanned (300 s per slice) to estimate the new distribution of tracer now comprising basal activity from the low dose and superimposed activity taken up during the activation task. The design of the experiment is shown in Fig. 1. The technique probably lends itself poorly to modification for systems employing rotating γ-cameras because of the much longer times required for data acquisition.

---

[1]MRC Brain Metabolism Unit, Royal Edinburgh Hospital, Morningside Park, Edinburgh, EH10 5HF, UK.

Imaging of the Brain in Psychiatry and Related Fields
Edited by K. Maurer

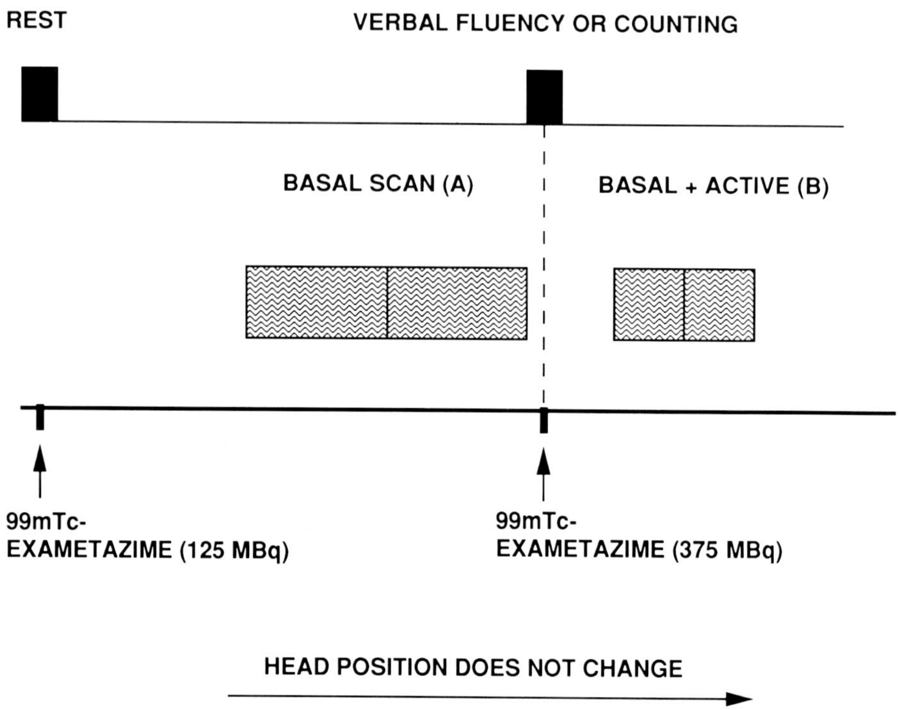

Fig. 1. The use of Tc 99m-exametazime for split-dose SPECT imaging. The initial low dose is injected at rest (basal) conditions. The second dose is injected during a cognitive task. The trapping of the tracer within the brain means that the first scan (*A*) can be delayed until convenient; the second scan (*B*) is obtained without the subject changing head position so that individual slices are fully comparable

The activation tasks were: (1) the verbal fluency test; the subject had to say out loud as many words as possible beginning with a specified letter (Borkowski et al. 1967). The first letter was F: after 1 min the subject was asked to switch to A and during this letter the second injection of tracer was made. The command letter was subsequently changed to R, L, S, and C at 1 min intervals. For counting, subjects were asked simply to count out loud for 6 min and injection was made during the second minute.

The pattern of tracer uptake in basal and activated phases was reconstructed as 12 mm slices with a transverse resolution of 10 mm. Quantitative estimates of tracer uptake (as mean counts per pixel) were determined in 14 regions of interest (ROIs) corresponding approximately to anatomical regions of the brain visualized in transverse section (Hunter et al. 1989).

Data Analysis

Activation was determined by the ratio of the mean counts of tracer uptake per pixel for each ROI from the cognitively activated scan (B) divided by the mean counts per pixel for the identical ROI from the basal scan (A). The resulting number (B/A) was dimensionless and, in the absence of a region-specific effect, should have shown random variation about the mean for each individual subject. B will be a composite of activity remaining from the first scan, A1, and the counts acquired in the second scan, B1. The component A1/A is a constant term derived from measures of the same basal distribution at two different times and B1/A reflects the change in relative distribution produced by the cognitive task. Any systematic change in the variance should reflect only changes in B1/A.

The ratios B/A are plotted in Fig. 2. Calcarine areas represent primary visual sensory cortex and in the absence of direct visual stimulation are unlikely to have changed glucose uptake or regional cerebral blood flow (rCBF) between basal and activated conditions (Roland et al. 1987). The ratios for calcarine areas are therefore taken to estimate the null condition and are used in preference to a global mean as a reference baseline in Fig. 2.

In counting, most areas show prominent activation compared with calcarine cortex. The areas showing the greatest increases in rCBF during counting were high frontal and parietal areas bilaterally. There were also increases in basal ganglia. During the fluency test, frontal and parietal regions showed similar trends to those seen in counting but were less prominent. Much more striking were the decrements in tracer uptake in the regions of the basal ganglia bilaterally during the fluency task. The left temporal cortex also showed a relative decrement during fluency compared with counting.

Discussion

The primary differences that were observed in uptake patterns show that fluency is associated with bilateral reduction of tracer uptake in the region of the basal ganglia and superior temporal cortex; these changes are the converse of those seen during counting. Using $^{15}O_2$ and positron emission tomography (PET), Seitz et al. (1990) have described a bilateral reduction in basal ganglia rCBF in a motor learning task. After training, there were increases in the same regions in association with identical motor output. This pattern of response is directly comparable with that seen here, suggesting that novelty or the development of a motor or cognitive strategy may be an important attribute of the verbal fluency task. The involvement of the basal ganglia in such tasks is extremely interesting in view of the association between subcortical pathology and disorders of motor or cognitive performance (Cummings 1986).

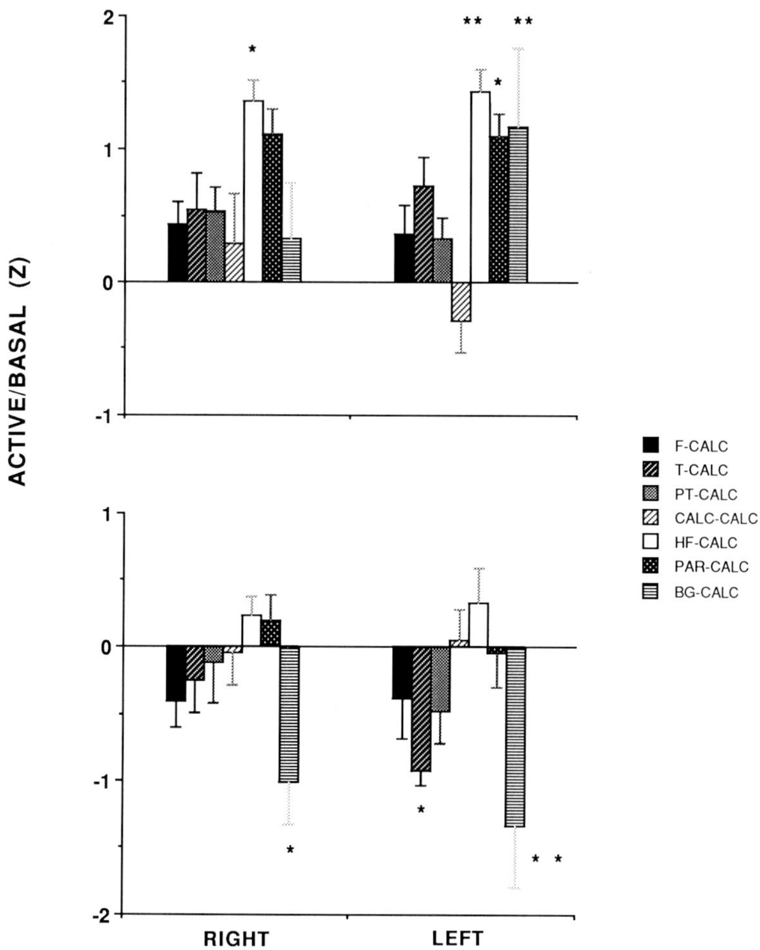

Fig. 2. Changes in regional uptake of Tc 99m-HMPAO during counting and verbal fluency. Ten subjects in each group. The mean of ratios (see text) for right and left calcarine areas has been subtracted from frontal (*F*), temporal (*T*), posterior temporal (*PT*), basal ganglia (*BG*), and calcarine (*CALC*) areas 5–6 cm above the orbitomeatal line (OML) on right and left. High frontal (*HF*) and parietal (*PAR*) areas were taken from a slice 7–8 cm above the OML. The ratios were Z transformed and the graphs show the patterns of cerebral activation during counting and fluency as Z scores for regions of interest (ROIs), grouped by cerebral hemisphere. ANOVA showed regional effects (counting $p < 0.001$, fluency $p < 0.0002$) and two-way analysis of variance was employed to compare fluency and counting conditions, with ROIs as repeated measures. The pattern observed with fluency was different from that seen with counting (interaction, $p = 0.0001$). One SD unit corresponds to about 5% modulation of mean uptake. For counting and fluency conditions, respectively, comparison was made between calcarine areas and the other ROIs of Z-transformed ratios using Dunnett's test: $^*p < 0.05$, $^{**}p < 0.01$

In all such studies some caution is required because of the potentially confusing effects or anxiety or arousal. PET studies suggest that extreme anxiety influences all brain areas equally perhaps via arterial hypocapnia (Mountz et al. 1989), but lower grade anxiety may show differential regional effects involving the basal nuclei and temporal lobes (Reiman et al. 1989). Anxiety or relaxation effects may interact with task performance in evaluating basal/activation differences.

A number of important issues are beyond the scope of the present discussion (Shedlack et al. 1991). These include the validity of using calcarine cortex as a reference area, the method for selection of ROIs, the physiological interpretation of reduced flow, and the relationship of tomographic data to that from planar techniques employing xenon.

The technical limitations of SPECT tend to be emphasized to the advantage of PET, but the genuine advantages of SPECT with Tc 99m-exametazime are the intravenous administration of tracer, the short functional sampling interval, and the dissociation of tracer uptake/task performance from real-time scanning. The split-dose SPECT technique employed in this study has several additional advantages: while minimizing radiation exposure, it permits multiple anatomically identical but metabolically distinct scans in individual subjects thus allowing the use of an intravenous SPECT ligand for a dynamic investigation of cerebral metabolic demand during normal cognitive processes. The method can be applied to the study of clinical syndromes, such as the dementias, neurodegenerative diseases, and psychiatric illness, in which abnormal performance on clinical neuropsychological tests is at present poorly explained by classical theories based on test results from patients with anatomically specific brain lesions.

Acknowledgements. We thank Norma Brearley for the careful preparation of this manuscript. We are also grateful to our volunteers who made the work possible and to Ms. M.T. Hansen for technical assistance. K.S. was an Ethel Dupont Warren Research Fellow, Harvard Medical School.

References

Borkowski JG, Benton AL, Spreen O (1967) Word fluency and brain damage. Neuropsychologia 5:135–140

Cummings JL (1986) Subcortical dementia: neuropsychology, neuropsychiatry and pathophysiology. Br J Psychiatry 149:682–697

Hunter R, McLuskie R, Wyper D, Patterson J, Christie JE, Brooks DN, McCulloch J, Fink G, Goodwin GM (1989) The pattern of function-related regional cerebral blood flow investigated by single photon emission tomography with 99mTc-HMPAO in patients with presenile Alzheimer's disease and Korsakoff's psychosis. Psychol Med 19:847–855

Mountz JM, Modell JG, Wilson MW, Curtis GC, Lee MA, Schmaltz S, Kuhl DE (1989) Positron emission tomographic evaluation of cerebral blood flow during state anxiety in simple phobia. Arch Gen Psychiatry 46:501–505

Neirinckx RD, Canning LR, Piper IM, Nowotnik DP, Pickett RD, Holmes RA, Volkert WA, Forster AM, Weisner PS, Marriott JA, Chaplin SB (1987) Technetium-99m D,1-HMPAO: a new radiopharmaceutical for SPECT imaging of regional cerebral blood perfusion. J Nucl Med 28:191–202

Reiman EM, Fusselman MJ, Fox PT, Raichle ME (1989) Neuroanatomical correlates of anticipatory anxiety. Science 243:1071–1074

Roland PE, Eriksson L, Stone-Elander S, Widen L (1987) Does mental activity change the oxidative metabolism of the brain? J Neurosci 7:2373–2389

Seitz RJ, Roland PE, Bohm C, Greitz T, Stone-Elander S (1990) Motor learning in man: a positron emission tomographic study. Neuro Report 1:17–20

Shedlack KJ, Hunter R, Wyper D, McLuskie R, Fink G, Goodwin GM (1991) The pattern of cerebral activity underlying verbal fluency shown by split-dose single photon emission tomography (SPET or SPECT) in normal volunteers. Psychol Med 21:687–696

Regional Cerebral Blood Flow and Auditory Evoked Potential Studies in Childhood Autism

N. Bruneau[1], M. Zilbovicius, B. Garreau, C. Raynaud, B.M. Mazoyer, C. Barthélémy, A. Syrota, and G. Lelord

Introduction

An impairment of sensory modulation has been proposed as a putative brain dysfuntion in autism. All sensory modalities could be affected and the faulty modulation is manifest as either underreactivity or overreactivity to sensory stimuli (Ornitz 1985). These deficits are particularly evident in the auditory modality. Bruneau et al. (1987) studied evoked potentials to auditory stimulations varying in intensity and found normal and abnormal patterns of modulation in autistic children in relation to clinical features.

A functional approach of the brain is also available with single photon emission computerized tomography (SPECT), which allows quantitative measurements of regional cerebral blood flow (rCBF) at rest and during different types of activation.

The aim of this study was to investigate putative relationships between auditory evoked potential (AEP) responses recorded at temporal sites and rCBF modifications induced by auditory stimulations.

Methods

A total of 11 children (3 girls and 8 boys) diagnosed as autistic according to the DSM III-R criteria (APA 1987) were studied. The ages ranged from 5 to 9 years (mean = 6.8 years; SD = 1.4). They had normal CT or magnetic resonance imaging (MRI) findings and were free of medication at least 1 month prior to the examination.

AEPs were recorded at T3 and T4 sites referred to linked earlobes. The paradigm was detailed in Bruneau et al. (1987). The stimuli were tone bursts of 750 Hz and 200 ms duration. Each child was presented with a randomized series of tones varying in intensity (40, 50, 60, 70, 80 dB SPL) and in interstimulus interval (2.4–4 s.). AEPs were averaged from 40 trials at each intensity level.

[1] INSERM U 316, Explorations fonctionnelles psychopathologiques, Service Pr Lelord, CHRU Bretonneau, 37044 – Tours Cédex, France.

Imaging of the Brain in Psychiatry and Related Fields
Edited by K. Maurer

The rCBF measurements were performed with a brain-dedicated SPECT system (MEDIMATIC, Tomomatic 564), using xenon-133 inhalation and a computation method designed by Celsis et al. (1981). Five, 20 mm thick, continuous, axial slices were obtained parallel to the orbitomeatal line (plane resolution of approximately 14 mm). During the first minute of image acquisition, xenon-133 was inhaled using a concentration of 740 MBq/l (20 mCi/l). Studies were performed during sleep after premedication.

Two measurements were performed: at rest and during a simple auditory binaural stimulation (80 dB, 750 Hz, 200 ms) delivered at a rate of 1 per s.

Ten cortical brain regions were a priori included in the analysis, five on each hemisphere, based on the model of modular and hierarchic cortical organization proposed by Mesulam (1987): 1) sensory motor, SM (Brodmann's areas 1, 2, 3, 4 and 43, including Broca's area on the left side); 2) visual unimodal association, VIS (Brodmann's areas 20, 21 and 37); 3) auditory unimodal association, AUD (Brodmann's area 22, including Wernicke's area on the left side); 4) heteromodal association, PLURI (Brodmann's areas 7, 39 and 40) and 5) frontal areas (Brodmann's areas 10, 44, 45 and 46).

The anatomical localization of each region of interest was made using the corresponding CT scan slices obtained for each child and an anatomical brain atlas (Matsui and Hirano 1978).

Results

No left-right differences were found for the mean amplitude of temporal AEP responses (right side 15.8 ± 2.1 uV; left side 14.8 ± 2.0 uV; paired student t test = 0.47 ddl = 9; ns). The results indicated a very high interindividual variability for these left-right differences (mean of the differences = 0.97, SD = 6.49) with AEPs higher either on the right side (six patients) or on the left side (four patients).

Compared with resting conditions, rCBF changes brought about by auditory stimulations were not significant whatever the region of interest. These results were due to the high interindividual variability of the differences, indicating more or less important rCBF increases or decreases according to the subject.

Modifications of rCBF with auditory stimulations were considered at each region of interest according to the AEP amplitude measured at the temporal site. On the right side, AEP amplitudes showed a strong significant correlation with rCBF modifications observed on AUD ($r = -0.69$; $p = 0.02$), VIS ($r = -0.73$; $p = 0.01$), PLURI ($r = -0.63$; $p = 0.05$) and SM ($r = -0.84$; $p = 0.001$) but not with rCBF found at the frontal site ($r = -0.53$; $p = 0.11$). Negative correlations indicated that the larger the AEP, the higher the rCBF decrease with auditory stimulation and/or the smaller

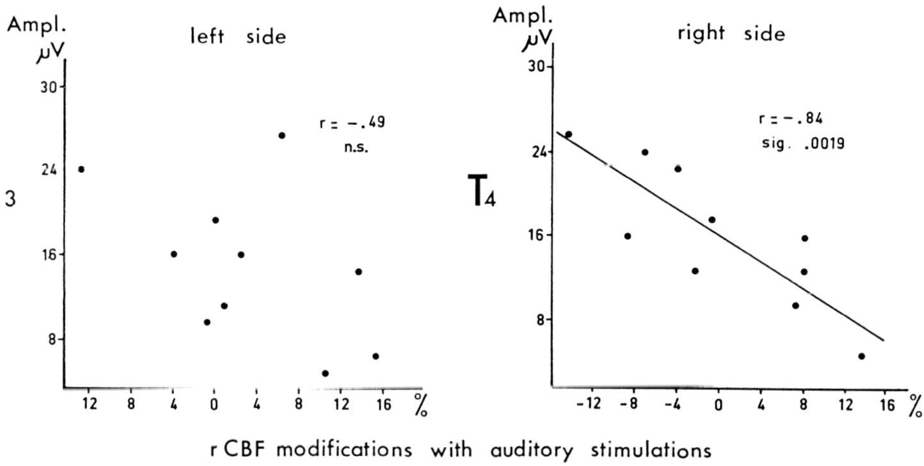

Fig. 1. Relationships between amplitudes of auditory evoked potential (AEP) responses and percent of regional cerebral blood flow (rCBF) modifications (rCBF stim – rCBF rest)/ rCBF rest during auditory stimulations

the AEP, the higher the rCBF increase with auditory stimulations (Fig. 1). Such relationships were weaker on the left side. Negative correlations were also found between the amplitude of left temporal AEPs and the rCBF modifications, but this was only significant with the PLURI region ($r = -0.65$; $p = 0.04$). Similar trends were also observed when considering VIS ($r = -0.61$; $p = 0.06$) and SM ($r = -0.57$; $p = 0.08$), whereas no relationship at all was found between AEP and frontal and auditory regions.

Discussion

Our results suggest that the amplitude of temporal responses evoked by auditory stimulations in autistic children could be indicative of the rCBF modifications induced by auditory stimulations in the temporoparietal regions of these children. In view of some methodological considerations (awake conditions for AEPs vs sleeping conditions for rCBF and some differences in stimulation paradigms), the interpretations of the relationships found (large AEP/rCBF decrease and small AEP/rCBF increase) would be very hazardous. To confirm these results, rCBF and AEP responses should be recorded simultaneously, i.e., under identical conditions. However, our results could support the assumption that the reactivity to auditory stimulations is rather different on each side of the brain. Further investigations on control groups are needed before concluding that these left-right differences are specific to autism and indicative of a physiopathological basis for this developmental disorder.

References

APA (American Psychiatric Association) (1987) Diagnostic and statistical manual of mental disorders, DSM-III-R, 3rd rev edn. APA, Washington DC

Bruneau N, Garreau B, Roux S, Lelord G (1987) Modulation of auditory evoked potentials with increasing stimulus intensity in autistic children. In: Johnson R Jr, Parasuraman R, Rohrbaugh JW (eds) Current trends in event-related potentials research. Electroencephalogr Clin Neurophysiol Suppl 40:609–616

Celsis P, Goldman T, Henriksen L, Lassen NA (1981) A method for calculating regional cerebral blood flow from emission computed tomography of inert gas concentrations. J Comput Assist Tomogr 5:641–645

Matsui T, Hirano A (1978) An atlas of human brain for computed tomography. Igaku-Shoin, New York

Mesulam MM (1987) Principles of behavioral neurology. Davis, Philadelphia

Ornitz EM (1985) Neurophysiology of infantile autism. J Am Acad Child Psychiatry 24:251–262

Hexamethylpropilene-amino-oxime Perfusion Scintigraphy in Brain Death

P. BERLIT[1], E. WETZEL, and P. VETTER

Introduction

Current criteria in the diagnosis of brain death are based upon:

1. Clinical history (exclusion of reversible conditions like hypothermia, intoxication)
2. Physical examination (coma, apnea, absence of brain stem function)
3. Adequate observation period (depending on the age of the patient and the underlying cause of the brain lesion).

In Germany neurophysiological examinations are accepted in documenting brain death. Angiography is believed to be a reliable method to prove cessation of the cerebral circulation, but this method is not legally acceptable because it is potentially dangerous for the patient (Gänshirt et al. 1985). While radionuclide imaging has been accepted as a method for brain death diagnosis in the USA (Goodman et al. 1969), this is not the case in Europe. We performed a scintigraphic evaluation of 22 consecutive patients in order to evaluate this method.

Patients and Methods

A total of 22 patients were investigated prospectively. The age range of the patients was 1.5–68 years. Causes of death in the group studied were craniocerebral injury (n = 18), subarachnoid hemorrhage (n = 3), and drug intoxication (flecainide; n = 1). In all cases there was clinical diagnosis of brain death with brainstem areflexia, a negative apnea test, and an observation time of at least 12 h. Additional neurophysiological examinations included electroencephalography (EEG) (isoelectric n = 16; focal cortical low activity still present n = 6) and auditory evoked potentials (AEP) (loss of peaks 2–6 in all patients).

[1] Neurologische Klinik am Alfried Krupp Krankenhaus, W-4300 Essen, FRG.

Imaging of the Brain in Psychiatry
and Related Fields
Edited by K. Maurer

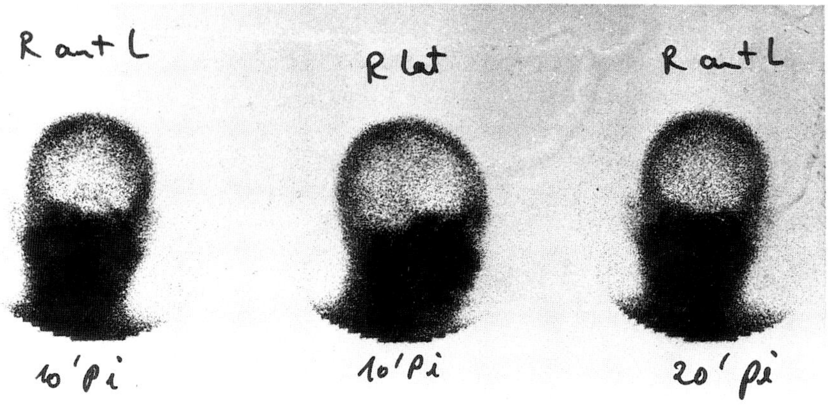

Fig. 1. HMPAO scintigraphy in a patient after clinical diagnosis of brain death. No perfusion was detectable

Neuroradiological studies included cerebral scintigraphy and digital subtraction angiography (DSA). Scintigraphic studies were performed with hexamethylpropylene-amine-oxime (HMPAO) – 370 MBq (10 mci) Tc 99m-HMPAO were given i.v. Sequential pictures were made (2/s) up to 60 s (anterior projection); anterior and lateral planar pictures 10 and 20 min. post injection, respectively. DSA was performed via the femoral artery with selective injection in all four brain-supporting vessels.

Results

HMPAO scintigraphy was performed in all patients (n = 22) after the clinical diagnosis of brain death. It was negative in 21 patients (Fig. 1). In one patient, discrete perfusion was still detectable; a control scintigraphy 6 h later was negative. An additional arterial DSA was performed in ten patients. It was negative in nine patients; in one patient the T segment of the internal carotid artery on one side was still visualized. Control angiography 6 h later showed no cerebral circulation. In this patient the scintigraphy had been negative at the time of the first DSA. Focal EEG activity was present in six patients. In all of them both scintigraphy and DSA were negative.

Conclusions

In this study HMPAO scintigraphy was a reliable noninvasive method to document the arrest of cerebral circulation. Arterial DSA revealed negative results in all but one patient, who showed no circulation 6 h later. Like angiography, scintigraphy studies are independent of the influence of barbiturates and transquilizers used in clinical practice on intensive care units. In contrast to angiography, however, scintigraphy is a noninvasive method without any risk for the patient. From the legal point of view, possibly dangerous methods must be avoided in brain death diagnosis (Gänshirt et al. 1985). In patients with persisting, focal, cortical activity in the EEG and negative AEP scintigraphy is especially helpful in diagnosing clinical brain death. In conflicting neurophysiological results like these, both scintigraphy *and* angiography seem to be necessary (Galaske et al. 1988). If both clinical and electrophysiological findings are consistent with the diagnosis of brain death, scintigraphy is the neuroradiological method of choice to document the loss of cerebral circulation (Goodman et al. 1985; Lee et al. 1987). In these cases, an additional DSA is not indicated. Perfusion scintigraphy should be officially accepted as a method for the documentation of brain death in Europe as it is in the USA.

References

Galaske RG, Schober O, Heyer R (1988) 99m Tc-HM-PAO and 123 I-amphetamine cerebral szintigraphy: a new non-invasive method in determination of brain death in children.

Gänshirt H, Berlit P, Haack G (eds) (1985) Kardiovaskuläre Erkrankungen und Nervensystem. Neurotoxikologie. Probleme des Hirntodes. Springer, Berlin Heidelberg New York (Verhandlungen der Deutschen Gesellschaft für Naurologie, vol 3)

Goodman JM, Mishkin FS, Dyken M (1969) Determination of death by isotope angiography. JAMA 290:1869

Goodman JM, Heck LL, Moore BD (1985) Confirmation of brain death with portable isotope angiography: a review of 204 consecutive cases. Neurosurgery 16:492–497

Lee VW, Hauck RM, Morrison MC, Peng TT, Fischer E, Carter A (1987) Scintigraphic evaluation of brain death: significance of sagittal sinus visualization. J Nucl Med 28:1279–1283

Concussion: Regional Cerebral Blood Flow and Associate Learning Ability

T. Pogačnik[1], B. Pečnik, and B. Žvan

Introduction

Commotio cerebri (a slight concussion of the brain) is a sudden, brief, traumatic impairment of cerebral function attended by loss of consciousness and/or amnesia and without a demonstrable anatomic lesion of the brain (Verjaal and Van't Hooft 1975).

The so-called postconcussion syndrome includes symptoms such as headache, vertigo, insomnia, excessive sweating, fatigue, poor concentration, memory impairment, irritability, intolerance for alcohol and heat, increased sensitivity to noise and weather changes, disturbances in sexual function, and visual symptoms. Clinical examination does not reveal any characteristic abnormalities. However, the occurrence of the syndrome in exactly the same form in patients of different ages, occupations, educational backgrounds, and social standing, along with the fact that it is encountered only after craniocerebral trauma and not after other injuries (e.g., to the extremities, abdomen, or chest), strongly suggest an organic cerebral basis for this syndrome (Kartin 1976). Among the numerous hypotheses those that take circulatory disorders in to account have an important place (Courville 1953; Overgaard and Tweed 1974; Miller 1981, 1982; Knežević et al. 1982). A century ago Roy and Sherrington (1890) suggested that cerebral blood flow (CBF) increases during functional activity of the brain and that this increase is related to an increased metabolic rate in the brain. This hypothesis was later supported by several authors. With the regional CBF (rCBF) method introduced by Lassen and Ingvar (1961, 1963), it became possible to measure changes in blood flow in fairly small cortical regions. In the normal human brain the rCBF is coupled to the regional cerebral oxygen consumption (Raichle et al. 1976; Roland et al. 1987). During physiological stimulation there is a linear correlation between changes in rCBF and changes in the regional oxidative metabolism (Roland et al. 1987).

[1] Department of Neurology, University Medical Centre Ljubljana, Zaloška 2, 61000 Ljubljana, Slovenia.

Imaging of the Brain in Psychiatry and Related Fields
Edited by K. Maurer

The aim of our study was to set the hypothesis that patients with postconcussion syndrome are unable to respond to increased metabolic demands by increasing to blood supply to the activated regions of the brain.

rCBF was measured while at rest and during enhanced functional activity using Wechsler's word pair learning and recall (WPLR) test. The results of earlier CBF measurements, using the recent visual memory test in one of our previous studies, supported our hypothesis that, in patients with concussion, the regulation of CBF is altered during enhanced functional activity (Pogačnik 1987, 1989).

Patients and Methods

Our study group comprised 19 patients who were selected according to the following criteria: (a) age 18–45 years; (b) history of cerebral concussion preceding the date of CBF measurement by no more than 4 months; (c) presence of symptoms consistent with postconcussion syndrome.

The control group was comprised of 19 healthy volunteers age 18–45 years (Hagstadius and Risberg 1983). The rCBF was measured while at rest and during enhanced functional activity (visual associative learning) using Wechsler's WPLR test. We evaluated the rCBF parameter ISI (initial slope index) (Risberg et al. 1975). The rCBF was measured by ^{133}Xe inhalation method using a Novo Cerebrograph 32C with 16 scintillation detectors. Statistical analysis was performed by using the student t test ($p < 0.01$) and the Wilcoxon signed rank test ($p < 0.01$).

Results

As noted briefly above, the study group was comprised of 19 patients with postconcussion syndrome (13 female, 6 male), aged 32.8 ± 7.5 years. The control group was comprised of 19 healthy volunteers (mostly medical staff) (14 females and 5 males) age 28.7 ± 5.4 years. The subjects of this study were all strictly right-handed. The groups did not differ significantly with respect to age and sex. The mean time from the date of cerebral concussion to the date of CBF measurement in our study group was 2.3 months.

Fig. 1. Regional cerebral blood flow (*rCBF*) values measured at rest and during visual associative learning (*VAL*) in the control and study groups. Ordinate rCBF: ml/100 mg/min; Abscissa. Control and study (*EXPER.*) groups. Location of detectors: F_1, anterior area of frontal region; F_2, superior area of frontal region; F_5, inferior area of frontal region; C_2, central region; T_1, anterior temporal region; T_3, posterior temporal region; P_3, parietal region; O_1, occipital region; R, right; L, left; □, Rest, ▨, VAL. $^{**}p < 0.01$ $^{*}0.01 < p < 0.02$

Graph 1
rCBF F1R and F1L

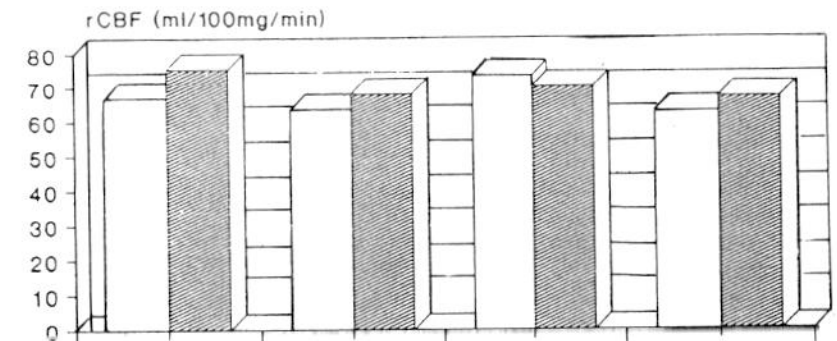

	CONTROL	EXPER.	CONTROL	EXPER.
REST	67	63.5	73.3	62.7
VAL	75.5	68	70.1	67

Graph 2
rCBF F2R and F2L

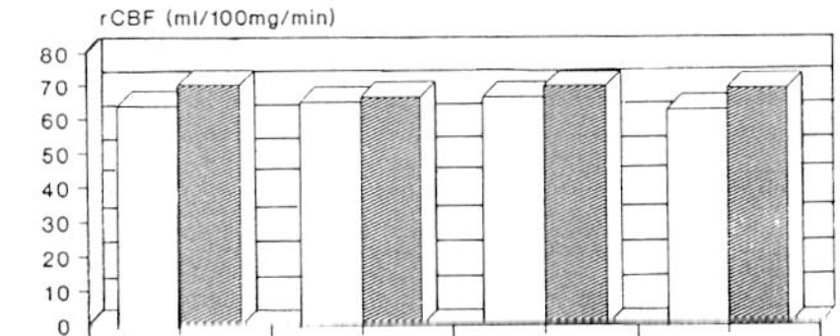

	CONTROL	EXPER.	CONTROL	EXPER.
REST	63.9	65.1	66.4	62.6
VAL	70.3	66.6	69.8	69.1

Graph 3
rCBF F5R and F5L

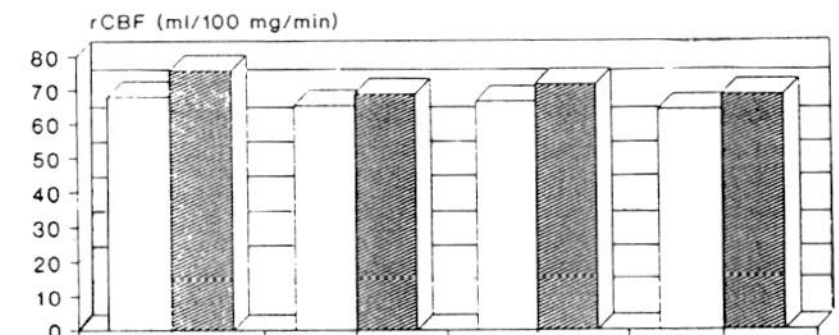

	CONTROL	EXPER.	CONTROL	EXPER.
REST	68	65.4	66.5	64.1
VAL	75.8	68.8	71.7	68.6

Graph 4
rCBF C2R and C2L

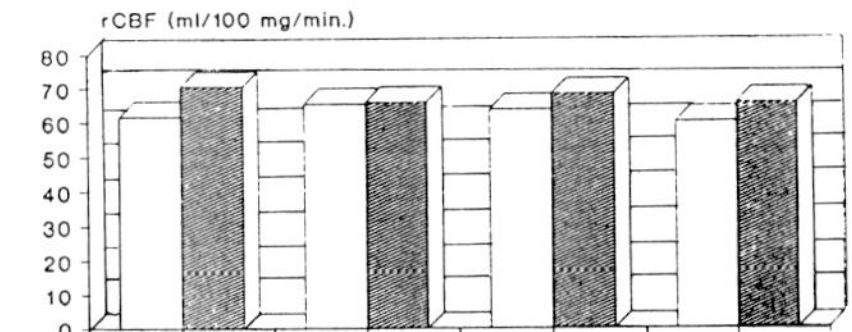

	CONTROL (••)	EXPER.	CONTROL	EXPER.
REST	61.7	65.4	63.6	60
VAL	70.6	65.9	68.1	64.2

Graph 5
rCBF T1R and T1L

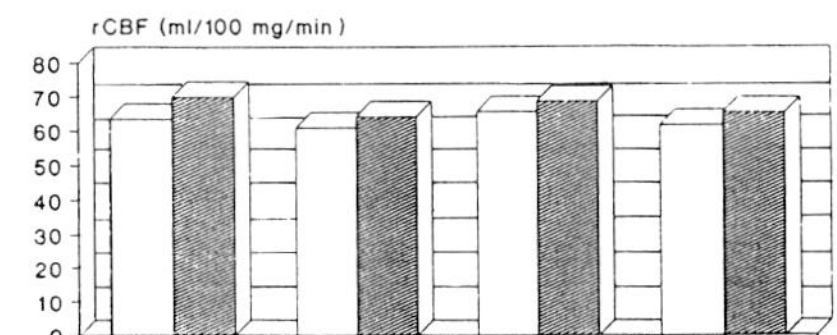

	CONTROL (•)	EXPER.	CONTROL	EXPER.
REST	63.5	60.9	65.5	61.4
VAL	70	64.1	68.6	65.2

Graph 6
rCBF T3R and T3L

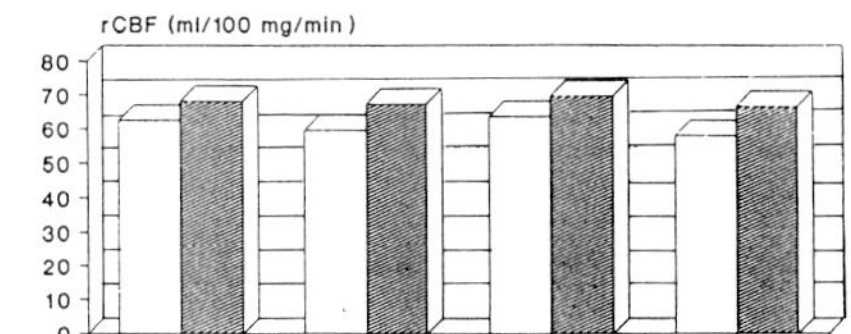

	CONTROL (••)	EXPER. (••)	CONTROL (••)	EXPER. (••)
REST	62.5	59.5	63.6	57.9
VAL	68.2	67.4	69.6	66.7

Graph 7
rCBF P3R and P3L

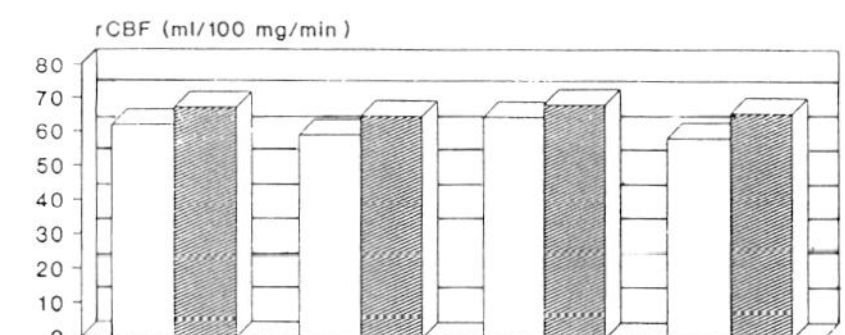

	CONTROL (•)	EXPER.	CONTROL	EXPER.
REST	62	59	64.4	58.2
VAL	67.2	64.6	68.2	65.6

Graph 8
rCBF O1R and O1L

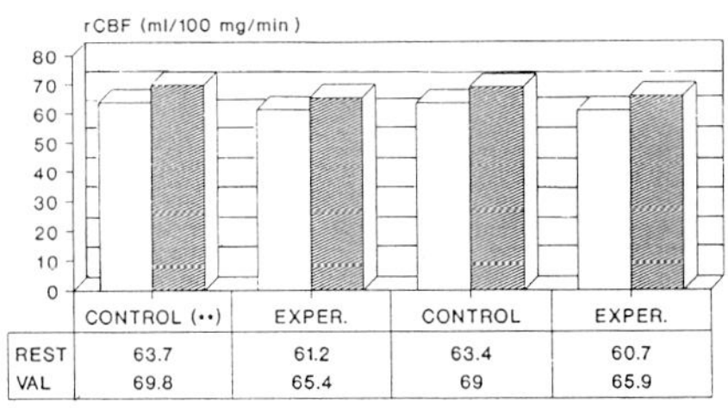

	CONTROL (••)	EXPER.	CONTROL	EXPER.
REST	63.7	61.2	63.4	60.7
VAL	69.8	65.4	69	65.9

Graph 9
rCBF HR and HL

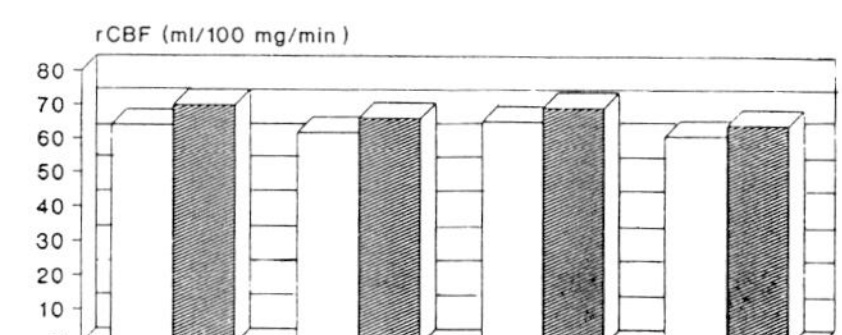

	CONTROL (••)	EXPER.	CONTROL	EXPER.
REST	64	61.8	65.2	61
VAL	69.9	66.2	69.4	64.3

The evaluation of WPLR test results revealed significant differences between both groups. Recall performance, tested after visual learning activation, was significantly lower than that found in healthy subjects ($0.01 < p < 0.02$). ISI values in the hemisphere and individual regions were normal in both groups while at rest. The activation procedure caused the mean blood flow to increase in the right hemisphere of healthy volunteers, whereas in the patients no such increase was observed in either hemisphere. Analysis of the results obtained during activation procedures revealed a difference between the control group and the patient group in the increased values obtained for several regions in the right hemisphere (central, anterior temporal, posterior temporal, occipital) and for the posterior temporal region of the left hemisphere in healthy volunteers. In patients, increased blood flow was recorded for both posterior temporal regions only. The regional and interhemispheric differences between the two groups are presented in Fig. 1.

Discussion

rCBF is coupled to regional cerebral metabolism, and changes in rCBF reflect changes in neuronal activity (Friberg and Roland 1988). It is known that variations in CBF occur mainly as a result of lesion of the cerebral parenchyma and changes in functional and metabolic activity of the brain. Higher blood flow is found in regions with higher functional activity (Ingvar et al. 1975; Risberg et al. 1977).

The results of rCBF measurements in both groups support our hypothesis that, in patients with postconcussion syndrome, during enhanced functional activity the regulation of CBF is altered. Whereas controls presented with right spatial flow increase, concussion subjects showed no interhemispheric asymmetry during the task.

Wechsler's WPLR test above all shows the capacity for associative learning and contains spatial elements. It therefore represents a very sensitive test for evaluation of organic lesions (Wechsler 1945).

Recall performance, tested after visual learning activation, was significantly lower than in healthy subjects. The combination of a low rCBF response to a specific mental task and poor performance could be used as an indication of neurofunctional impairment (Maximilian and Brawanski 1988). Impaired adaptability of rCBF to metabolic needs is thus one of the demonstrable functional disorders in patients with postconcussion syndrome. The possible role of this mechanism in the generation of clinical symptoms is still unclear.

References

Courville CB (1953) The cerebral circulation in concussion and the post-concussion state, commotio cerebri. San Lucas, Los Angeles

Friberg L, Roland PE (1988) Functional activation and inhibition of regional cerebral blood flow and metabolism. In: Olesen J, Edvinsson L (eds) Basic mechanisms of headache. Elsevier, New York

Hagstadius S, Risberg J (1983) The effects of normal aging on rCBF during resting and functional activation. Reg Cereb Blood Flow Bull 6:116

Ingvar DH, Risberg J, Schwartz MS (1975) Evidence of subnormal function of association cortex in presenile dementia. Neurology 25:964–974

Kartin, P (1976) Tako imenovani postkomocionalni sindrom. Zdrav Vestn 45:277–280

Knežević S, Zurak N, Gubarev N (1982) Regional cerebral blood flow in patients following post-concussion and minor head trauma. Reg Cereb Blood Flow Bull 5:101

Lassen NA, Ingvar DH (1961) The blood flow of the cerebral cortex determined by radioactive Krypton-85. Experienta 17:42–43

Lassen NA, Ingvar DH (1963) Regional cerebral blood flow measurements in man. Arch Neurol Psychiatry 9:615–622

Maximilian VA, Brawanski A (1988) Functional and vascular challenge procedures during noninvasive rCBF measurement. In: Knežević S et al. (eds) Handbook of regional cerebral blood flow. Erlbaum, Hillsdale, pp 79–121

Miller JD (1981) Cerebral blood flow, reduced perfusion pressure and head injury. In: Minderhound JM (ed) Cerebral blood flow: basic knowledge and clinical implications. Excerpta Medica, Amsterdam

Miller JD (1982) Disorders of cerebral blood flow and intracranial pressure after head injury. Clin Neurosurg 29:162

Overgaard J, Tweed WA (1974) Cerebral circulation after head injury: part I. Cerebral blood flow and its regulation after closed head injury with emphasis on clinical correlations. J Neurosurg 41:531

Pogačnik T (1987) Lastnosti možganskega pretoka krvi pri bolnikih s postkomocijskim sindromom. Thesis, Medical faculty, University of Zagreb

Pogačnik T (1989) Characteristics of regional cerebral blood flow in patients with concussion. Psychiatry Res 29:313–316

Raichle ME, Grubb RL, Gado MH, Eichling JO, Ter-Pogossian MM (1976) Correlation between regional cerebral blood flow and oxidative metabolism. Arch Neurol 33:523–526

Risberg J, Ali Z, Wilson EM, Wills EL, Halsey JH (1975) Regional cerebral blood flow by 133 Xe inhalation. Stroke 6:142–148

Risberg J, Maximilian A, Prohovnik I (1977) Changes of cortical activity patterns during habituation to reasoning test. Neuropsychologia 15:793

Roland PE, Eriksson L, Stone-Elander S, Widen L (1987) Does mental activity change the oxidative metabolism of the brain? J Neurosci 7:2373–2389

Roy CS, Sherrington CS (1890) On regulation of the blood supply of the brain. J Physiol (Lond) 11:85–108

Verjaal A, Van't Hooft F (1975) Commotio and contusio cerebri. In: Vinken PJ, Bruyn GW (eds) Handbook of clinical neurology. North-Holland, Amsterdam

Wechsler D (1945) A standardized memory scale for clinical use. J Psychol 19:87

Functional Imaging Methods (Positron Emission Tomography)

Imaging Neuroreceptors with Positron Emission Tomography: A New Strategy for Measuring Pharmacological Activity in the Treatment of Schizophrenia

J.D. Brodie[1], S.L. Dewey, A.P. Wolf, and G.S. Smith

Introduction

Among the major problems which must be faced in the study of schizophrenia is the lack of an objective set of biological discriptors which can be used to define the syndrome and thus the response to treatment. The advent of positron emission tomography (PET) in the early 1970s offered a new opportunity to directly visualize aspects of cerebral function. PET is a medical imaging technique which measures the concentration of a positron emitting radioisotope in a volume element of tissue. When an appropriately radiolabeled ligand is used, PET provides functional images of the target tissue. Interpretation of these images in a meaningful way is dependent upon an understanding of the underlying biochemistry and physiology of the tissue and characterization of the binding of the radioligand. This involves a knowledge of the process to be traced and the kinetics of that process, since the tomograph only measures but does not attach biological significance to radioactive events.

When [^{18}F]fluorodeoxyglucose (FDG) is used as a radiotracer, the process visualized represents cerebral glucose metabolism. The earliest studies of schizophrenics with PET and FDG attempted to measure regional brain glucose metabolism in patients with the schizophrenic syndrome at rest (Farkas et al. 1981, 1984; Buchsbaum et al. 1982). Later, the technique was applied to measure changes in glucose metabolism in response to treatment with neuroleptics. It is well known that a high percentage of schizophrenic patients are resistant to neuroleptic treatment. In order to understand the mechanism of treatment resistance, one must first attempt to define measurable biological responses to pharmacological intervention. A number of reports which have used this approach to study the metabolic effects of treatment have yielded conflicting results (Wolkin et al. 1985; DeLisi et al. 1985; Gur et al. 1987; Szechtman et al. 1988). There are many reasons for the reported discrepancies. Included in these are subject selection, duration of illness, effects of prior treatment, and differences in the treatment regi-

[1] Dept. of Psychiatry, New York University Medical Center, New York, NY 10016, USA.

Imaging of the Brain in Psychiatry
and Related Fields
Edited by K. Maurer

men (that is, the choice of neuroleptic, dose, time of treatment, ancillary medication). Until recently (Bartlett et al. 1988; Tyler et al. 1988) there has been a lack of data on the stability of the method and only limited information on the effects of treatment on cerebral metabolism in normal subjects. In addition, interpretation of the findings has been complicated by technical factors, such as the resolution of the tomograph, and by image analysis strategies and statistical issues.

The use of radioligands which bind selectively to specific neurotransmitter receptors allows brain activity to be viewed from another perspective. Here, the process visualized may reflect the binding, distribution, concentration, and kinetic properties of a particular receptor. Subject to the limitations of sensitivity and kinetic modeling, the resulting images can be nonetheless quite striking (e.g., Wagner et al. 1983). The quantitation and interpretation of these images is subject to significant impediments in the light of the effects of cerebral blood flow, receptor density, and endogenous competing ligands. Nevertheless, as we shall show, the application of this approach can already lead to meaningful answers to questions of particular clinical relevance such as: is the drug delivered to the brain and, if so, what is its pharmacological effect, if any?

The main purpose of this article is to describe a novel strategy currently under investigation in our laboratory for the assessment of therapeutic efficacy of neuroleptics in schizophrenia using PET. By measuring changes in receptor activity as a *direct* index of drug activity in the brain, we believe an in vivo assay of pharmacological intervention can be established. Using the unique capabilities of PET, such an assay should:

1. Establish validity by showing that the measurement is due and sensitive to the intervention
2. Establish reliability by showing that the reference measurement is stable in repeated measurement over the time course of the assay
3. Prove that the drug is delivered to the target and in relation to the administered dose
4. Delineate the dose-response relationship and time course
5. Give results which can be correlated with an independent relevant outcome measurement

Strategy for Measuring Neurotransmitter Activity

One promising approach is to administer an antipsychotic agent and measure alterations in a neurotransmitter system that is functionally linked to the drug receptor. This would offer a more direct assessment of pharmacological activity than might be provided by glucose utilization which reflects the energy required to support all physiological processes of living cells. The general strategy is analogous to the use of a coupled enzyme assay to measure the activity of an enzyme whose product is not readily measured. Hence, we propose to observe the activity of the neuron of interest by observing changes in the binding characteristics of a receptor which is located on a different neuron but functionally coupled to it. By this approach, the change in *activity* caused by the specific binding of a drug to its receptor can be visualized in vivo. An example of such a strategy is the measurement of binding of a cholinergic ligand to the striatal *cholinergic* receptors for the purpose of measuring *dopaminergic* activity. In this case, the product of the activity at the dopaminergic receptor (located on the cholinergic neuron) is visualized by its effect on the cholinergic receptor (located on the GABAergic neuron) which is linked to the dopamine receptor. After establishing the anatomic distribution of the cholinergic receptors, it is desirable to define control regions in which the connections between these two systems are minimal or absent and to subclassify the distribution of cholinergic receptor subtypes with a suitable ligand(s).

A suitable PET ligand for assessing the neurochemical product of drug action should have the following characteristics: high receptor specificity (low nonspecific binding), saturability, reversibility, stereoselectivity, moderate stability of the receptor ligand complex (adequate time to image), ease of labeling, high specific activity, limited metabolism of the label and no reentry of the labeled metabolites from the plasma, adequate uptake in the brain, tolerable side effects under experimental conditions, and relatively high affinity. The notion of using the binding of a ligand to a receptor as a measure of the activity of a preceding synaptic event has the following implications: a labeled ligand with a high K_D (lower affinity) has the advantage of increased sensitivity to perturbation with the disadvantage of its binding being susceptible to competition with endogenous ligands (Seeman et al. 1989). A PET ligand with a low K_D (higher affinity) has the advantage of increased stability of the measurement with decreased competition from endogenous transmitters at the expense of a relative insensitivity to the perturbation one is trying to assay. We may conclude that there is no single ligand for measuring neurotransmitter activity that is ideal under all conditions.

A classical biochemical approach to evaluate the activity of a biological system is to perturb the system and measure either the ensuing change in the product concentration or, if that is too rapid, to measure the return to the preexisting equilibrium, as the perturbation is extinguished. When studying the dopaminergic system, it follows that the perturbing agent should be highly specific for the D_2 or D_1 (or other) receptor and tolerable to the subject under the range of experimental conditions with readily reversible side effects. Its concentration should be readily measured in vivo and in vitro (for determinations of protein binding, metabolites, etc.) and its binding to the dopamine receptor should be irreversible in the time frame of the experiment, in order that physiological changes in endogenous ligand (dopamine) concentration are not propagated through the system while it is being measured. Finally, it must cause a measurable change in functionally coupled neuronal activity under the experimental conditions.

In order to use changes in binding of a radioligand to the cholinergic receptor as a measure of dopaminergic activity, it must first be shown that this binding is reproducible in the unperturbed state. It must then be demonstrated that perturbation with both cholinergic agonists and antagonists causes predicted changes in the binding of the radioligand to the cholinergic receptor system which exceed the variance of the unperturbed state. If the outcome measure is not sufficiently sensitive to these perturbations, then a different cholinergic radioligand with lower affinity should be employed. In order to measure changes in dopaminergic activity caused by a drug, it is necessary to establish the quantitative relationship between binding of the radioligand to the cholinergic receptor and dopaminergic activity. This may not be a simple function of ligand concentration in the plasma, since neuronal activity will reflect endogenous ligand, relative affinities, the kinetic form of the competition, and the effective concentrations (activity) of these compounds at the synaptic cleft. It is even possible that the changes in binding to the cholinergic system will be observed as an all or none process. Since the brain is a highly interconnected system of biochemically distinguishable neurons, it is also desirable to show that changes in the binding to the cholinergic receptor reflect the direct connection to the dopaminergic system within the experimental time frame.

With these considerations in mind, we are in a position to measure dopaminergic activity in vivo by measuring binding of a suitable labeled cholinergic ligand to the acetylcholine (ACh) receptor in the presence of pharmacological amounts of appropriate D_1 and D_2 ligands. Indeed, the same strategy can be extended to examine the possible interaction of D_1 and D_2 receptors by using an appropriate D_2 ligand such as raclopride or remoxipride. An important control for such experiments is to show that an unrelated neurotransmitter system either does not change under these conditions or does not effect outcome.

Visualization of Neurotransmitter-Specific Receptors

Our initial efforts to establish the above mentioned in vivo assay of pharmacological intervention involved the visualization of relevant neurotransmitter specific receptors and their properties. Since the dopaminergic (DA) hypothesis of the pathophysiology of schizophrenia was in part derived from the observation that antipsychotic drugs blocked the DA system, we chose the dopaminergic system to establish such an assay.

Human DA receptors were initially visualized with PET by using [^{11}C]N- methyl spiperone (NMSP) and subsequently [^{11}C]raclopride (Wagner et al. 1983; Farde et al. 1985). We then further defined some of the properties of the striatal dopamine receptors in chronic schizophrenics with the use of [^{18}F]NMSP: first, the time course of DA receptor blockade following neuroleptic administration; second, the relationship of receptor occupancy to the plasma concentration of the administered neuroleptic; and finally the presence or absence of receptor blockade in the case of clinical nonresponse.

In our first report we used a competitive ligand binding approach to determine the length of time required for striatal DA receptors to become available for radiotracer ([^{18}F]NMSP)binding following the last dose administered of an ongoing neuroleptic treatment regimen (Smith et al. 1988). We found that the *availability* of the striatal DA receptors returned to that found in control subjects following 1 week of washout. These data should not be confused with a finding that there may still be a significant amount of neuroleptic in the brain (Farde 1989). Nor should the clearing of neuroleptic from the receptor be necessarily equated with a disappearance of the biochemical and pharmacological *effects* attendant to prior blockade.

In the following study, we administered daily as much as 80–100 mg of haloperidol per subject. Using a slightly different strategy we assessed how much haloperidol would be sufficient to achieve a clinical effect if clinical outcome was related to dopamine blockade (Wolkin et al. 1989a). We measured the relationship between the availability of DA receptors and plasma haloperidol concentration with 36 different measurements in 25 subjects and found that maximal DA blockade occurred at a plasma haloperidol concentration of 10–15 ng/ml. Increasing the haloperidol concentration had no effect on the blockade of [^{18}F]NMSP binding. In spite of the limitations of our approach, we were able to show a quantitative relationship between plasma neuroleptic concentration and blockade of central DA receptors. A similar finding was reported by Cambon et al. (1987).

In the above studies, our approach was limited to the evaluation of striatal DA receptors. While PET receptor ligands, however, may be quite specific for the DA system, commonly used antipsychotic drugs are not. Haloperidol, a widely used neuroleptic drug, binds to receptors other than the DA receptor. Nevertheless, with PET, we have been able to take advantage of the relative specificity of NMSP to measure the specific effects of haloperidol on the DA system. The next experiment addressed the question of whether clinical nonresponse to haloperidol was due to a failure in drug delivery or a failure of drug activity. To that end we examined the ability of haloperidol to block the striatal DA receptors in two groups of schizophrenics. One group clinically responded to treatment, the other did not. Before treatment, both groups showed a similarly high availability of binding by the PET ligand [^{18}F]NMSP. After treatment with high dose haloperidol for up to 6 weeks, both groups showed identical blockade of NMSP binding *despite the difference in clinical outcome* (Wolkin et al. 1989b). We concluded that nonresponse is due to a failure of drug activity but is not due to a failure of haloperidol to block the DA receptor.

Since it is clear from these experiments that haloperidol was transported to the brain dopamine sites, we chose to assess the feasibility of the coupled receptor assay approach in the nigrostriatal pathway since animal studies have suggested the presence of multisynaptic feedback loops that directly link DA neurons to cholinergic neurons (McGeer et al. 1987). This finding is consistent with the clinical observation that anticholinergic drugs relieve the extrapyramidal signs induced by dopamine blockade.

Prior to our examination of dopaminergic-cholinergic interactions, it was necessary to develop a PET ligand suitable for investigations of the muscarinic-cholinergic system. Benztropine was selected and initial results suggest that this ligand is adequate to establish the feasibility of PET for assessing neurotransmitter interactions in vivo (Dewey et al. 1988, 1990a). For further evaluation of [^{11}C]benztropine as a specific cholinergic antagonist, we measured in baboons the effect of coadministration of unlabeled benztropine or scopolamine (antagonist) or pilocarpine (agonist). All decreased the incorporation of [^{11}C]benztropine in the various brain regions with a high concentration of cholinergic receptors (Dewey et al. 1990a).

Finally, it was necessary to show that the pharmacological effect of benztropine would reflect this multisynaptic loop and not be complicated by the reuptake of dopamine into presynaptic terminals (Coyle and Snyder 1969). In order to determine what component of the PET image of labeled benztropine was due its binding to this specific site, we pretreated animals with nomifensine, a potent dopamine reuptake blocker, and were unable to demonstrate any decrease in [^{11}C]benztropine uptake. This could mean that benztropine and nomifensine bind to different sites on the dopamine transporter and each interfere with dopamine reuptake in an uncompetitive manner. However, the simplest interpretation of this experiment is that the PET images of labeled benztropine represent binding to the muscarinic-cholinergic receptor wtihout a significant dopamine reuptake component.

Interactions

With this preliminary information, we began to address whether PET could be effective in the in vivo study of the interactions demonstrated for the nigrostriatal loop. This loop is shown in Fig. 1. This model predicts that unlabeled benztropine should decrease the striatal uptake of [^{18}F]NMSP since benztropine would stimulate the release of endogenous dopamine which would effectively compete with NMSP for postsynaptic dopamine binding sites. Similarly, blockade of the dopamine receptor with NMSP would relieve the tonic inhibition of the cholinergic neuron on which this receptor resides, resulting in an increase in the concentration of endogenous ACh and serve to decrease the uptake of [^{11}C]benztropine. When these experiments were performed in baboons, the results confirmed our assumptions (Dewey et al. 1990b). In normal human subjects, the predicted effect

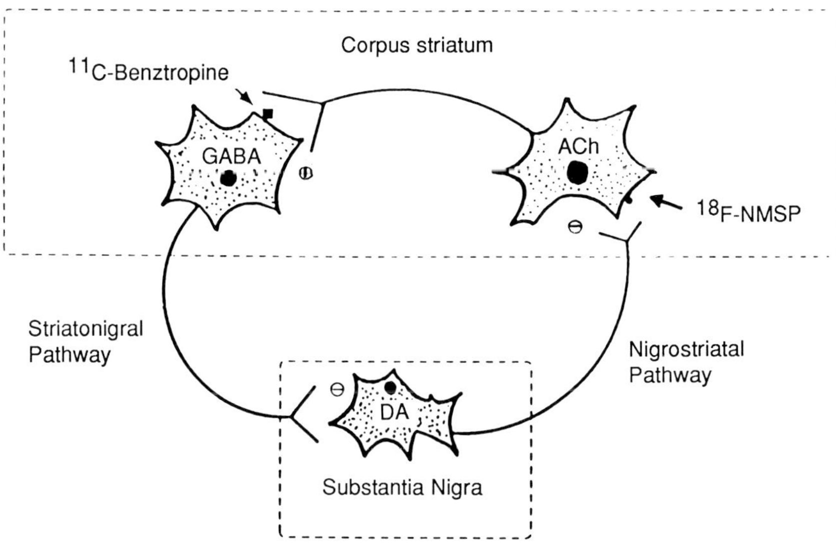

Fig. 1. The nigrostriatal loop

of diminished striatal uptake o [^{18}F]NMSP upon administration of benztropine was also realized. In this series of seven subjects (Dewey et al. 1988), the diminution ranged up to 70%, a finding consistent with the notion that the resting activity of the dopamine system is not necessarily constant in different individuals. The comparable experiments with an unlabeled neuroleptic and [^{11}C]benztropine are in progress with human subjects.

It would appear from these early studies that PET can be used to examine the activity of virtually any pharmacological agent which works in the central nervous system, using a strategy of coupled receptor assay to measure the *activity* of a given receptor system by measuring changes in the apparent binding parameters of linked postsynaptic receptors. Indeed, the underlying principle for this approach is that the change in apparent binding properties of a functionally linked receptor is a direct index of pharmacological *activity* and can be assessed independently from such final common path measures as behavior and energy utilization. Clearly, an assay which measures neurotransmitter activity would provide different and complementary data to the existing emphasis on determining the number of available binding sites (B_{max}). Certainly it seems that both kinds of information would be important in evaluating the potential response to therapy.

Conclusion

We have tried to illustrate the reasoning which led us to believe that a strategy of using in vivo neurotransmitter interactions as an outcome measure of pharmacological activity can be generally applied to the development of new pharmaceutical agents in schizophrenia and any other psychiatric disorder. This approach lends itself to the experimental determination of the critical site of drug resistance so that alternative treatment strategies can be formulated. Our preliminary results suggest that this approach is a feasible alternative to the use of clinical descriptors for the measurement of pharmacological activity in vivo. At the present time, the minimal criteria for adequate quantitation have not been fulfilled in any series of studies of which we are aware. Nevertheless, it appears that these criteria can be met by suitable experiments with PET methodology. Indeed, what we emphasize is that such dynamic information can be applied to measure pharmacological activity in vivo in the dopamine and other neurotransmitter systems. Application of the information obtained to the treatment of disabling psychiatric illness should then follow.

References

Bartlett EJ, Brodie JD, Wolf AP, Christman DR, Laska E, Meissner M (1988) Reproducibility of cerebral glucose metabolic measurements in resting human subjects. J Cereb Blood Flow Metab 8:502–512

Buchsbaum MS, Ingvar DH, Kessler R, Waters RN, Cappelletti J, van Kammen DP, King AC, Johnson JL, Manning RG, Flynn RW, Mann LS, Bunney WE Jr, Sokoloff L (1982) Cerebral glucography with positron tomography: use in normal subjects and in patients with schizophrenia. Arch Gen Psychiatry 39:251–259

Cambon H, Baron JC, Boulenger JP, Loc'h C, Zarifian E, Maziere B (1987) In vivo assay for neuroleptic receptor binding in the striatum. Positron tomography in humans. Br J Psychiatry 151:824

Coyle JT, Snyder SH (1969) Antiparkinsonian drugs: inhibition of dopamine uptake in the corpus striatum as a possible mechanism of action. Science 166:809–811

DeLisi LE, Holcomb HH, Cohen RM, Pickar D, Carpenter W et al. (1985) Positron emission tomography in schizophrenic patients with and without neuroleptic medication. J Cereb Blood Flow Metab 5:201–206

Dewey SL, Wolf AP, Fowler JS, Brodie JD, Shiue C-Y, Alavi A, Hiesiger E, Schlyer DJ, Volkow ND, Raulli R, Christman D (1988) The effects of central cholinergic blockade on [^{18}F]-N-methylspiroperidol binding in human brain using PET. XVI CINP Congress

Dewey SL, MacGregor RR, Brodie JD, Bendriem B, King PT, Volkow ND, Schlyer DJ, Fowler JS, Wolf AP, Gatley SJ, Hitzeman R (1990a) Mapping muscarine receptors in human and baboon brain using [N-^{11}C-methyl]benztropine. Synapse 5:213–223

Dewey SL, Brodie JD, Fowler JS, MacGregor RR, Schlyer DJ, King PT, Alexoff DL, Volkow ND, Shiue C-Y, Wolf AP, Bendriem B (1990b) Positron emission tomography (PET) studies of dopaminergic/cholinergic interactions in the baboon brain. Synapse 6:321–327

Farde L, Ehrin E, Eriksson L, Greitz TY, Hall H, Hedstrom CG, Litton JE, Sedvall G (1985) Substituted benzamides as ligands for visualization of dopamine receptor binding in the human brain by positron emission tomography. Proc Natl Acad Sci USA 82:3863

Farde L, Wiesel F-A, Halldin C, Sedvall G, Nilsson L (1989) Dopamine receptor occupancy and plasma haloperidol levels: in reply. Arch Gen Psychiatry 46: 483–4

Farkas T, Wolf AP, Fowler J, MacGregor R, Brodie JD, Christman D, Cancro R, Brill R, Goldman A (1981) Regional brain glucose metabolism in schizophrenia. J Cereb Blood Flow Metabol 1 [Suppl 1]:496

Farkas T, Wolf AP, Jaeger J, Brodie JD, Christman D, Fowler JS (1984) Regional brain glucose metabolism in chronic schizophrenia. Arch Gen Psychiatry 41:293–300

Gur RE, Resnick SM, Gur RC, Alavi A, Caroff S, Kushner M, Reivich M (1987) Regional brain function in schizophrenia. Arch Gen Psychiatry: 44:119–125

McGeer PL, Eccles JC, McGeer EG (1987) Molecular neurobiology of the mammalian brain. Plenum, New York

Seeman P, Guan H-C, Nizik HB (1989) Endogenous dopamine lowers the dopamine D2 receptor density as measured by [^{3}H]raclopride: implications for positron tomography of the human brain. Synapse 3:96–97

Smith M, Wolf AP, Brodie JD, Arnett CD, Barouche F, Shiue CY, Fowler JS, Russell JAG, MacGregor RR, Wolkin A, Angrist B, Rotrosen J, Peselow E (1988) Serial 18F-N-Methylspiroperidol PET studies to measure changes in antipsychotic drug D2 receptor occupancy in schizophrenic patients. Biol Psychiatry 23:653–663

Szechtman H, Nachmias C, Garnett ES, Firnaue G, Brown GM, Kaplan RD, Cleghorn JM (1988) Effects of neuroleptics on altered cerebral glucose metabolism in schizophrenia. Arch Gen Psychiatry 45:523–532

Tyler JL, Strother SZ, Zatorre RJ, Alivisatos B, Worsley KJ, Diksie M, Yamamoto YL (1988) Stability of regional cerebral glucose metabolism in the normal human brain measured by positron emission tomography. J Nucl Med 29:631

Wagner HN Jr, Burns HD, Dannals RF, Wong DF, Langstrom B, Duelfer T, Frost JJ, Ravert HT, Links JM, Rosenbloom SB, Lukas SE, Kramer AV, Kuhar MJ (1983) Imaging dopamine receptors in the human brain by positron tomography. Science 221:1264–1266

Wolkin A, Jaeger J, Brodie JD, Wolf AP, Fowler J, Rotrosen J, Gomez-Mont F, Cancro R (1985) Peristence of cerebral metabolic abnormalities in chronic schizophrenia as determined by positron emission tomography. Am J Psychiatry 142:564–571

Wolkin A, Brodie JD, Barouche F, Rotrosen J, Wolf AP, Cooper T (1989a) Dopamine receptor occupancy and plasma haloperidol levels. Arch Gen Psychiatry 46:482–483

Wolkin A, Barouche F, Wolf AP, Rotrosen J, Fowler JS, Shiue CY, Cooper TB, Brodie JD (1989b) Dopamine blockade and clinical response: evidence for two biological subgroups of schizophrenia. Am J Psychiatry 146:905–908

Bimodal Distribution of Brain Dopamine D_2 Receptors in Schizophrenic Patients Explained by In Vivo Binding Studies*

J. Korf[1], S. Zijlstra, J.A.A. Swart, and J.W. Louwerens

Introduction

The so-called dopamine hypothesis in schizophrenia can be divided into two subhypotheses: one involving pathogenetic aspects of the dopamine systems in the brain and the other the mode of action of antipsychotic drugs (Carlsson 1988). In particular, the D_2 type dopamine receptor has been studied both in vitro (e.g., Seeman et al. 1984, 1987; Kornhuber et al. 1989) and very recently in vivo (e.g., Wong et al. 1986; Farde et al. 1987, 1988; Sedvall et al. 1986). Reports showing a pathogenetically increased dopamine D_2 type receptor density in vivo (e.g., Seeman et al. 1984, 1987; Kornhuber et al. 1989, and references therein) have been challenged as being the result of long-term antipsychotic medication (e.g., Kornhuber et al. 1989). In the most extensive report on in vitro D_2 receptor investigations, published by Seeman and collaborators (1984, 1987), more than 100 schizophrenic brain specimens were analyzed. There appeared to be a bimodal distribution in the density in three brain areas: caudate nucleus and putamen, structures belonging to the extrapyramidal system, and the nucleus accumbens, a limbic structure. Interestingly, the mean densities of the two modes differed by twofold and the lowest density was rather similar to that of controls or of nonschizophrenic patients treated with antipsychotic medication.

Recent in vivo techniques for studying central dopamine receptors using positron emission tomography (PET) revealed either a normal (Farde et al. 1990; Martionot et al. 1990) or an increased dopamine D_2 type receptor density in schizophrenia (Wong et al. 1986). The reported increase may have to be attributed to the complicated mathematical model applied to quantify D_2 receptor density (Swart and Korf 1989). A recent attempt to replicate the findings of Wong et al. (1986) by the original authors was only partly successful (Schizophrenia Meeting Badgastein, Austria, February 1990). Taken together, the present in vivo studies favor the idea that

* These studies were supported by the Netherlands Organization of Pure Research, The University Hospital of Groningen and the J.K. de Cock Stichting.

[1] Department of Biological Psychiatry, Psychiatric University Clinic, Oostersingel 59, 9713 EZ Groningen, The Netherlands.

Imaging of the Brain in Psychiatry and Related Fields
Edited by K. Maurer

an increased D_2 type dopamine receptor density is not characteristic of schizophrenia.

In contrast to the lack of evidence for a possible pathogenetic role of dopamine dysfunction in schizophrenia, there is overwhelming support for the antidopaminergic effects of the present generation of antipsychotic drugs, not only from animal research in vivo and in vitro but also from human in vivo investigations. As an example of the latter conclusion, recent PET studies have shown that all neuroleptics occupy to a signficant degree (between 65% and 95%) cerebral dopamine D_2 receptors during normal dose treatment (Baron et al. 1989; Farde et al. 1987, 1988; Coppens et al. 1991; Sedvall et al. 1986; Wolkin et al. 1989). In a few patients D_2 receptor occupancy was correlated with therapeutic effect (Farde et al. 1987), but in therapy resistent patients high receptor occupancy has been noticed as well (Wolkin et al. 1989; Coppens et al. 1991). These results may also indicate that blockade of cerebral D_2 type dopamine receptors is necessary but not sufficient to achieve therapeutic response.

Both the postmortem studies and the in vivo studies using PET do not substantiate the idea that an increased density of dopamine receptors is the cause of schizophrenia. If indeed an excess of D_2 type dopamine receptors is not the cause of schizophrenia or related psychoses, but rather the result of the antipsychotic treatment, the question remains why, in the best documented postmortem investigation, is the density of the cerebral dopamine receptors bimodally distributed? We hypothesize that this finding is an artifact of the in vitro approach and due to the loss of dopamine receptors during tissue fragmentation necessary for in vitro assay. For the development of our argument we followed three experimental approaches: (1) quantification of dopamine receptor D_2 type density in vivo in the rat; (2) relation of receptor occupation in the rat determined in vivo with postsynaptic effects; and (3) postmortem analysis of the human brain in relation to neuroleptic treatment.

In Vivo Binding Studies in the Rat Brain

Quantification and Location

In a series of in vivo studies Van der Werf et al. (1983, 1984a,b), Korf et al. (1985), Korf and Sebens (1987), and Swart et al. (1990) estimated the density of D_2 receptor binding in several rat brain areas with an antagonist (spiperone) or an agonist (*N*-*n*-propylapomorphine, NPA) of dopamine D_2 type receptors. Complete saturation curves were made by plotting the cerebellar radioactivity (or dose, blood or plasma radioactivity: x axis) versus the radioactivity of the area of interest (striatum, accumbens, tuberculum olfactorium: y axis) 1 (NPA) or 2 (spiperone) h after intravenous injection. Such a curve showed saturation at relatively low doses and was linear at high doses. In this method the values of x are independent from the values of y and not – as was contended by Seeman (1987) – that the x values were subtracted from the y values. Receptor densities were estimated either by graphical or by nonlinear procedures and were relatively high as compared to densities reported with in vitro assays. Interestingly, the density of spiperone binding sites was about twice that of NPA in the striatum but somewhat less than twice in the nucleus accumbens and the olfactory tubercle. A similar ratio of binding densities between NPA and spiperone was reported by Battaglia and Titeler (1982) using an in vitro method. Destruction of striatal neurons with a local injection of kainate resulted in disappearance of twice as many spiperone binding sites as of NPA ones (Van der Werf et al. 1984a,b).

The in vivo distribution of NPA was studied in considerable detail using an ex vivo autoradiographic method (Loopuijt 1989; Loopuijt et al. 1988). The distribution of NPA binding sites was essentially what has been reported for D_2 receptors: a dorsal to ventral gradient and less in the striosomes than in the matrix in the dorsal striatum; the distribution coincides with that of acetylcholinesterase activity. Of interest may also be the extremely high density in the islands of Calleja, localized at the ventrocaudal part of the striatal-accumbens complex. Recently, another dopamine receptor was postulated: the D_3 receptor to which apomorphine had a high affinity (Sokoloff et al. 1990). This receptor was also abundantly localized in the islands of Calleja. Thus, it might be postulated that, in vivo, NPA also binds to the D_3 dopamine receptor. This could explain our in vivo observation that in the limbic structures the number of NPA binding sites found was somewhat less than twice that of spiperone, thus suggesting that the D_3 receptor has a single binding site for NPA, spiperone, and iodosupiride (the ligand used by Sokoloff et al. 1990). The in vivo binding studies together suggest that in the rat striatum (and possibly in limbic brain areas as well) there are multiple binding sites for the dopamine D_2 recptor, of which NPA binds to one site and spiperone (and possibly other classical neuroleptics) binds to twice as many sites.

Receptor Stability

In studies based on irreversible binding of D_2 receptors (with *N*-ethoxycarbonyl-2-ethoxy-1, 2-dihydroquinoline, EEDQ) neuroleptics protected receptor deterioration (Van der Weide 1988; Meller et al. 1985). In addition, acute treatment with a neuroleptic resulted in higher receptor density than found in vitro, thus receptor supersensitivity had not occurred yet. (J. Van der Weide, unpublished).

In a postmortem study Kornhuber et al. (1989) showed that high receptor density was seen only in those patients treated with antipsychotic drugs until death, whereas in patients who were withdrawn from drugs before death lower values were found a few days after withdrawal. It may be of interest to notice that some authors of Kornhuber's study were also involved in the study of Seeman et al. (1984), suggesting that the latter study included patients treated with neuroleptics until death. From rat studies, the half-life of the striatal dopamine D_2 receptor was estimated to be approximately 4 days (Meller et al. 1985; Loopuijt et al. 1988). Thus, if the human turnover rates of the receptor are of a similar magnitude, the increase in receptor density in Kornhuber's study cannot be explained by the normal receptor turn over. Instead, together these findings may indicate the possible enhancement by (some) neuroleptic drugs of the stability of the D_2 type dopamine receptors during in vitro processing.

Receptor Binding In Vivo and Postsynaptic Effects

The relatively high D_2 receptor densities found with spiperone in vivo might be attributed to binding to nonfunctional sites. Therefore in some studies the direct consequence of receptor occupation for a post-synaptic marker was assessed. A major consequence of D_2 dopamine receptor blockade in the rat striatum is the decrease of acetylcholine levels, possibly due to a disinhibition of cholinergic neurons. Occupation with an antagonist, such as spiperone, results in a linear relationship between receptor occupation and acetylcholine level (Korf et al. 1985; Korf and Sebens 1987), indicating that virtually all specific binding in the striatum is representative for D_2 type binding. Such results do not, however, prove that all the specific binding of spiperone is confined to cholinergic neurons. The subpopulation of the D_2 receptors involved in the regulation of cholinergic transmission seems to have similar binding properties as other D_2 type receptors of the rat striatum. A strong relationship between recepor occupation and cholinergic parameters was maintained after long-term treatment with haloperidol but, per occupied receptor, a smaller decrease in acetylcholine levels was seen, possibly due to the increase in receptor density (Korf and Sebens 1987). The linearity of the relationship between receptor binding and acetylcholine was lost after denervation of the dopaminergic input, indicating that the blockade was dependent upon the presence of dopamine in the striatum (Korf and Sebens 1987).

There was little if any relationship between receptor occupation with NPA and cholinergic parameters, which may be attributed to either an almost maximal occupation of dopamine receptors with endogenous dopamine or to the fact that NPA is not a full agonist (Korf et al. 1985). Indeed, acute depletion of dopamine increases NPA binding given at tracer dose, suggesting that NPA may serve as a marker for receptor occupation. Thus, if suitable PET ligands could be developed in vivo, agonist binding has the potency to provide information about the state of the D_2 receptor in vivo. Recently we explored [^{11}C]apomorphine for this purpose, but the specific binding of the compound was probably too low to be clinically useful (S. Zijlstra, H. van der Worp. T. Wiegman, W. Vaalurg, and J. Korf, unpublished).

Final Comments

In the rat striatum, the number of D_2 dopamine receptor blocker binding sites is about twice that for a (partial) dopamine agonist. The occupancy of the spiperone binding sites correlates highly with changes in acetylcholine levels of the rat striatum and these changes were only found in the presence of dopamine. Binding in human post mortem tissue is higher (about twice) during than shortly after neuroleptic treatment and cannot be attributed to thc normal turnover of the receptor. These observations together may explain the reported bimodality of D_2 receptors in schizophrenia (Seeman et al. 1984, 1987) as an artifact of the in vitro assay.

References

Baron JC, Martinot JL, Cambon H, Boulenger JP, Poirer MF, Blin J, Huret JD, Loc'h C, Maziere B (1989) Striatal dopamine receptor occupancy during and following withdrawal from neuroleptic treatment: correlative evaluation by positron emission tomography and plasma prolactin levels. Psychopharmacology 99:463

Battaglia G, Titeler M (1982) [^{3}H]n-propylapomorphine and [^{3}H]spiperone binding in brain indicate two states of the D_2-dopamine receptor. Eur J Pharmacol 81:493

Carlsson A (1988) The current status of the dopamine receptor hypothesis of schizophrenia. Neuropsychopharmacology 1:179

Coppens HJ, Slooff CJ, Paans AMJ, Wiegman T, Vaalburg W, Korf J (1991) High central D2-dopamine receptor occupancy as assessed with positron emission tomography in medicated but therapy resistant schizophrenic patients. Biol Psychiatry 29:429

Farde L, Halldin C, Stone-Elander S, Sedvall G (1987) PET analysis of human dopamine receptor subtypes using ^{11}C-SCH 23390 and ^{11}C-raclopride. Psychopharmacology 92:278–284

Farde L, Wiesel F-A, Halldin C, Sedvall G (1988) Central D2-dopamine receptor occupancy in schizophrenic patiens treted with antipsychotic drugs. Arch Gen Psychiatry 45:71–76

Farde L, Wiesel FA, Stone-Elander S, Halldin C, Nordstöm AL, Hall H, Sedvall G (1990) D_2-dopamine receptors in neuroleptic-naive schizophrenic patients. Arch Gen Psychiatry 47:213–219

Korf J, Sebens JB (1987) Relationship between dopamine receptor occupation by spiperone and acetylcholine: levels in the rat striatum after long-term haloperidol treatment depend upon dopamine innervation. J Neurochem 48:516–521

Korf J, Sebens JB, Flentge F, VanderWerf JF (1985) Occupation of dopamine receptors with *N-n*-propylnorapomorphine or spiperone and acetylcholine levels. J Neurochem 44:314–318

Kornhuber J, Riederer P, Reynolds GP, Beckman H, Jellinger K, Gabriel E (1989) ^{3}H-spipeone binding sites in post-mortem brains from schizophrenic patients: relationship to neuroleptic treatment, abnormal movements, and positive symptoms. J Neural Transm 75:1–10

Loopuijt LD (1989) Distribution of dopamine D-2 receptors in the rat striatal complex and its comparison with acetylcholinesterase. Brain Res Bull 22:805–817

Loopuijt LD, Sebens JB, Korf J (1988) Regional differences in reappearance of D2-dopamine receptors in the rat caudate-putamen complex after irrevesible inactivation. Brain Res 456:263–270

Martinot JL, Peron-Magnan P, Huret JD, Mazoyer B, Baron JC, Boulenger JP, Loc'h C, Maziere B, Caillard V, Loo H, Syrota A (1990) Striatal D_2 dopaminergic receptors assessed with positron emission tomography and ^{76}Br-bromospiperone in untreated schizophrenic patients. Am J Psychiatry 147:44–50

Meller E, Bohmaker K, Golstein M, Friedhoff AJ (1985) Inactivation of D1 and D2 recptors by *N*-ethoxycarbonyl-2-ethoxy-1, 2-dihydroquinoline in vivo. J Pharmacol Exp Ther 233:656–662

Sedvall G, Farde L, Persson A, Wiesel FA (1986) Imaging of neurotransmitter receptors in the living human brain. Arch Gen Psychiatry 43:995–1005

Seeman P (1987) The absolute density of neurotransmitter receptors in the brain: example for dopamine receptors. J Pharmacol Methods 17:347–360

Seeman P, Ulpian C, Bergeron C, Riederer P, Jellinger K, Gabriel E, Reynolds GP, Tourtelotte WW (1984) Bimodal distribution of dopamine densities in brains of schizophrenics. Science 225:728–731

Seeman P, Bzowej N, Guan HC, Bergeron C, Reynolds GP, Bird ED, Riederer P, Jellinger K, Tourtellotte WW (1987) Human brain D1 and D2 dopamine receptors in schizophrenia, Alzheimer's, Parkinson's and Huntington's diseases. Neuropsychopharmacology 1:5–15

Sokoloff P, Giros B, Martres M-P, Bouthenet M-L, Schwartz J-C (1990) Molecular cloning and characterization of a novel dopamine receptor (D3) as a target for neuroleptics. Nature 347:146–151

Swart JAA, Korf J (1989) Quantification of dopamine D2-receptors by irreversible tracer binding in the living human brain: the model-dependent correction of metabolites. J Cereb Blood Flow Metab 9:906–908

Swart JAA, Van der Werf JF, Wiegman T, Paans AM, Vaalburg W, Korf J (1990) In vivo binding of spiperone and *N*-methylspiperone to dopaminergic and serotonergic sites in the rat brain: multiple modelling and implications for PET scanning. J Cereb Blood Flow Metab 10:297–306

Van der Weide J (1988) Determination of the pharmacological profile of the dopamine agonist N-0437. Thesis, University of Groningen, pp 1–142

Van der Werf JF, Sebens JB, Vaalburg W, Korf J (1983) In vivo binding of *N-n*-propylnorapomorphine in the rat brain: regional localization, quantification in striatum and lack of correlation with dopamine metabolism. Eur J Pharmacol 87:259–270

Van der Werf JF, Sebens JB, Korf J (1984a) In vivo binding of *N-n*-propylnorapomorphine in the rat striatum: quantification after lesions produced by kainate, 6-hydroxydopamine and decortication. Eur J Pharmacol 102:251–259

Van der Werf JF, Van het Schip F, Sebens JB, Korf J (1984b) Quantification of in vivo spiperone binding in the rat striatum after lesions produced by kainate or decortication. Eur J Pharmacol 102:387–399

Wolkin A, Barouche F, Wolf AP, Rotrosen J, Fowler JS, Shiue C-Y, Cooper TB, Brodie JD (1989) Dopamine blockade and clinical response: evidence for two biological subgroups of schizophrenia. Am J Psychiatry 46:905–908

Wong DF, Wagner HN, Larry ET, Dannals RF, Pearlson GD, Links GM, Tamminga CA, Bronssolle EP, Ravert HT, Wilson AA, Toang JKT, Malot J, Williams JA, O'Tuama LA, Snyder SH, Kuhar MJ, Gjedde A (1986) Positron emission tomography reveals elevated D2 dopamine receptors in drug naive schizophrenics. Science 234:1558–1563

Age-Dependent Changes of the Metabolic Pattern in Patients with Alzheimer's Disease*

R. Mielke[1], M. Grond, K. Herholz, J. Kessler, and W.D. Heiss

Introduction

Since the first description of Alzheimer's disease (AD) by Alois Alzheimer (1910) and its introduction by Kraepelin in 1910, the influence of age on the background of different psychopathological and apparative criteria has been discussed. Whether AD should be considered as a uniform manifestation or classified into a presenile and a senile type as a possible means of differentiation of subtypes by age remains controversial. Even Alzheimer waived this concept of presenile disease and applied his term to all presenile and senile disease types showing the characteristic typical macroscopic and microscopic pattern (Alzheimer 1911). Nonetheless, the terms dementia of Alzheimer type and senile dementia of Alzheimer type (DAT and SDAT) were introduced (Katzman 1976) with an arbitrary cutoff age of 65 years.

Manifold parameters have been analyzed with respect to influence of age. Apart from psychopathometric and other clinical results, epidemiological, neuropathological, biochemical, and genetic parameters have been evaluated with different results concerning homogeneity between presenile and senile disease. Nowadays, the quantitative imaging of regional cerebral glucose metabolism by means of positron emission tomography (PET) is a reliable method to analyze the typical metabolic pattern of degenerative dementia and to show either AD subtype. In contrast with other functional diagnostic methods, e.g., single photon emission computerized tomography, which yields information on certain aspects of cerebral hemodynamics only, PET permits the investigation of cerebral energy metabolism. Thus it may be better suited for assessment of abnormal functional neuroanatomy, even in regions showing no gross structural abnormality or only mild atrophy. Quantitative imaging of the metabolic changes occurring in AD has shown that reductions of glucose metabolism are most prominent in the temporoparietal and frontal association cortices while metabolism of

*Supported by the Bundesministerium für Forschung und Technologie, No. 0701763A.

[1] Max-Planck Institut für Neurologische Forschung, Gleueler-Strasse 50, W-5000 Köln 41, FRG.

Imaging of the Brain in Psychiatry and Related Fields
Edited by K. Maurer

primary sensorimotor and visual cortices, basal ganglia, and cerebellum is relatively preserved (Benson et al. 1983; Duara et al. 1986; Foster et al. 1983; Friedland et al. 1983; McGeer et al. 1986). This metabolic pattern has proved to be relatively specific for AD (Herholz et al. 1990). Recently, it was reported that temporoparietal hypometabolism is not as prominent in SDAT as in DAT (Grady et al. 1987; Small et al. 1989). In the following study we therefore investigated the influence of age on metabolic pattern in patients with AD.

Patients and Methods

A total of 38 patients, 13 males and 25 females, with probable AD according to NINCDS-ADRDA criteria (McKhann et al. 1984) were included in this study. The average age was 66.5 ± 7.6 years (range 47–81 years). Laboratory tests included erythrocyte sedimentation rate, complete blood count, serum levels of glucose, bilirubin, urea, creatinine, sodium, potassium, calcium, total protein, lipids, liver enzymes, lactate dehydrogenase (LDH), thyroid function, and *Treponema pallidum* hemagglutination assay (TPHA). Computerized tomography (CT) or magnetic resonance imaging (MRI) was performed on each patient to rule out ischemic or tumorous lesions. The modified Haschinsky score of Rosen (1980) was below 3. A history of intellectual deficits such as memory loss and loss of abstractive ability lasted from 6 months until 6 years with an average duration of disease of 2.5 ± 1.3 years. The degree of mental deterioration was quantified by standardized rating scales and psychometric tests, i.e., the mini-mental state test (MMSE) (Folstein et al. 1975) and the global deterioration scale (GDS) (Reisberg et al. 1982). Average scores were: MMSE, 16.2 ± 6.0 (3–27); GDS, 4.2 ± 1.0 (3–6).

A group of 59 normal individuals without a history of cognitive deficits, without evidence of neurological disease, and a totally normal clinical and neuropsychological examination served as controls. The average age was 43.8 ± 18.7 years (range 16–77 years).

The [^{18}F]fluorodeoxyglucose (^{18}FDG) method was applied according to a standard measurement protocol (Heiss et al. 1984) and under resting conditions for determination of regional cerebral glucose metabolic rates (rCMRGlu), which were calculated according to the procedure described by Wienhard et al. (1985) 30–50 min after tracer injection. Some 14 levels parallel to the canthomeatal plane were scanned with a slice thickness of 11 mm and a center to center distance of 7 mm. Regions of interest were adapted to major functional-anatomical structures according to a standard scheme using an interactive, computer assisted, mapping procedure (Herholz et al. 1985). rCMRGlu was averaged over several slices yielding a total of 192 standardized brain regions for quantitative evaluation. The plane with the basal ganglia served as a reference for anatomical localization of cortical

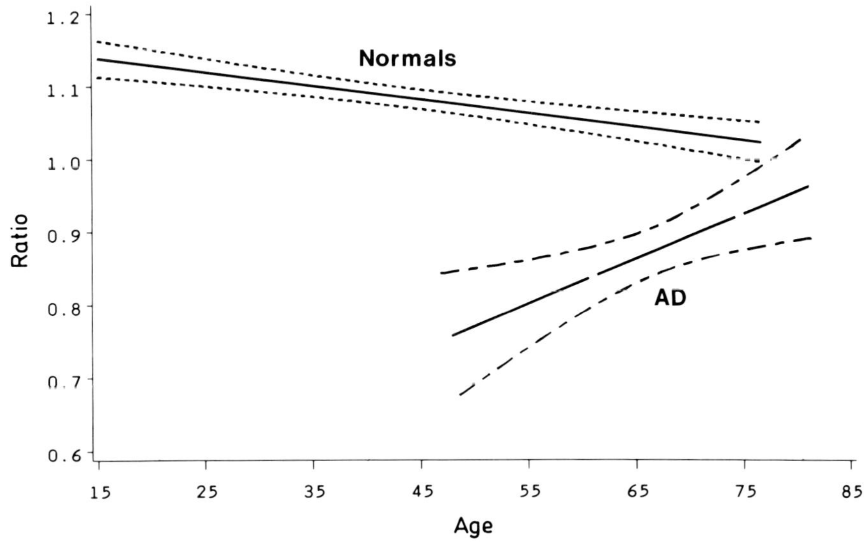

Fig. 1. Relationship between the ratio (regional cerebral glucose metabolic rates of regions typically affected in Alzheimer's disease divided by those of not affected regions) of patients and normals indicated by the regression line and 95% confidence limits. While the ratios are quite different in presenile age individuals, with increasing age they approach an approximation of the metabolic pattern seen in normal elderly subjects

regions. A ratio consisting of rCMRGlu of regions typically affected in AD (temporoparietal and frontal areas) divided by rCMRGlu of regions typically not affected (cerebellum, brainstem, lentiform nucleus, visual and sensorimotor cortex) was calculated as described previously (Herholz et al. 1990).

All statistical analysis was performed using the SAS software package (SAS Institute, Cary, NC, USA).

Results

The correlation of the ratio and the MMSE score, as an indicator of the degree of dementia severity, was significant ($p < 0.001$; $r = 0.52$). In this context the obvious relationship of the MMSE score and the metabolism of regions typically affected in AD has to be mentioned, i.e., the frontal associative cortex ($p < 0.05$; $r = 0.4$) and the temporoparietal cortex ($p < 0.05$; $r = 0.35$).

There was a positive correlation between the ratio and the age of persons suffering from AD ($p < 0.005$; $r = 0.48$; Fig. 1). This means that the regional distribution pattern of the pathological metabolism is markedly less in patient's with SDAT than in those with DAT. In contrast the ratio of the 59 normals was significantly inversely correlated with age ($p < 0.0005$; $r = -0.57$; Fig.1). Differences between the ratios of patients with AD and the control group are therefore less obvious in elderly (SDAT) patients.

Discussion

In this systematic analysis of rCMRGlu in patients with AD, the preferential affection of glucose metabolism in frontal and temporoparietal association areas, as pointed out by other authors (Benson et al. 1983; Duara et al. 1986; Foster et al. 1983; Friedland et al. 1983; Herholz et al. 1990; McGeer et al. 1986), was demonstrated by PET. We found age-dependent changes in the metabolic pattern. The quotient of rCMRGlu of regions typically affected divided by those without primary affection by the disease was markedly lower in patients with DAT than in those with SDAT. The diagnostic power of this quotient has been tested in another study (Herholz et al. 1990). In previous reports similar but not identical ratios (i.e., parietal/basal ganglia metabolic ratio) have been tested to characterize the metabolic pattern in AD (Kuhl et al. 1982) or in relation to the effects of gender and age (Small et al. 1989). In the latter study, the observed heterogeneity was used to separate patients with early onset AD from those with late onset disease. The authors (Small et al. 1989) referred to a significantly lower left parietal ratio (left posterior parietal region divided by the hemispheric average) as a distinguishing feature between these groups.

To illustrate rCMRGlu changes in patients with AD we compared the rCMRGlu ratio (typically affected regions divided by typically not affected regions) of AD patients with that of normals. While the ratios showed an enormous gap at presenile age (<45) they approached each other in older patients. These findings are consistent with the fact that, in PET images from presenile demented people, a pattern can often be observed which is typical for AD patients but which is missing in SDAT patients, except for the reduced global metabolism. Although we have still not been able to obtain autopsy data that confirm our diagnosis, it is possible to achieve a high degree of accuracy with respect to clinical diagnosis by strict selection criteria (Morris et al. 1988). Thus, our data indicate a more localized expression of AD in younger patients while, in SDAT, less specific factors may contribute to the development of dementia.

References

Alzheimer A (1907) Über eine eigenartige Erkrankung der Hirnrinde. Allg Z Psychiatr 64:146–148

Alzheimer A (1911) Über eigenartige Krankheitsfälle des späteren Alters. Z Ges Neurol Psychiatr 4:356–360

Benson DF, Kuhl DE, Hawkins RA, Phelps ME, Cummings JL, Tsai SY (1983) The fluorodeoxyglucose ^{18}F scan in Alzheimer's disease and multi-infarct dementia. Arch Neurol 40:711–714

Duara R, Grady C, Haxby J, Sundaram M, Cutler NR, Heston L, Moore A, Schlageter N, Larson S, Rapoport SI (1986) Positron emission tomography in Alzheimer's disease. Neurology 36:879–887

Folstein MF, Folstein SE, McHugh PR (1975) Mini-mental state. J Psychiatr Res 12:189–198

Foster NL, Chase TN, Fedio P, Patronas NJ, Brooks RA, DiChiro G (1983) Alzheimer's disease: focal cortical changes shown by positron emission tomography. Neurology 33:961–965

Friendland RP, Budinger TF, Ganz E, Yano Y, Mathis CA, Koss B, Ober BO, Huesman RH, Derenzo SE (1983) Regional cerebral metabolic alterations in dementia of the Alzheimer's type: positron emission tomography with (^{18}F)fluorodeoxyglucose. J Comput Assist Tomogr 7:5590–5598

Grady CL, Haxby JV, Horwitz B, Berg G, Rapoport SI (1987) Neuropsychological and cerebral metabolic function in early vs late onset dementia of the Alzheimer type. Neuropsychologia 25:807–816

Heiss WD, Pawlik G, Herholz K, Wagner R, Göldner H, Wienhard K (1984) Regional kinetic constants and cerebral metabolic rate for glucose in normal human volunteers determined by dynamic positron emission tomography of (^{18}F)-2-fluoro-2-deoxy-D-glucose. J Cereb Blood Flow Metab 4:212–223

Herholz K, Pawlik G, Wienhard K, Heiss WD (1985) Computer assisted mapping in quantitative analysis of cerebral positron emission tomography. J Comput Assist Tomogr 9:154–161

Herholz K, Adams R, Kessler J, Szelies B, Grond M, Heiss WD (1990) Criteria for the diagnosis of Alzheimer's disease with positron emission tomography. Dementia 1:156–164

Katzman R (1976) The prevalence and malignancy of Alzheimer's disease. Arch Neurol 33:217–218

Kraepelin E (1910) Psychiatrie, ein Lehrbuch für Studierende und Ärzte, vol II/1, 8th edn. Barth, Leipzig

Kuhl DE, Metter EJ, Riege WH, Phelps ME (1982) Effects of human aging on patterns of local cerebral glucose utilization determined by the [^{18}F]fluorodeoxyglucose method. J Cereb Blood Flow Metab 2:163–171

McGeer PL, Kamo H, Harrop R (1986) Positron emission tomography in patients with clinical diagnosed Alzheimer's disease. Can Med Assoc J 134:597–607

McKhann G, Drachman D, Folstein M, Katzman R, Price D, Stadlan EM (1984) Clinical diagnosis of Alzheimer's disease: report of the NINCDS-ADRDA work group under the auspices of Department of Health and Human Services Task Force on Alzheimer's disease. Neurology 19:939–944

Morris JC, McKeel DW Jr, Fulling K, Torack RM, Berg L (1988) Validation of clinical diagnostic criteria for Alzheimer's disease. Ann Neurol 24:17–22

Reisberg B, Ferris SH, De Leon MJ, Crook T (1982) The global deterioration scale for assessment of primary degenerative dementia. Am J Psychiatry 139:1136–1139

Rosen WG, Terry RD, Fuld PA, Katzman R, Peck A (1980) Pathological verification of ischemia score in differentiation of dementias. Ann Neurol 7:486–488

Small GW, Kuhl DE, Riege WH, Fujikawa DG, Ashford JW, Metter EJ, Mazziotta JC (1989) Cerebral glucose metabolic patterns in Alzheimer's disease. Effect of gender and age at dementia onset. Arch Gen Psychiatry 46:527–532

Wienhard K, Pawlik G, Herholz K, Wagner R, Heiss WD (1985) Estimation of local cerebral glucose utilization by positron emission tomography of (^{18}F)-2-fluoro-2-deoxy-D-glucose: a critical appraisal of optimization procedures. J Cereb Blood Flow Metab 5:115–125

Activity Changes in the Human Brain Due to Vibratory Stimulation of the Hand Studied with Positron Emission Tomography

R.J. SEITZ[1] and P.E. ROLAND

Introduction

With positron emission tomography (PET) one can measure the activity of neuronal populations in the human brain indirectly by measurements of the regional cerebral blood flow (rCBF) or of the regional metabolic rate of glucose (rCMRGlu) or oxygen (rCMRO_2) (Raichle 1987). The accurate localization of functional information in the PET images demands, however, integration with additional anatomical information from computerized tomography (CT) or magnetic resonance imaging (MRI). Usually, the changes in rCBF or rCMRGlu that are specifically induced by physiological or psychological stimulation are compared with the resting control state (Roland and Larsen 1976; Mazziotta et al. 1981). Rest is, however, also a specific functional state of brain activity, which in the electroencephalogram is characterized by the expression of α-activity in the parietooccipital leads and in rCBF measurements by high flow in prefrontal areas (Ingvar 1979). Furthermore, PET studies have shown that in rest the mean global CBF and CMRGlu are higher than during sleep (Heiss et al. 1985; Marquet et al. 1990) but lower than during cognitive tasks (Cameron et al. 1990; Roland et al. 1987) and unchanged during simple motor and sensory activation tasks (Fox and Raichle 1984; Fox et al. 1987). These observations raise two questions: (1) Does brain work activate numerous regions? (2) Does brain work depress the activity of neuronal populations?

Patients and Methods

We addressed these questions in a study of vibratory stimulation of the right hand in five adult healthy male volunteers (age range 20–35 years). Vibratory stimulation is a robust somatosensory stimulation that does not

[1] Abt. für Neurologie, Heinrich-Heine-Universität Düsseldorf, Moorenstr. 5, W-4000 Düsseldorf 1, FRG.

Imaging of the Brain in Psychiatry
and Related Fields
Edited by K. Maurer

involve active exploration (Ibanez et al. 1989). However, the subjects had to observe if changes of the vibratory frequency occurred. The rCBF was measured with bolus inhalation of [^{11}C]-fluoromethane as described in detail previously (Roland et al. 1987). For the measurements of the rCMRO$_2$ we applied the approach of (Mintun et al. 1984). The measurements were performed during vibratory stimulation and rest with the Scanditronix PC384-7B PET camera (Litton et al. 1984). The functional PET images were adjusted to a common PaCO$_2$ level and spatially standardized by use of the computerized brain atlas program as described in detail elsewhere (Seitz et al. 1990a). Out of the spatially standardized PET images, mean images, images of the standard error of the mean across subjects (SEM), t-maps, and images of the percent changes compared to rest were calculated voxel by voxel. Only mean changes with a t value >2.78 ($p < 0.05$, 4 degrees of freedom, two-tailed t test) in adjacent voxels with a spatial extent of an area of at least $7.6 \times 7.6 \times 13.5\,\text{mm}^3$ were accepted as significant (Seitz et al. 1990a,b, 1991).

Results and Discussion

Vibratory stimulation of the right hand led to a significant increase of the mean rCBF (16.3 ± 4.6 SD ml/100 g per minute) in the left sensory hand area. As depicted in Fig. 1a, the mean rCBF increase in percent clearly exceeded the corresponding mean rCMRO$_2$ increase (0.42 ± 0.12 SD ml/100 g/min) in accordance with an earlier report from our laboratory (Eriksson et al. 1989). However, the percent changes of the mean rCBF and rCMRO$_2$ expanded in an area of identical magnitude. In a voxel by voxel plot, the mean rCBF and mean rCMRO$_2$ were strongly correlated (Fig. 1b). In variance with a report by Fox et al. (1987), in the left secondary somatosensory area (16%) and the left inferior parietal cortex (18%) significant mean rCBF increases were also observed. The additional mean rCBF increases in the left motor hand area (24%) and the left supplementary motor area (13%) were probably related to reflectory finger flexion due to the vibratory stimulus (Ibanez et al. 1989). Thus, even this passively perceived physiological stimulation activated numerous cortical areas (Fig. 2).

In addition to these increases, there were also coupled decreases of the mean rCBF and rCMRO$_2$ in a number of cortical and subcortical structures during right hand vibratory stimulation (Fig. 1b). The cortical areas with significant rCBF decreases are also depicted in Fig. 2. These decreases occurred in the left superior parietal lobule (−15%), the right superior parietal lobule (−18%), the left supplementary sensory area (−18%), the right superior prefrontal gyrus (−12%), the left temporal pole (−15%), and the left posterior cingular gyrus (−14%).

The mean global CBF during vibratory stimulation was 54.4 ± 8.6 (SD) ml/100 g/min and was unchanged compared to a series of 26 healthy subjects

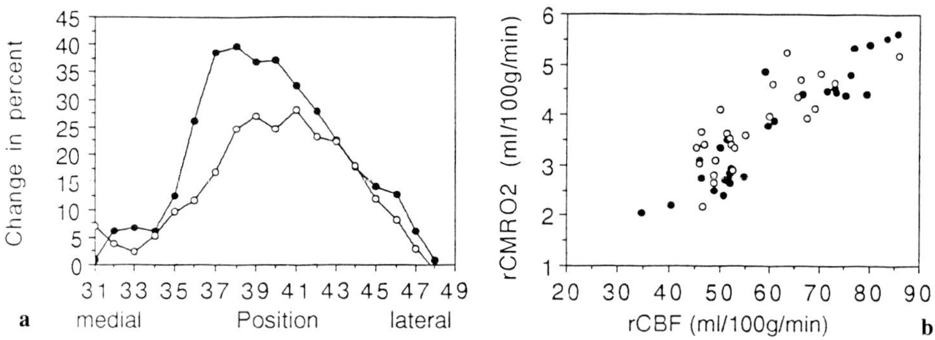

Fig. 1. **a** Mean changes of the rCBF (●) and $rCMRO_2$ (○) in the left sensory hand area due to vibratory stimulation of the right hand. Shown are coronal profiles through the images of the mean percent changes compared to rest. **b** Correlation ($r = 0.90$) of the mean rCBF and the mean $rCMRO_2$ during vibratory stimulation in individual voxels; ● rCBF increases; ○ rCBF decreases

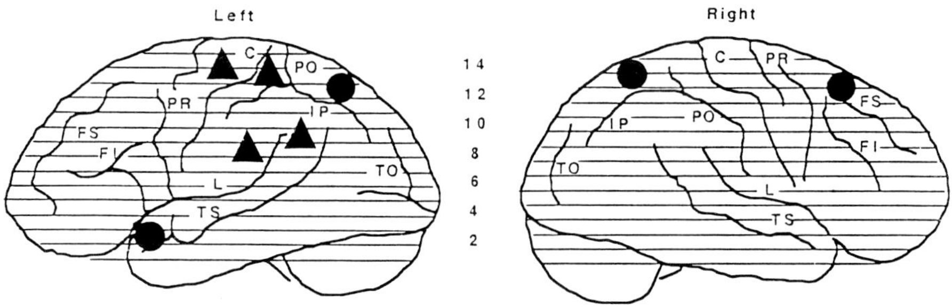

Fig. 2. Lateral aspects of the atlas brain (Greitz et al. 1991) with the major sulci and the levels of the mean PET images. Indicated are the areas with the significant mean rCBF increases (▲) and decreases (●). Modified after Seitz and Roland (1992)

of similar age studied at rest (54.2 ± 9.5 SD ml/100 g per minute) (Seitz et al. 1990a). Similarly, the mean global CBF was unchanged compared to rest during performance of sequential finger movements (55.1 ± 8.8 SD ml/100 g per minute) (Seitz et al. 1990b) and slightly decreased during visual stimulation with colored, standardized, geometric patterns (51.2 ± 5.8 SD ml/100 g per minute) (Roland et al. 1990). In contrast, mean global CBF was significantly elevated in the route finding task (59.5 ± 6.7 SD ml/100 g per minute). In this task, numerous cortical areas, including the prefrontal and remote visual association areas in the parietal lobe, were significantly activated (Roland et al. 1987). Also, during somatosensory discrimination of rectangular parallelepipeds, the mean global CBF (66.7 ± 12.6 SD ml/100 g per minute) was significantly higher than at rest. In this task, motor areas that were engaged for the execution and control of the exploratory finger movements, somatosensory and sensory association areas that were activated for processing of the sampled sensory information, and prefrontal and paralimbic areas that were related to working memory and decision making exhibited significant mean rCBF increases (Seitz et al. 1991). Finally, recent results from our laboratory indicate that the mean global CBF in subjects who had the PET measurement at rest as the first experiment (unadapted rest, 59.2 ± 10.2 SD ml/100 g per minute) was significantly higher than in subjects who had the PET measurement at rest after a preceding physiological stimulation (51.5 ± 8.2 SD ml/100 g per minute). This difference resulted from a significantly higher mean rCBF in the parietal association areas and the prefrontal and paralimbic cortices in unadapted rest. All these structures were related to fear and attention (Reiman et al. 1989; Reivich et al. 1983).

The use of the computerized brain atlas program (Greitz et al. 1991; Seitz et al. 1990a) made it possible to accurately determine the activity changes in the human brain voxel by voxel. Our results showed that, during simple sensory stimulation and during the motor activation task, the rCBF and the $rCMRO_2$ were decreased compared to rest in the higher order cortical association areas. Thus, the mean rCBF increases and the mean rCBF decreases were balanced so that the mean global CBF did not change. We interpret the observed coupled decreases of the rCBF and $rCMRO_2$ as regional depressions of synaptic activity. From electrophysiological studies there is evidence for reduced activity of neuronal populations in the superior temporal cortex during the production of speech compared to rest (Creutzfeldt et al. 1989). A further argument for an assumed reduction of synaptic activity in structures with decreases of the mean rCBF was that in the same structures increases of the mean rCBF occurred during other stimulation tasks. For instance, the mean rCBF in the temporal poles was decreased during visual and vibration stimulation and the motor sequences but increased during unadapted rest. Moreover, in the midsector of the putamen-pallidus complex, mean rCBF decreases were observed during learning of a finger movement sequence, while there were mean rCBF increases during skilled performance of sequential finger movements (Seitz et al. 1990b, 1991). These differences in the mean rCBF in these two examples were statistically significant ($p < 0.05$, two-tailed t test). In contrast, in more complex cognitive processes, the activity was raised in numerous cerebral structures compared to rest. The mean global CBF, $CMRO_2$, and CMRGlu, measured with PET, but probably also the rCBF measurements performed with the Kety-Schmidt and single photon techniques, therefore reflect the mean amount of ongoing neuronal activity in the entire brain. One of the challenging perspectives of PET is to reveal abnormal patterns of the rCBF, rCMRGlu, and $rCMRO_2$ in rest and during stimulation in neurological and psychiatric diseases (Volkow et al. 1987).

References

Cameron OG, Modell JG, Hichwa RD, Agranoff BW, Koeppe RA (1990) Changes in sensory-cognitive input: effects on cerebral blood flow. J Cereb Blood Flow Metab 10:38–42

Creutzfeldt O, Ojemann G, Lettich E (1989) Neuronal activity in the human lateral temporal lobe. II. Responses to the subjects own voice. Exp Brain Res 77:476–489

Eriksson L, Roland P, Dahlbom M, Blomqvist G, Widén L (1989) Coupling between regional cerebral oxidative metabolism and regional cerebral blood flow during physiological stimulation. J Cereb Blood Flow Metab 9 [Suppl 1]:S578

Fox PT, Raichle ME (1984) Stimulus rate dependence of regional cerebral blood flow in human striate cortex demonstrated by positron emission tomography. J Neurophysiol 51:1109–1120

Fox PT, Burton H, Raichle ME (1987) Mapping human somatosensory cortex with positron emission tomography. J Neurosurg 67:34–43

Greitz T, Bohm C, Holtc S, Eriksson L (1991) A computerized brain atlas: construction, anatomical content, and some applications. J Comp Ass Tomogr 15:26–38

Heiss W-D, Pawlik G, Herholz K, Wagner R, Wienhard K (1985) Regional cerebral glucose metabolism in man during wakefulness, sleep, and dreaming. Brain Res 327:362–366

Ibanez V, Deiber MP, Mauguière F (1989) Interference of vibrations with input transmission in dorsal horn and cuneate nucleus in man: a study of somatosensory evoked potentials (SEPs) to electrical stimulation of median nerve and fingers. Exp Brain Res 75:599–610

Ingvar DH (1979) "Hyperfrontal" distribution of the cerebral grey matter flow in resting wakefulness; on the functional anatomy of the conscious state. Acta Neurol Scand 60:12–25

Litton J, Bergström M, Eriksson L, Bohm C, Blomqvist G, Kesselberg M (1984) Performance study of the Pc-384 positron camera system for emission tomography of the brain. J Comput Assist Tomogr 8:74–87

Maquet P, Dive D, Salmon E, Sadzot B, Franco G, Poirrier R, von Frenckell R, Franck G (1990) Cerebral glucose utilization during sleep-wake cycle in man determined with positron emission tomography and [^{18}F]2-fluoro-2-deoxy-D-glucose method. Brain Res 513:136–143

Mazziotta JC, Phelps ME, Miller J, Kuhl DE (1981) Tomographic mapping of human cerebral metabolism: normal unstimulated state. Neurology 31:503–516

Mintun MA, Raichle ME, Martin WRW, Herscovitch P (1984) Brain oxygen utilization measured with O-15 radiotracers and positron emission tomography. J Nucl Med 25:177–187

Raichle ME (1987) Circulatory and metabolic correlates of brain function in normal humans. In: Plum F (ed) Handbook of physiology: sect 1; the nervous system, vol 5. Oxford University Press, New York, pp 643–674

Reiman EM, Fusselman MJ, Fox PT, Raichle ME (1989) Neuroanatomical correlates of anticipatory anxiety. Science 243:1071–1243

Reivich M, Gur R, Alavi A (1983) Positron emission tomographic studies of sensory stimuli, cognitive processes and anxiety. Hum Neurobiol 2:25–33

Roland PE, Larsen B (1976) Focal increase of cerebral blood flow during stereognostic testing in man. Arch Neurol 33:551–558

Roland PE, Eriksson L, Stone-Elander S, Widén L (1987) Does mental brain activity change the oxidative metabolism in the human brain. J Neurosci 7:2373–2389

Roland PE, Gulyás B, Seitz RJ, Bohm C, Stone-Elander S (1990) Functional anatomy of storage, recall and recognition of a visual pattern in man. Neuroreport 1:53–56

Seitz RJ, Bohm C, Greitz T, Roland PE, Eriksson L, Blomqvist G, Nordell B, Rosenkvist G (1990a) Accuracy and precision of the computerized brain atlas programme (CBA) for localization and quantification in positron emission tomography. J Cereb Blood Flow Metab 10:443–457

Seitz RJ, Roland PE, Bohm C, Greitz T, Stone-Elander S (1990b) Motor learning in man: a positron emission tomographic study. Neuroreport 1:57–60

Seitz RJ, Roland PE, Bohm C, Greitz T, Stone-Elander S (1991) Somatosensory discrimination of shape: tactile exploration and cerebral activation. Eur J Neurosci 3:481–492

Seitz RJ, Roland PE (1992) Vibratory stimulation increases and decreases the regional cerebral blood flow and oxidative metabolism: a positron emission tomography (PET) study. Acta Neurol Scand 86:60–67

Volkow ND, Wolf AP, VanGelder P, Brodie JD, Overall JE, Cancro R, Gomez-Mont F (1987) Phenomenological correlates of metabolic activity in 18 patients with chronic schizophrenia. Am J Psychiatry 144:151–158

Functional Imaging Methods (Magnetoencephalography)

The Use of Magnetoencephalography in Psychiatry

P. Fenwick[1], A. Ioannides, and J. Lumsden

Introduction

In the 1950s, as EEG became widely available, psychiatrists hoped that at last a tool had been found which would give them insight into those cerebral processes which underpin mental illness. Apart from major neurological units, EEG machines were placed mainly in psychiatric hospitals. There was a directive in the UK which advocated the purchasing and training of personnel in EEG technology for all prisons. That was a time of great optimism; not only would this new technology help with the eradication of mental illness, but also with the eradication of crime by the insights that it would give into brain function. Our prisons came to be more like hospitals. Disillusion set in over the next decade. By the end of the 1960s neurologists were claiming that EEG was no more than a toy. A stethoscope on the wall outside a football match was the current phrase, trying to establish how the players were placed on the field. Had it not been for the absence of neuroimaging and the advent of evoked potentials, particularly visual evoked potentials, and their relationship to the diagnosis of multiple sclerosis, EEG might have remained simply a research tool.

The birth of magnetoencephalography (MEG) in the 1970s and its development in the 1980s came at a time when computed tomography (CT) scans and magnetic resonance imaging (MRI) scans were able to give an excellent structural image of the brain. Brain pathology could be easily and accurately identified, so the psychiatrist was not looking for further diagnostic tools. The early single channel MEG systems, which required filling with liquid helium every 3 days, were difficult to run. Measurement times to achieve even the simplest magnetic map ran into several hours, during which the patient had to keep still. This limited its usefulness significantly.

The first multichannel systems to come on the market in the mid-1980s were even more cumbersome to operate, and because of the increased complexity of the technology, they could not be used outside a screened room. Thus the cost of these systems increased. Although eight- and ten-channel systems are able to acquire data at a greater rate than a single

[1] Institute of Psychiatry, De Crespigny Park, Denmark Hill, London SE5 8AF, UK.

Imaging of the Brain in Psychiatry
and Related Fields
Edited by K. Maurer

channel system, the compromises in their design still significantly limit the signals they can measure. The usual design configuration allows for the measurement of superficial rather than deep sources. Another reason that clinicians are not yet falling over themselves to install MEG units in their hospitals is that they see no immediate clinical application (Fenwick 1987).

The current generation of machines, with nearly 40 MEG channels, have already provided a unique view of brain dynamics, and a sample from these studies will be discussed in the next few sections. However, the full potential of the technique can only be realised with the introduction of even bigger sensor arrays which can cover both hemispheres simultaneously. Such probes, with 100 MEG channels, will be in production soon. The increase in the number of channels, and a modification in the design so that a greater number of signal sources of different depths can be detected, will mean that these systems may have an application in a much greater range of neurological and psychiatric diseases, and they may then start to play a part in the clinical examination of patients.

Investigation of Brain Activity

Clinical Acceptability of MEG

If it is to be accepted clinically, and used widely, MEG must be seen to give a quick and accurate answer to clinical problems. It should provide information that other tests cannot easily obtain. It is very important that the information gained should have consequences for the treatment of the patient. The capital costs of the installation must be reasonable, and the technique must be cost-effective. The technique should fit into a branch of clinical medicine where there is already expertise to interpret the results. Finally, it should be acceptable to the patient. How does MEG compare with other brain imaging methods available?

CT Scanning

CT scanning was immediately recognised by the clinical community as being a method which provided enormous help with the diagnosis and treatment of clinical disease. The cost of a fourth generation CT scanner is between 1.5 and 2 million pounds, which makes it expensive to install, although it forms the basic workhorse of any X-ray department. But despite the cost, within 2 years of the successful demonstration of the principle, most major neurological centres throughout the world had initiated campaigns to raise funding for CT installation. Compare this to the reaction to MEG of the medical establishment, which has consistently maintained that it has little to offer psychiatry.

Since the late 1970s and early 1980s there has been an explosion in imaging methods. MRI has enhanced the structural resolution of brain images. Positron emission tomography (PET) and in a less significant way, single photon emission computed tomography (SPECT), have produced dynamic images of brain function. However, the time resolution of these two methods is in the range of a few minutes. There is still the need for an imaging system that can give functional information on a millisecond by millisecond basis. The only methods at present available are those which analyse the electrical activity of the brain. Thus the EEG and MEG, if they can be used to image the activity in both cortical and deep structures, must become one of the major research tools of the future.

MEG Versus EEG

As any MEG or EEG enthusiast will tell you, however committed they are to their field, they accept the Clark Maxwell equations. Thus, in the limit, there should be no inconsistency between MEG imaging and EEG imaging, although some differences are expected because the signal in each case carries complementary information. However, there are at present considerable difficulties, firstly because of our understanding and models, which represent brain, skull and scalp structure, and because of the measuring instruments that we are currently using. From the point of view of the EEG, the conductance of the brain, skull and scalp are poorly known. The way the conductance varies in the presence of a pathological condition such as tumour, or close to brain ventricles or the frontal air sinuses, is still obscure. The EEG technology is not yet as highly advanced as MEG and no EEG systems either have sufficient channels or the mechanism for recording the exact position of electrode placements and their relationship to the brain.

This means that at the present time EEG is unlikely to be as effective in modelling activity in either superficial or deep regions of the brain as is MEG. Only one limited study is so far available on the comparative accuracy of MEG and EEG in locating artificial electrical sources within the brain (Cohen et al. 1983; Cohen et al. 1990). Unfortunately, for various technical reasons this does not represent the obtainable accuracy of either method, and so it will be necessary for these studies to be repeated before an accurate assessment can be given. Furthermore the nature of two generators in the brain is known to be distributed and very different to the one used in this study.

The Analysis of the Cortical Spike in Neuropsychiatric Populations

For many years research workers have recorded a relationship between cortical spike activity and psychiatric morbidity. The precise definition of where these spikes are arising and to what structures they can be attributed is likely to expand our understanding of psychiatric illness.

Spike activity does not necessarily represent an epileptogenic cortical lesion (Stevens 1977). EEG spike activity has been reported in children with psychiatric disorders and disappeared as the children's psychiatric condition improved (Lairy et al. 1967). Hill and Parr (1963) and other authors have reported the presence of "larval" spike and spike and wave in the EEG of patients with schizophrenia, particularly those with catatonia. In all these studies there is a definite correlation between the presence of EEG spikes, increased cortical excitability, and behaviour disorders, the EEG normalising as the abnormal behaviour improves. By defining the generators for these spike foci, MEG should be able to define more accurately the areas of cortex from which they come and their magnetic field maps. This information would help further our understanding of the electrophysiological processes underlying their generation.

There is also a relationship between cortical spikes and patients who show impulsive thinking and behaviour but do not have epilepsy. Small (1970) found an increase in the number of spikes in patients who attempted suicide and in those undergoing psychotic depressive episodes. Those with spikes showed some degree of psychomotor retardation, more mood swings, anxiety, feelings of hopelessness, morbid thoughts, concentration difficulties and insomnia, compared to psychiatric patients who had normal records. This group also had more psychiatric hospital admissions, suicidal attempts, and a family history of depression. Small et al. (1975), in a further study, showed that small sharp spikes were significantly related to a positive family history of affective disorder, raising the possibility that there may be some kind of genetic marker in bipolar affective disorder. MEG measurement of the spike fields might therefore more accurately characterise the generators giving rise to spikes and their likely location within the cortex.

Struve et al. (1977) found a relationship between spikes and suicidal ideation, probably related to change in cortical excitability resulting from an alteration in neurotransmitter balance (for a review, Fenwick et al. 1983). However, Fenton (1986) in a review chapter suggests that disturbance of the calcium flux in cerebral neurones can provide the link between spikes and affective disorder.

The association between paroxysmal EEG features and antisocial behaviour can be seen in particular in respect of posterior temporal slow waves (Hill 1952; Fenton et al. 1974). The likelihood that MEG can provide reasonable localisations of slow wave paroxysms is strong, particularly if a distributed source analysis is used. Slow wave phenomena are likely to be generated by discrete cortical areas, such as damaged tissue. Precise localisations of these abnormal discharges would enable biochemical and cytoarchitectural investigations into these disorders.

The relationship between different neurotransmitter systems and behaviour could potentially be revolutionised using the MEG technique. The possibilities of some type of functional biochemical tomography, with the manipulation of levels of different neurotransmitters in normal populations and in pathological populations is worth considering here. Already changes in slow potentials have been demonstrated following acute drug administrations (Tecce and Cole 1974; Howard et al. 1982; Thompson et al. 1978), and other significant effects are seen in pathological populations (Amabile et al. 1986).

There is increasing evidence that impairment of serotonergic function impairs avoidance learning and releases hyperactivity, aggression and sexual behaviour. Some pathological populations have been shown to be depleted in 5-hydroxytryptamine (5-HT). Other populations have been demonstrated with acquired 5-HT depletion, such as chronic alcohol users (Ballenger et al. 1979).

The use of MEG to map the activation of different functional systems mediated by different neurotransmitters onto discrete structures in the brain is now possible. (Fenwick et al. 1992).

The Possible Use of MEG in Paroxysmal Disorders of Behaviour

Ever since the discovery of the EEG it was realised that scalp potentials would probably reveal only a fraction of the ongoing cerebral discharges. Numerous animal studies in the 1950s showed an imperfect relationship between electrical discharges in the depth and discharges on the surface. However, it was not possible to verify this relationship in humans experimentally because of the difficulty of implanting electrodes in these subjects.

Because of far field effects, all EEG discharges in the depth must show potential changes on the surface of the scalp, unless there is some cancellation of their electrical fields. In the 1960s, it was standard teaching in the UK that an epileptic seizure was always accompanied by an alteration in cortical rhythms. Alterations in behaviour not accompanied by such changes were thought *not* to be due to epilepsy. This view has been very powerful in shaping attitudes to paroxysmal disorders of behaviour. In an attempt to change this words such as epileptoid, epileptic equivalent, etc. which had been employed for many years (Schwab 1951; Wilson and Kinnie 1935; Hill 1981 (review)) were used to describe these disorders of behaviour. This attempt to gain credibility failed because there was insufficient data to show that these disorders were caused by true epileptic seizures in the depth and not by psychological causes.

In the 1950s Heath (1986) embarked on a programme of depth electrode implantation which led him to the recognition that discharges in the amygdala, hippocampus, and septal region were at times correlated with paroxysmal changes in behaviour. Monroe (1970) proposed a specific syndrome, called episodic dyscontrol (Fenwick 1986), based on the ob-

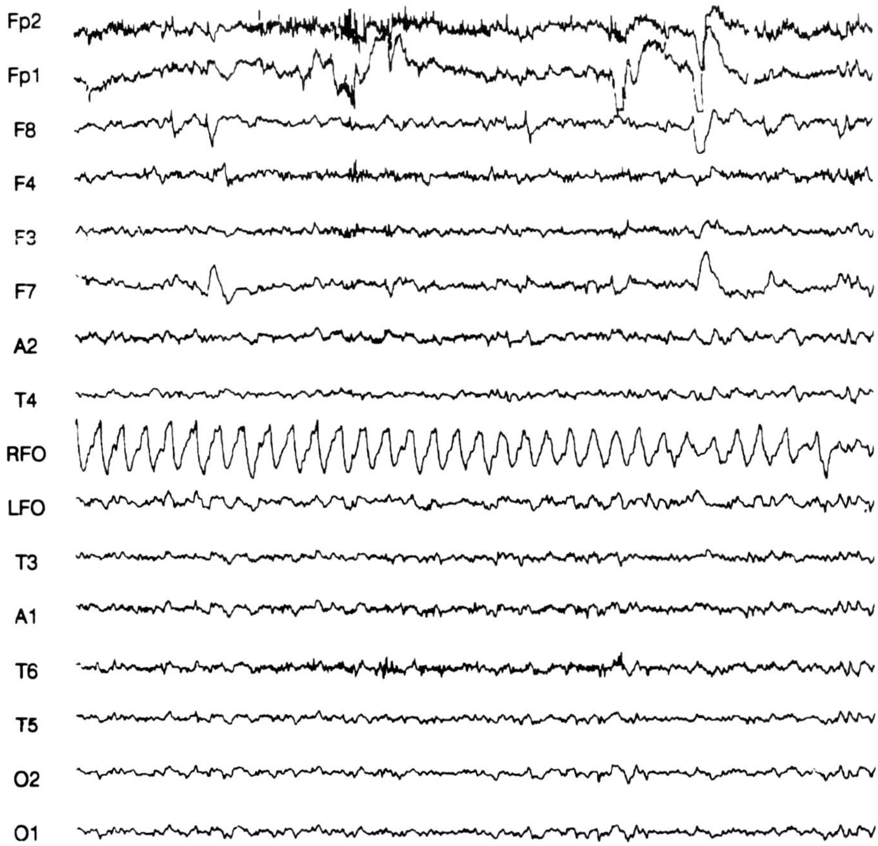

Fig. 1. High-voltage seizure within the limbic structures, as recorded from a foramen ovale electrode, producing disturbed behavior but not affecting cortical rhythms to any degree. (Recordings thanks to Dr. Birnie)

servation that paroxysmal disorders of behaviour arose when there were paroxysmal discharges in subcortical structures which were not necessarily recorded by the EEG on the surface of the cortex. (Heath and Mickle 1960; Sem-Jacobson 1968).

In the mid 1970s, many different units started to implant depth electrodes in patients who were to undergo temporal lobectomy. It soon became apparent that it was not uncommon for paroxysmal seizure discharges to involve the limbic structures, the amygdala and hippocampus, without noticeable spread to the cortex. (Hitchcock and Cairns 1973; Mark and Ervin 1970; Wieser 1983; Fenwick 1986). It is now accepted that seizure discharges within the depth do not necessarily have to propagate to the surface at easily observable amplitudes, and that *some* of these limbic discharges *may* be accompanied by changes in behaviour.

One of the difficulties in the diagnosis of paroxysmal disorders of behaviour has been the impossibility of measuring deep discharges confined to the limbic system with scalp EEG electrodes (Fig. 1). MEG technology is eminently suited to this problem, as it has the capacity to pick up discharges from the depth. With this in mind we have recently started in our MEG unit (Chris Guy and Simon Walker at Imperial College) a programme of exploration and measurement of deep limbic discharges in patients from the Maudsley Hospital who are undergoing investigation for temporal lobe epilepsy and are being considered for temporal lobe surgery. By implanting foramen ovale electrodes discharges arising in medial temporal structures can be compared with those on the scalp, and those appearing in the MEG. We have found that it is possible to monitor deep discharges from the limbic system which do not appear in the scalp EEG. Only a small number of discharges appear at the foramen ovale and in the MEG but not in the scalp EEG. There are also differences in phase relationships between the MEG and the electrical discharges, which could be due either to the sampling of a different neuronal population or to the orientation of the generator, leading to only part of the complex appearing in the MEG. It will not be possible to use averaging with this data, as within the average, phase information is lost. However, there are severe limitations in assessing deep activity with only a few MEG channels, as it is impossible to obtain a significantly large sample of the scalp magnetic field for any single event in the depth. It is now becoming apparent that with modern multichannel probes with 37 or so channels and some powerful analysis it is possible to localise accurately superficial activity and to identify deep generators (Ioannides et al. 1991; Ioannides 1992).

The Required Contribution of MEG to Schizophrenia

Whether spike activity is necessarily pathological has been questioned by many authors. There is certainly evidence that spikes in the EEG are found in many nonepileptic conditions, for example sleep, and thus spikes recorded from limbic structures in humans may be part of normal function. So the occurrence of spike activity in the depth in the absence of a clear epileptic condition should be interpreted with caution. However, three fundamental principles have been clearly established. Firstly, that epileptic activity in the depth need not necessarily be accompanied by changes in scalp activity; secondly, that these discharges may be accompanied by paroxysmal changes in behaviour; thirdly, that epileptic (like) discharges in the limbic system can

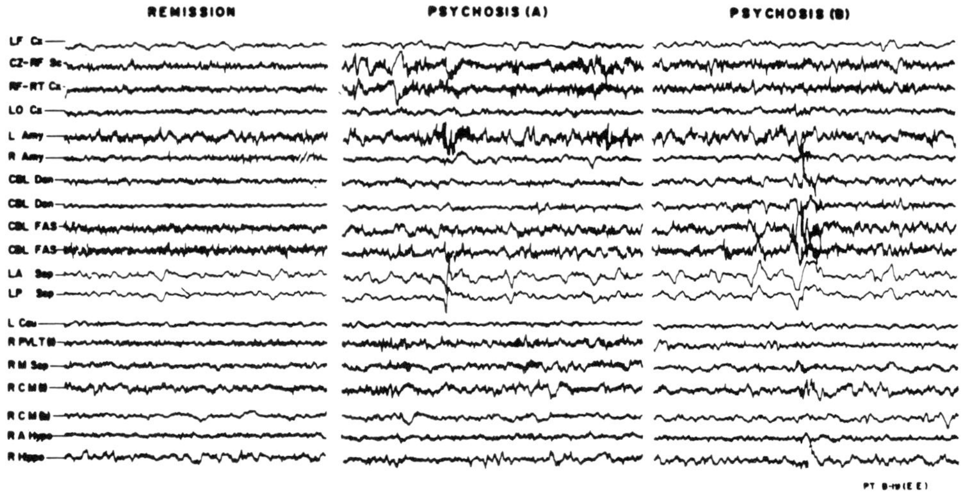

Fig. 2. Recordings from a schizophrenic patient when his symptoms had remitted and when he was psychotic. Abbreviations used in figures: *AMY*, amygdala; *CAU*, caudate nucleus; *CM*, centro median thalamus; *CX*, cortex; *CZ*, central zero – scalp; *DEN*, dentate nucleus; *F*, frontal; *FAS*, fastigal nucleus of the cerebellum; *GENIC*, geniculate; *HIP. HIPPO*, hippoeampus; *HYP. HYPO*, hypothalamus; *L*, left; *M*, medial; *O. OCC*, occipital; *PALL*, pallidum; *PAR*, parietal; *PVL*, posterior ventral lateral; *R*, right; *SEP*, septal region; *SUP*, superior; *T. TEMP*, temporal; *THAL*, thalamus

be associated with abnormal mental states. The MEG should be an ideal instrument for detecting deep discharges within the brain in patients with a clinical diagnosis of schizophrenia.

In the 1950s and 1960s Heath implanted electrodes in patients diagnosed as suffering from schizophrenia but who did not have epilepsy. He reported that they showed epileptiform activity in the form of spikes and noted a relationship between this spiking in the depth and hallucinatory experiences (Fig. 2). At that time the diagnosis of schizophrenia lacked methodological precision, so there must be some doubt about the exact diagnostic category of Heath's patients. However, there is little doubt that the observations relating to deep discharges within the amygdala, hippocampus and septal regions and the occurrence of hallucinatory behaviour are valid.

In a recent review, Heath (1986) describes these early studies: "The psychotic behaviour of patients with deep electrodes was consistently correlated with a recording abnormality in the form of spike and slow wave activity in the rostral-septal region . . . In those patients who had electrodes in the lateral amygdala, the recording abnormality also appeared there . . . But the significant correlation was with the abnormal activity in the septal region. Despite the dramatic changes in deep recordings, no changes were seen in scalp recording. Most of the psychotic patients in our series were schizophrenics, but the recording correlation was consistent with psychotic behaviour regardless of its underlying aetiology . . .".

"During interictal periods, numerous epileptic patients without complicating psychotic behaviour showed spike and slow wave activity predominantly in the hippocampus with no involvement of the septal region. A few epileptic patients had episodes of psychotic behaviour. On those occasions, spiking and slow wave activity appeared in recordings of the septal region as well as the hippocampus." (Heath and Walker 1985; Heath 1962; Mickle and Heath 1957).

Gibbs (1952) in a remarkable but relatively unknown paper, described the results of implanting over 50 patients who had schizophrenia but not epilepsy. He found that both the schizophrenics and the nonschizophrenic patients with temporal lobe epilepsy showed a similar distribution of epileptiform spikes over the temporal cortex and in deep temporal structures.

Heath's demonstration that spike activity in the septum correlated with hallucinatory behaviour has given rise to the speculation that these structures may be involved in schizophrenia, and that deep spike foci may be part of the pathology of schizophrenia. This model of schizophrenia has been extended by Stevens who noted "similarities in the auras and automatisms of psychomotor epilepsy and the subjective symptoms and stereotypes of schizophrenia. We have been particularly interested in dopamine regulation and the mesolimbic system, which originates in the ventral tegmental nucleii of midbrain and terminates in limbic striatal structures that receive projections from amygdala, hippocampus and temporal cortex . . ." (Stevens 1977, p. 193). Stimulation by a reduction of inhibitory feed-back in the ventral-tegmental in waking, unrestrained cats, produced "behavioural states of hypervigilance, searching, hiding, fear, and repeated orientating activity, during which spikes are recorded from the ipsilateral nucleus accumbens, essentially the same region from which Heath recorded spike activity in schizophrenic man . . . Similarly spike activity and changed behaviour were also induced after kindling of ventral tegmental area (in cats)" (Stevens 1977).

Several studies in the literature demonstrate a deterioration in behaviour and the development of psychosis in patients who have undergone epilepsy surgery. In the case of frontal lobe surgery this is understandable, as the surgery may interfere with the neural functioning responsible for an intact personality and the execution of socially acceptable behaviour. However, in the case of patients undergoing temporal lobe surgery it is not always possible to predict preoperatively which patients will develop psychiatric illness postoperatively. There are certainly some pointers; for example, it is known that patients whose epilepsy has been caused by meningitis do worse after temporal lobectomy than those whose epilepsy is caused by mesial temporal scleroisis following febrile convulsions. The psychiatric state apears to be independent of seizure remission. It has also been found that patients with hamatomas in the left temporal lobe are more likely to develop a psychosis after temporal lobectomy than those whose epilepsy has other causes (Fenwick 1991). It is thus imperative that presurgery more information is gained concerning the seizure focus and discharges, which will allow a more accurate prediction of psychiatric state postoperatively.

Recent Studies in Schizophrenia

Reite (1990) and co-workers have been studying the auditory evoked response in both normal individuals and schizophrenic patients. They looked at the M50 component of the auditory evoked response (the peak identified between 35–65 ms) in six normal subjects and in six schizophrenic men. Their modelling programme calculated the position of the dipole midway between the two extremes of the field generated by the M50. They then estimated the depth of the field using the method of Williamson and Kaufman (1981) and plotted out the putative sources on MRI scan slices. They estimated the M50 source to lie in the planum temporale bilaterally, slightly posterior to the primary auditory cortex of Heschl's gyrus. They suggested that the field arose from pyramidal cells in the cortex of the temporal planum. There was, however, an asymmetry between the two sides, with the sources being significantly higher with respect to the nasion–inion line over the left as compared with the right hemisphere. This suggested a different structure to the planum temporale on the left side.

Schizophrenic patients showed a different pattern. The M50 was in the same position as in normal subjects but the schizophrenics did not show the interhemispheric asymmetry of the normal subjects. These findings suggested that there was a different structure and/or function of the left temporal planum in schizophrenia.

M100

The M100 peak of the auditory evoked response was estimated in both normal and schizophrenic men. A single current dipole was calculated and its position within the brain was noted. "In normal subjects left hemnisphere dipoles were significantly further posterior than were right hemisphere dipoles, whereas in the schizophrenics there were no significant differences between left and right hemispheres" (Reite 1990). Dipole orientation was similar in the schizophrenics, unlike the normals, and schizophrenic dipoles were tilted more posteriorly in the left hemisphere than were those of normal subjects. They again argue for slight differences in the left temporal region of the brain in patients with schizophrenia.

Reite concludes that MEG may make substantial contributions to our understanding of psychiatric disorders by the further study of the M300 and intrahemisphere transfer deficits.

Cortical Excitability and Abnormal Behaviour

Poor impulse control is known to be related to brain dysfunction (Fenwick 1989). Drugs which change neurohumoral transmission within the brain are frequently used to modify episodes of violent and abnormal behaviour. Fenwick et al. (1983) suggested a relationship between poor impulse control and changes in brain catecholamines. This hypothesis is based on the behaviour inhibitory system (BIS) of Gray (1979) which controls activity in the hippocampus and projects to the frontal and septal regions of the forebrain. The BIS is enervated by the dorsal noradrenergic tracts originating in the nucleus coerelius and mediates the passive avoidance behaviour which Gray suggests is equated with anxiety. Howard et al. (1982) and Fenwick et al. 1983 suggested that lack of passive avoidance in an animal model can also be equated with behavioural impulsiveness, and that in humans this system mediates not only anxiety but impulse control. In several experiments and various populations of patients they showed that changes in cortical excitabilities (represented by differentiation of the contingent negative variation, CNV, GO/NO GO amplitudes) correlates with poor impulse control. They also showed that drugs which modify the action of the BIS by decreasing passive avoidance also decrease the CNV differentiation (Figs. 3 and 4).

Figure 3 shows GO/NO GO CNV averages in a population of controls and patients from Broadmoor Special Hospital. Sixteen trials are averaged in each condition. It can be seen that those with personality disorders who were highly impulsive show poor differentiation of the GO/NO GO response, whereas those who showed low impulsiveness showed a greater differentiation.

Figure 4 shows the difference of the 12 CNV points between GO/NO GO responses in the patient groups shown in Fig. 3. Highly significant differences can be seen between the differentiations of the highly impulsive personality disorders and the controls, whereas there are no significant differences between the low impulsive personality disorders and the controls (*$p < 0.05$, +$p < 0.01$).

On the basis of these observations they suggested that poor impulse control and episodic violent behaviour in humans is mediated by a noradrenergic system, the BIS of Gray. Episodes of disordered behaviour which characterise the dyscontrol system can arise either from a modification of activity in the mesolimbic or septral regions or from a change in impulse control by the frontal cortex. Depletion of noradrenaline will lead to an increase in cortical excitability, an increase in impulsiveness and a decrease in CNV differentiation.

They also showed that the activity of this system can be measured by using the CNV. Further information confirming these results has recently been found in a population of normal subjects. Poor GO/NO GO differentiation was found to correlate with impulsiveness on Eysenck's I5 questionnaire. This suggested that the findings are not limited only to pathological

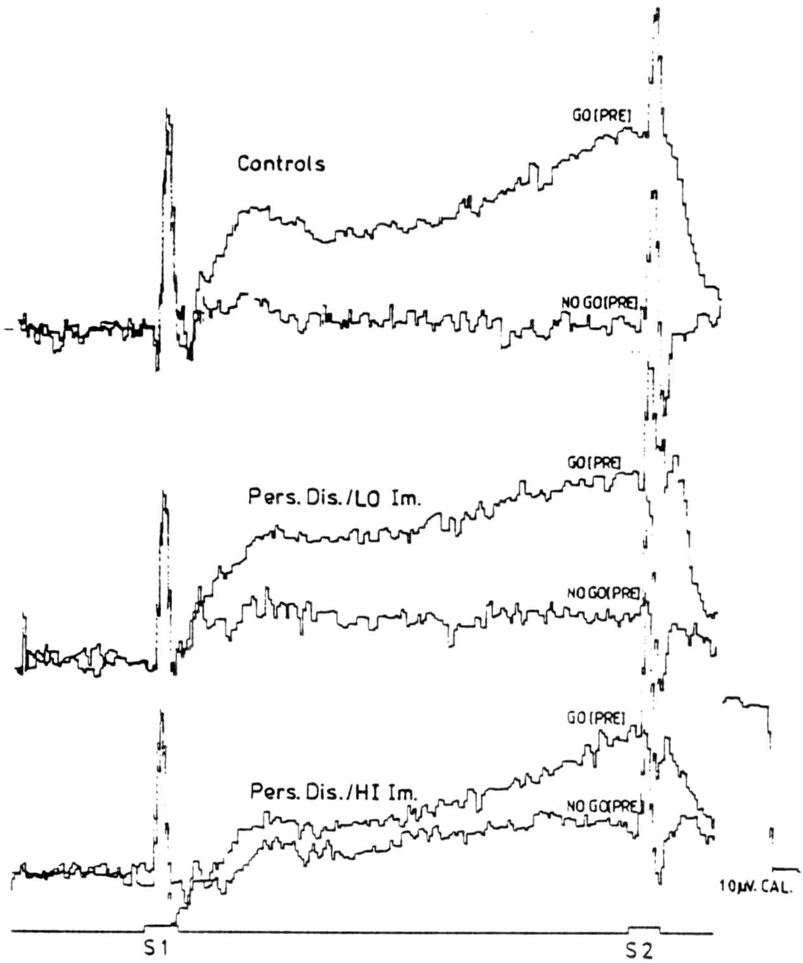

Fig. 3.

populations, but reflect quite generally a system which underpins the mechanism of impulsiveness (Brown et al. 1987).

Recent MEG Studies with Distributed Source Models – Magnetic Field Tomography

The distributed source model developed at the Open University (UK) produces an estimate of the *expectation value of the current density* (Ioannides et al. 1990; Ioannides 1991). The primary current density is constrained within the region of space, the source space, to which the measurements are

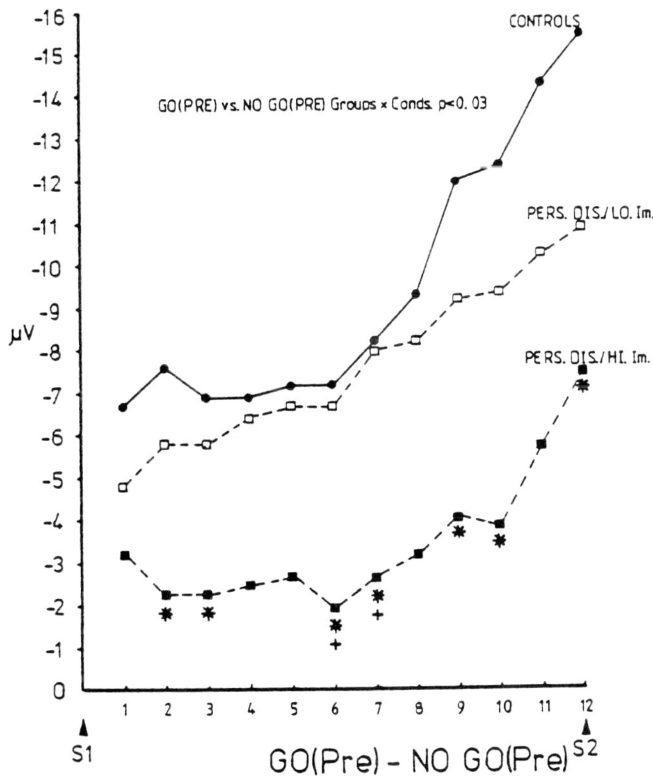

Fig. 4.

sensitive. In the case of MEG signals recorded with modern multichannel probes (e.g. the SIEMENS AG KRENIKON or the BTi MAGNES, both with 37 channels), this region is well defined. It is roughly the cortical area facing the sensor arrangement up to a depth (usually a few centimeters) which depends on the details of the sensor geometry and the level of noise in the measurements. In all recent applications a cylindrical source space has been used; a contour plot of intensity (square of the current density) obtained along a slice cut at a right angle to the symmetry axis of the cylinder is used to display the activity at a given depth. Magnetic field tomography (MFT) uses a sequence of subcontour plots, with the nost superficial slice placed at the top of the page and successive slices displayed below with depth from the cortical surface increasing down the page. An MFT column thus provides a three-dimensional description of the activity at one instant in time. These maps of activity are shown with background anatomical details if MRI or other structural images are available. Solutions at successive time instances are then printed next to each other with time increasing from left to right, yielding a representation of the evolution of activity in both space and time. The first application of MFT to real data (Ribary et al. 1991) was used to visualise the origin of a spatiotemporally organised pattern of coherence 40 Hz electrical activity (Ribary et al. 1991). This coherence, initially observed during auditory input, was proposed to be generated by recurrent corticothalamic oscillation (Llinas 1990). The MFT estimates provided support of this hypothesis, revealing a well-defined corticosubcortical sequence of activation with a time shift that is consistent with thalamocortical conduction times. In addition, studies on Alzheimer patients indicate that the cortical amplitude of this 40-Hz response is markedly reduced in these subjects (Ribary et al. 1991).

In a separate study, MFT estimates were obtained for interictal epileptic activity (Ioannides 1992). The signals were obtained with the SIEMENS 37-channel magnetoencephalograph KRENIKON (Schneider et al. 1990) at Erlangen, FRG. These signals were recorded from the left temporal area of a patient with pharmacoresistant epilepsy and partial complex seizures (Helstrand et al. 1991). A spatiotemporal correlation template technique (Abraham-Fuchs et al. 1990) was applied to the filtered data to identify an average 39 sharp wave candidate events, yielding the emphasised average signal. Comparison of equivalent current dipole and MFT solutions obtained from the average signals close to the peak of the sharp wave have shown that reliable current dipole solutions are obtained when a very high cross correlation coefficient is calculated between the measurements and the field produced by the current dipole solution, typically in excess of 0.97. In general, the evolution of activity in the distributed source solutions is more stable than the current dipole solution. Divergence of agreement between the two methods often shows as movement in the current dipole solution when the distributed source solution begins to develop activity at more than one centre (Ioannides et al. 1991). The MFT estimates for unaveraged signals (Ioannides 1992) show a continuous interplay between cortical and subcortical activity, including a high frequency modulation in both superficial and deep levels and irregular interruptions of activity in the deep end of the cylinder. The MFT analysis of the averaged signal shows instead an explosive build up of activity at the deep end of the cylinder, leading to the peak of the sharp wave. The appearance of an explosive buildup in the average signal is probably due to the increased likelihood of a strong cycle of activity close to the last peak. The true millisecond by millisecond evolution in a single epoch suggests that interictal activity is made up of transient bursts of activity followed by relatively long silent periods. The picture that emerges is one of recurrent, intermittent failure, over a rather large brain volume.

The rhythmical interplay between cortical and subcortical activity illustrated by the above-mentioned two studies is likely to be modified in psychiatric conditions. MFT is well suited to explore these possibilities.

The final example of MFT analysis is the first multichannel MEG/CNV study carried out using the 39-channel KRENIKON magnetometer in a shielded room in Erlangen, FRG, With the aid of Jorgen Veith and co-workers we recorded the CMV in a GO/NO GO paradigm. A 2000-Hz tone indicated the GO trials and a 1000-Hz stimulus the NO GO trials. There was a 3.5-ms interstimulus interval with a random intertrial interval of 5–20 s. fifty trials were averaged in each condition. The EEG was sampled at 250 Hz, with a low pass filter of 30 Hz and a time constant of 4.5 s. The subject was required to make a mandatory button press with his right hand to the GO trials and if he failed to do so within a time window of 270 ms after S2 he would receive 90 decibels of white noise. The stimulus and white noise were delivered to the right ear.

Epochs with large eye movement artefacts were removed, and the final CNV record was obtained from the average of 50 artefact free epochs for each condition. The resulting average MEG signal was analysed at the Open University using the distributed current density of (Ioannides et al. 1990). MFT estimates of activity were superimposed onto outlines of the subjects brain traced from MRI images. It was thus possible to follow the evolution of activity in distinct brain regions throughout the 4 s of interest. During this time responses were found in regions of the brain implicated with hearing the stimulus, task engagement and motor output As the GO and NO GO trials are interleaved randomly, the only difference between GO and NO GO is the inhibitory significance of the low-pitched tone compared to the active significance of the high-pitched tone. Clear differences are seen in the evolution of this potential in the different conditions.

For the first 200 ms the activity is very similar, apart from the tonotopic differences in the location of the activity for the different tone pitches in the two conditions. After 400 ms for the GO condition, activity is seen in the deep slices which go through the temporal poles until approximately 1400 ms. This is the first CMV component. This is not seen in the NO GO condition during the same period. Thus the GO condition appears to activate right temporal structures. For the second CMV component, between 2100 and 3500 ms, well-defined activations are seen at different cortical levels in the GO condition, while in the NO GO condition some sustained, possibly inhibitory activity, is seen at both the superior and deep levels between 2500 and 3500 ms.

It would thus appear that there are clear differences in excitation and inhibition in both superficial and deep brain structures as the CMV evolves. As the GO/NO GO CNV differences are known to be related to impulsivity, and impulsivity is one of the cardinal indices which differentiates primary from secondary psychopaths, these changes may give further insights into the brain function in psychopathy and also in criminal offendess.

Conclusion

The detailed information of brain processes provided by MEG analysis of brain rhythms suggests that it will become an exceedingly important tool in the analysis of the cerebral causes of mental illness. It is quite clear that the current technology is sufficiently developed to be able to give insights into the function of both the cortex and deep brain structures. It is thus likely that within the next few years MEG technology will have significantly contributed to our understanding of brain dysfunction in mental illness.

References

Abraham-Fuchs K, Harer W, Schneider S, Stefan H (1990) Pattern recognition in biomagnetic signals by spatio-temporal correlation and applications to the localisation of propoagating neural activity. Med Biol Eng Comput 28:398–406

Fenwick P (1987) The inverse problem: a medical perspective. Phys Med Biol 32:5–9

Fenwick P (1989) Dyscontrol. In: Reynolds E, Trimble M (eds) The bridge between neurology and psychiatry. Churchill Livingstone, Edinburgh, pp 263–287

Fenwick, P (1991) Long term psychiatric outcome after epilepsy surgery. Epilepsy Surgery, Raven Press, New York, ed. Hans Otto Luders, Ch. 72, pp 647–652

Fenwick P, Howard R, Fenton G (1983) Review of cortical excitability, neurohumeral transmission and the dyscontrol syndrome. In: Parsonage M, Grant R, Garcia A, Ward A (eds) Advances in epileptology, XIVth epilepsy international symposium. Raven, New York, pp 181–191

Fenwick P, Howard R, Brown D, Norton R (1992) Relationship between CNV asymmetries and individual differences in cognitive performance, personality and gender. Intern J Psychophysiol (in press)

Fenwick P, Ioannides A, Fenton G et al. (1992) Estimates of brain activity using magnetic field tomography in a GO/NO GO avoidance paradigm. Brain Topogr (submitted)

Gibbs FA (1951) Ictal and non-ictal psychiatric disorders in temporal lobe epilepsy. Journal of Nervous and Mental Disease 113:522–528

Gray J (1979) A neuropsychological theory of anxiety. In: Izard (ed) Emotions in personality and psychopathology, vol 10. Plenum, New York, pp 303–331

Heath RG (1962) Common characteristics of epilepsy and schizophrenia: clinical observation and depth electrode studies. Amer J Psychiat 118:1018–1026

Heath RG (1986) Studies with deep electrodes in patients intractably ill with epilepsy and other disorders. In: Reynolds E, Trimble M (eds) What is epilepsy? Churchill Livingstone, Edinburgh, pp 126–138

Heath RG, Mickle WA (1960) Evaluation of seven years experience with depth electrode studies in human patients. In: Ramey ER, O'Doherty D (eds) Electrical studies of the unanaesthetised brain. Hober, New York, pp 214–247

Heath RG, Walker CF (1985) Correlations of deep and surface electroencephalograms with psychosis and hallucinations in schizophrenics. A report of two cases. Biol Psychiatry 20:669–674

Helstrand E, Abraham-Fuchs K, Schneider S (1991) Magnetoencephalographic localisation of epileptic dipolar activity along gyrus cinguli in patients with pharmacoresistant epilepsy. Proceedings of the 8th international conference on biomagnetism, Munster, pp 37–38

Hill D (1981) Historical review. In: Reynolds E, Trimble M (eds) Epilepsy and psychiatry. Churchill Livingstone, Edinburgh, pp 1–11

Hill D, Parr G (1963) The EEG in psychiatry. In: Electroencephalography. A symposium of its various aspects, 2nd edn. Macdonald, London, pp 360–428

Hitchcock E, Cairns V (1973) Amygdalotomy. Postgraduate Medical Journal 49: 894–904

Howard RC, Fenton GW, Fenwick P (1982) Event related brain potentials in psychiatry and psychopathology: a Pavlovian approach. Wiley, Chichester

Ioannides A (1991) Comparison of MEG with other functional imaging techniques. Clinical Phys Physiol Meas [Suppl A] 12:23–28

Ioannides A (1992) Studies of evoked responses in interictal epileptic activity using magnetic field tomography. In: Fenwick P (ed) COMAC Cambridge Epilepsy meeting (in Press)

Ioannides A, Bolton J, Hasson R, Clarke C (1989) Localised and distributed source solutions for the biomagnetic inverse problem II. (Reprints available from the first author, Physics Department, the Open University, Milton Keynes, MK7 6AA, UK

Ioannides A, Bolton J, Clarke C (1990) Continuous probabilistic solutions to the biomagnetic inverse problem. Inverse Problems 6:523–542

Ioannides A, Bolton J, Hasson R, Clarke C (1990) Localised a distributed source solutions for the biomagnetic inverse problem II. Proceedings of the New York Biomagnetism Conference, August 1989. Williamson SJ (ed) Plenum Press. New York

Ioannides A, Helstrand E, Abraham-Fuchs K (1991) Distributed current density analysis of interictal epileptic activity. Proceedings of the 8th international conference on biomagnetism, Munster, pp 431–432

Lairy GC (1967) L'EEG comme moyen de investigation des-modalités individualles d'adaption aux situations de stress. Electroencephalogy Clin Neurophysiol [Suppl] 25:282–297

Llinus R (1990) Intrinsic electrical properties of mammalian neurones and CNS function. Raven, New York, pp 175–326 (Fidia Research Foundation. Neuroscience award lectures, vol 4)

Mark VH, Ervin F (1970) Violence and the brain. Harper and Rowe, New York

Mickle WA, Heath RG (1957) Electrical activity from subcortical, cortical and scalp electrodes, before and during clinical epileptic seizures. Trans Am Neurol Assoc 82:63

Monroe R (1970) Episodic behavioural disorders. Harvard University Press, Cambridge

Reite M (1990) Magnetoencephalography in the study of mental illness. Adv Neurol 54:207–222

Ribary U, Ioannides A, Hasson R et al. (1991) Magnetic field tomography (MFT) of coherent thalamo-cortical 40 Hz oscillations in humans. Proc Natl Acad Sci USA 88:11037–11041

Schneider S, Hoenig B, Reichenberger H et al. (1990) Multichannel biomagnetic systems for the study of electrical activity in the brain and heart. Radiology 176:825–830

Schwab RS (1951) Electroencephalography. Saunders, London

Sem-Jacobson CW (1968) Vegetative changes in response to electrical brain stimulation. Electroencephalogr Clin Neurophysiol 24:88

Small JG (1970) Small sharp spikes in the psychiatric population. Arch Gen Psychiatry 22:277–284

Small JG, Small IF, Milstein V, Moore DF (1975) Familial associations with EEG variance in manic depressive disease. Arch Gen Psychiatry 32:43–48

Stevens J (1977) All that spikes is not fits. In: Shagass C, Gershon S, Friedhof A (eds) Psychopathology and brain dysfunction. Raven, New York, pp 183–198 (reprinted (1986) in: Trimble M, Reynolds EH (eds) What is epilepsy? Churchill Livingstone, Edinburgh, pp 97–109)

Struve FA, Kishore RS, Arko RS, Klein DF, Becker D (1977) Relationship between paroxysmal electroencephalographic dysrhythmia and suicide ideation and attempts in psychiatric patients. In: Shagass C, Gershon S, Friedhof AJ (eds). Psychopathology and brain dysfunction. Raven, New York, pp 199–221

Tecce JJ, Cole JO (1974) Amphetamine effect in man. Paradoxical drowsiness and lowered electrical brain activity (CNV). Science 185:451–453

Thompson J, Newton P, Pocock P, Cooper R, Crow H, McCallum W, Papakostopoulous D (1978) Preliminary study of pharmacology of contingent negative variation in man. In: Otto DA (ed) A multidisciplinary perspective in event related brain potential research. US Government, Washington

Wieser HG (1983) Depth recorded limbic seizures and psychopathology. Neurosci Biobehav Rev 7/3:427–440

Williamson S, Kaufman L (1981) Magnetic fields of the cerebral cortex. In: Erne S, Hahlbohm H, Lubbig H (eds) Biomagnetism. de Gruyter, Berlin, pp 353–402

Wilson SA, Kinnie F (1935) The epilepsies. Springer, Berlin, pp 1–84 (Handbuch der Neurologie, vol 9)

Comparison of Single-Channel and Multichannel Magnetoencephalogram Recordings

J. VIETH[1]

Introduction

The neuronal intracellular currents which produce magnetic fields (Okada 1989; Wikswo et al. 1981) can be detected outside the head by a sensitive magnetometer, the SQUID (super conducting quantum interference device) (Zimmerman et al. 1970). The record of the spontaneous or evoked magnetic fields is called the magnetoencephalogram (MEG) and of the electric recording, the electroencephalogram (EEG). The main difference between EEG and MEG is that the magnetic field of the MEG – in contrast to the EEG – is almost never influenced by the different conductivities of different tissues, such as brain, cerebrospinal fluid, or bone (Peters and de Munck 1990); thus the MEG has advantages over the EEG.

There is now a discussion on the degree of error of the MEG compared to that of the EEG. It was reported that the degree of error with respect to cortical sources is 3 mm measured by the MEG (Yamamoto et al. 1988) and 20–25 mm measured by the EEG (Smith et al. 1985). Others claim that the average degree of error of the MEG is 8 mm and of the EEG 10 mm (Cohen et al. 1990). Objections to this claim have been made (Hari et al. 1991). Further studies and basic experiments are needed.

Our interest in MEG was mainly influenced by earlier work showing the ability of the MEG to locate focal sources of electrical activity better than the EEG (Barth et al. 1982; Romani et al. 1982). Thus, the MEG might be a valuable tool to localize functional lesions, such as epileptic foci or clinically silent TIAs (transient ischemic attacks), when anatomical lesions are absent. Before this can be done, however, the accuracy and reliability of the MEG must be tested using previously verified brain lesions.

In January 1987, we started MEG recordings without a magnetic shield in a magnetically relatively silent environment using a purchased single-channel DC-SQUID magnetometer (Biomagnetic Technologies Inc. San Diego, CA, USA model 601). These recordings showed the need for more channels because with single channel systems the recording times are very

[1] Abt. für experimentelle Neuropsychiatrie, Universität Erlangen-Nürnberg, Schwabachanlage 6, W-8520 Erlangen, FRG.

Imaging of the Brain in Psychiatry
and Related Fields
Edited by K. Maurer

long and no simultaneous recording is possible. The recordings also showed the need for a shielded room, due to magnetic disturbances from the environment. Thus, recordings with a tolerable amount of artifacts (between 0 and 8 per minute) only could be obtained after normal business hours or on the weekend.

In the meantime Siemens (Erlangen, Germany) developed a multichannel biomagnetic instrument with 37 channels, the KRENIKON®, to which we have had access since 1989. We were thus able to record in the factory in a shielded room (Gudden et al. 1989). In October 1990 Siemens installed a 37 channel system in our hospital.

The goal of our research was to evaluated the accuracy of the MEG by locating brain lesions which were previously verified by magnetic resonance imaging (MRI) or by computerized tomography (CT). Such lesions included angiomas, cysts, and brain infarctions with spontaneous abnormal interictal epileptic spike activity or slow wave activity. The source model was a single-current dipole and the head model a sphere fitted to the surface of the brain as obtained from MRI or CT. The coordinates found were fitted with the morphology obtained by MRI slices; if a CT had been done then CT slices were also used.

Single-Channel MEG

The main disadvantage of using a single-channel system is the need for consecutive sampling at all measuring points. Therefore the spontaneous changes in source strength during the recording time must be minimized or compensated for. Epileptic activity can be averaged (Barth et al. 1982) and spontaneous slow wave activity can be processed by the relative covariance method (Chapman et al. 1983).

Our studies were done on 22 patients. One group contained 12 patients with abnormal slow wave and interictal epileptic activity, in 9 due to a

→

Fig. 1a,b. Single-channel magnetoencephalogram (MEG) recordings. Localization of single-current dipoles of abnormal, interictal, magnetic spike activity combined with slow wave activity produced by epileptic foci recorded sequentially with a single-channel SQUID system at 55 measuring points. The point distance was 2 cm. The field distribution at the peak of the spike was mapped and the relative covariance frequency peak at 2 Hz was determined. The dipoles were inserted into schematic brain sections derived from X-ray images into which the head model was fitted. **a** A 25 year old male with drug resistant, complex partial seizures. Standard EEG: right temporal spike and δ-wave focus. No lesion was seen by CT or MRI. **b** A 23 year old male with drug resistant, complex partial seizures. Standard EEG: right temporal spike and δ-wave focus. Angiography: right temporal angioma (*hatched area*). Some 7 months after resection no seizures, EEG focus, or MEG dipole was detected. A, Dipole at the peak of the spike; C, dipole of 2Hz activity (obtained by rel. covariance)

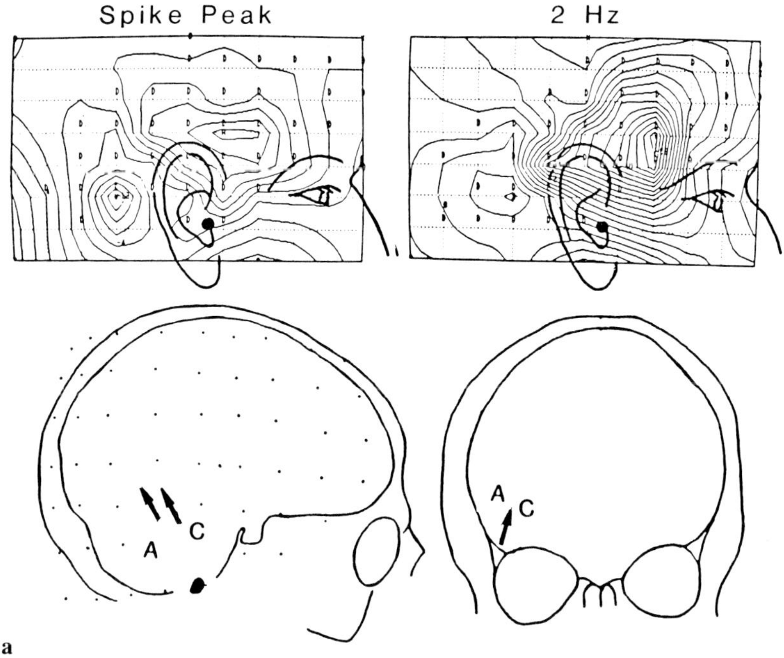

a

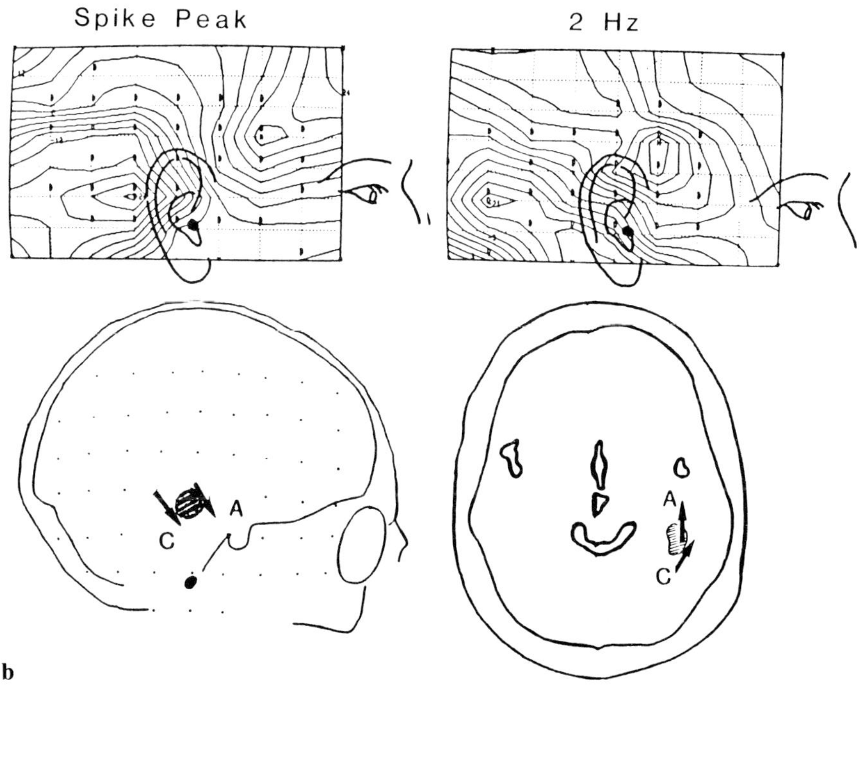

b

Table 1. Single-channel recordings

Patient	Lesion	Location	Map	Dipole location
			Slow/spike	Slow/spike
1[a]	Angioma, epilepsy	Right temporal	++/++	Close/close
2[b]	Epidermal cyst, epilepsy	Left temporal (1977, 1985 resected)	++/not done	Near/not done
3	Epilepsy	Grand mal	+/NA	Right temporal +/NA
4	Epilepsy	Complex partial right hemisphere	++/++	Rigth temporal close/close
5	Epilepsy	Complex partial left hemisphere	+/not done	Left temporal Close/close
6	Tumor	Left temporal	+/NA	Close/NA
7	Tumor (metastatic)	Left frontal	+/NA	Two dipoles Near/NA
8	Arachnoid cyst	Right temporal, polar	++/NA	Close/NA
9	Arachnoid cyst	Left temporal	+/NA	Close/NA
10	Multiple angioma	Right parietal concentration	One extremum/NA	Not done/ NA
11	Astrocytoma 3 years post-surgery	Left temporal defect	+/NA	Near/NA
12	Porencephalic cyst	Right temporal	++/NA	Close/NA

Comparison of the location of verified (by CT or MRI or by the clinical seizure classification) brain lesions (lesion location) with the dipole location of abnormal epileptic spike and/or slow wave brain activity.
Quality of maps: ++, not or only slightly distorted; +, light to moderately distorted but still two extremes; −, distorted map, single or two dipole localization not done. NA, not applicable.
[a] 7 months after resection there were no seizures, or dipoles but distorted maps.
[b] 8 months later nearly the same maps and the same dipole were detectable.

verified tumor, cyst, or angioma. Figure 1 shows two examples. As can be seen in Table 1, the locations of the estimated dipoles were close to the lesions if the source was not too deep or if no multiple sources were assumed (Vieth 1990a; Vieth et al. 1988, 1990b). The other group contained 11 patients with abnormal slow wave activity associated with ischemic lesions, i.e., brain infarctions, TIAs, and hemorrhages. Again, the estimated dipoles were found close to the lesions if the source was not too deep (Vieth

1990a; Vieth et al. 1988, 1990b). Other examples and a list of the results are published elsewhere (Vieth 1990a).

In this study we were able to demonstrate for the first time the localization of a purely functional ischemic lesion, the TIA. We could still localize TIAs more than 1 week after the short-lasting neurological deficit of a few minutes or hours (Vieth 1990a). Thus a basis exists for diagnosing clinically silent TIAs. Also, based on our epilepsy research we were able to detect, for the first time, very slow magnetic field changes (DC-coupled) associated with epileptic seizures (Vieth and Schüler 1989; Vieth et al. 1992).

The 37-Channel MEG

When using a 37-channel MEG system, activity can be recorded at all the necessary measuring points simultaneously. Thus, the recording time is very short compared to single- or few-channel systems. More importantly, the spatial spread of brain activity is preserved with a high resolution in time of the electric processes (Vieth 1990a).

Dipole Pathways

In studying slow wave activity associated with brain lesions (ten patients with brain infarctions, TIAs, hemorrhages), we first of all used the dipole pathway method (Vieth 1990a). These pathways result from the connection of the centers of consecutively (every 10 ms) estimated dipoles of selected (manually or automatically) slow wave sections with a sufficient signal to noise (S/N) ratio. The dipoles of almost all of the many pathways were concentrated near one side of the lesion (Table 2). The pathway pattern itself was typically a zigzag of up to several centimeters. An example is shown in Fig. 2. These patterns indicate that they are the result of multiple pathological sources and/or are combined with background activity (Vieth 1990a).

The possible distortion of the pathways by background activity can be assumed as the dipole pathways of pure (bandpass filtered) α background activity may "migrate" up to 4 cm during one α-wave (Grummich et al. 1991). Therefore we used a digital filter to eliminate the α portion (0.5–6 Hz). In addition, we recorded with the eyes of the patients open to decrease the α content in the signal.

Dipole Density Plot

To separate pathological from background activity we used the dipole density plot (DDP) (Vieth 1990b; Vieth et al. 1990a). During the analysis

Table 2. Multichannel MEG recordings

Patient	Lesion	Lesion location	Dipole locations Pathways/DDP
1	Infarction	Left temporal	Concentrated near lesion/not done
2	Infarction	Left temporal	Concentrated near lesion/not done
3	Hemorrhage	Left parietal, occipital	Concentrated near lesion/not done
4	TIA	Left temporal	Concentrated/not done
5	Hemorrhage	Left parietal	Breathing artifacts
6	Lymphoma	Left temporal (extensive edema)	Concentrated near lesion/not done
7	Infarction	Left frontal, temporal	Near/not done
8	Epilepsy	Left temporal, EEG focus	Left temporal concentration/not done
9	Infarction	Right occipital	Concentrated near lesion/close
10	Hemorrhage	Right parietal	Concentrated near lesion/close

Comparison of the location of verified (by CT or MRI or in TIA by clinical symptoms) brain lesions (lesion location) with the dipole locations of abnormal slow wave brain activity.
MEG, magnetoencephalogram; DDP, dipole density plot.

(60 s), the DDP reveals the concentration of estimated dipoles around a focus of abnormal activity. The concentrating effect can be adjusted by filtering, by the limit of the minimal S/N ratio, by the size of the volume unit, and by the density limit of dipoles per unit volume. Similar to CT, the method uses a density plot of dipoles in a given spatial unit. Figure 3 shows two examples; they are also listed in Table 2.

Basically, the DDP also can be applied to epileptic activity. Thus Sato (1991) used as a "prestep" a scatter plot of dipole locations of epileptic spike activity, as recorded by a 37-channel system (Biomagnetic Technologies Inc., San Diego, CA, USA), to demonstrate the area of spike generation.

The next step was the application of multidipole models. We started by making use of the α-rhythm as a model. Early results showed two main components (right and left occipital) as determined by factor analysis (Grummich et al. 1991).

Summary

The MEG seems to be a valuable tool to localize electrical, focal, abnormal, brain activity. Using a single-channel MEG system the localization of focal

Functional Imaging Methods (Computerized Electroencephalographic Topography)

Psychiatry and Microstates of the Brain's Electric Field: Towards the "Atoms of Thought and Emotion"

D. LEHMANN[1]

A primary characteristic of conscious private experiences is their sequential occurrence; one thought or idea is followed by the next one. The speed of this sequence varies and in extreme stages might become a hallmark of psychopathology. The apparent "size" of the momentary private experience, i.e., the magnitude (in terms of chunks of information, or better, in terms of topics) of what is being held in consciousness at a given moment in time appears to be limited. There are the famous 7 ± 2 items which can be held in short-term memory. One cannot pay full conscious attention to several things simultaneously (the "party conversation problem"). It thus appears that, in normal states, one cannot mentally treat several problems simultaneously. Aberrations from this rule, for instance coexistence of several hallucinatory experiences or coexistence of reality-induced and hallucinatory experiences, are recognized as typical of hypnagogic states at sleep onset ("synesthesia") or as pathological.

These considerations refer to subjectively identifiable thoughts, i.e., as one is inclined to say, "complete thoughts," and do not refer to some putative steps within thoughts. We assume steps must exist because: (1) information processing necessarily is a time-dependent process, and might well consist of concatenated sub-procedures, (2) there are indications of "steps" in cleverly designed motor reaction time experiments and, (3) there are suggestions of "steps" in studies of brain electric event-related data (see, e.g., Brandeis and Lehmann 1989; Pfurtscheller and Klimesch 1990).

In fact, "step"-type parts of thoughts are not thoughts any more. Using a crude metaphor: the parts of an automobile are not the automobile – many parts of an automobile could be parts of something very different from an automobile, for instance, floor mats, screws, bulbs, fuses, wheels, or even the engine. Soon, such simple allegories fail in the details. However, I wish to focus on the idea that a conscious thought is a phenomenon that consists of the sequential (not only parallel) occurrence and presence of very many subevents and local brain processes, from the molecular level to the level of local neuronal discharges, without any single one of them constituting by itself the thought. Only the complete description of all relationships (in

[1] Abt. für Neurologie, Universitätsspital Zürich, 8091 Zürich, Switzerland.

Imaging of the Brain in Psychiatry and Related Fields
Edited by K. Maurer

space and time) between all participating parts will be a correct representation of the thought. However, a description which uses lower level parts but adds all relationships between parts obviously is no longer a description of the lower level any more, even though the parts by themselves are on a level which is lower than that of the described phenomenon (in our case the thought). In addition, in order to deal with high level phenomena it might be uneconomical to resort to lower levels. The classical example for this consideration is the measurement of temperative in a room: measuring Brownian movement with sophisticated equipment leads to the possibility to work out the room temperature – information that can also be obtained by reading a thermometer bought across the street in a supermarket.

The question is whether there are adequate means to measure the brain's functional state on a level of objective phenomena that corresponds to the level of thought on the side of private conscious experiences. The brain's electromagnetic field appears to be a prime candidate for this: (1) It offers an extremely high temporal resolution, down to fractions of milliseconds, so that hypothetical thought representations in the subsecond range are expected to be resolvable. (2) It offers a very high sensitivity to changes in brain state, as documented in the extensive literature on effects of age, vigilance, presented information, medications, and diseases as determined by a multitude of spontaneous and event-related electroencephalogram (EEG) and magnetoencephalogram (MEG) measurements (e.g., Itil and Itil 1986; Koukkou and Manske 1986; John et al. 1989; Saletu 1989). (3) It is a homogeneous sum (even though it has detailed local structure) that invites treatment as a whole and thus is reminiscent of consciousness that presents as an undivisible entity of varying prominence (even though it is present only if a large set of conditions is met).

The brain electric field exhibits varying configurations over time; its scalp-measured "landscape" keeps changing (Lehmann et al. 1987). Multichannel EEG or MEG brain mapping demonstrates this most impressively. The momentary field's configuration is determined by the geometry of the neural elements which are momentarily active. It is reasonable to say that the electric landscape constituted by the field as measured on the scalp reflects the geometry of the momentarily active neural elements. Accordingly, if this landscape changes, a set of at least partially different electric elements must have become active. The activity of different elements, however, can reasonably be assumed to be associated with a different function of information processing executed by the brain.

It follows from the above that, in order to monitor cognition and to identify the conditions when cognition deviates from the norm, one could say that all one has to do is to establish a complete catalogue of the brain electric states, map the landscapes, i.e., the brain, and identify these states with cognitive/emotional/perceptional states. In theory, it is of no relevance how many parallel and local substates contribute to a given global state; the number of possible substates would only increase the number of possible global states. In practice, the number of possible global states quickly becomes very large with increasing numbers of substates. Hereby, the practical possibility to identify them all using scalp EEG data diminishes with increasing numbers of local substates. The prime questions thus are heuristic: Is it possible to identify different global functional states of the brain using the recordable electric landscape on the scalp? Is it possible to identify such states with subjectively experienced cognition/emotion/perception? How good is the resolution of the states, i.e., do the practical constraints permit the description of a useful set of different global states?

The putative, global, functional states of the brain discussed here refer, in the extreme case, to instantaneous states, since conceivably the configuration of the brain electric field might change at a very high rate. The actual rate of change will be discussed below. Before we do this, let me back up to survey classical observations on brain states. I wish to clarify in the following that the presently discussed instantaneous microstates are conceived as embedded into the conventional, longer-lasting macrostates defined by different EEG "wave" frequencies:

The most common example of spontaneously changing brain states is the change between attention, relaxed wakefulness, drowsiness, and sleep in a normal adult. It is clear that very different behaviors are associated with these states; particularly well known are the different types of mentation such as focused attention, thinking in logical categories in wakefulness, "day dreaming" in decreased vigilance, "hypnagogic hallucinations" with relaxed logic constraints during drowsiness leading to full-fledged dreams consisting of thought concatenations without reality checking and associated with possibly inadequate emotions (see also Koukkou and Lehmann 1983). The classical observation is that these different states are associated with very characteristically different EEG patterns in the time domain, i.e., with different dominant EEG wave frequencies detectable in single-channel EEG recording. These frequency patterns have proven to be very sensitive indicators of the different functional states, normal, pathological, and medication-induced (Itil and Itil 1986; Koukkou and Manske 1986; John et al. 1989; Saletu 1989), slower frequencies typically and systematically being associated with less vigilant, more sleep-like states.

Since these are patterns in the time domain, they naturally require a certain minimum time for recognition. Traditional work on EEG patterns analyzed epochs in the several minutes to seconds range, typically examining the data after transformation into the frequency domain (e.g., via Fourier transform). When methods for adaptive segmentation were utilized, the minimal time resolution came down to about a second, and with these minimal durations it was seen that quasistationary states defined with this time resolution might last for many seconds but might also be very short. Different states defined by this approach were associated with different motor reaction times (Gath et al. 1983). We think that this realm of state description is a very adequate approach to brain mechanisms, as obviously (and as also supported by our very different space-oriented approaches to EEG analysis) one basic aspect of brain electric mechanisms is their inherent periodicity. However, we propose to call the states that are recognized by their dominant temporal frequency or temporal pattern "global functional macrostates." These time-extending functional macrostates might consist of sequences of the putative "global functional microstates" which were proposed above. These are defined by the momentary electric landscape and conceptually require to time extension as a minimal requirement for recognition.

In several studies, we have examined the questions that I have formulated above about these putative momentary functional microstates. First, we investigated whether the microstates, defined by momentary map electric landscapes, persisted for recognizable epochs (Lehmann et al. 1987). Considering the basically periodic nature of brain electric activity, map polarity had to be disregarded and only landscape configuration was considered (accepting periodic reversing polarity). Six normal young subjects showed an average duration of quasistationary map landscape of 210 ms when we investigated the EEG alpha frequency band during relaxed wakefulness, but 50% of the analysis time was covered by microstates of stable landscape that were longer than 323 ms and 25% of the time by microstates that persisted for more than 508 ms. In summary, in terms of persisting momentary electric landscapes, microstates of varying durations can be observed. Their durations appear to be short enough to make them serious candidates for the building blocks of (conscious) cognition and emotion, for the "atoms of thought." We hypothesized, in 1987, that psychopathological conditions might be associated with aberrant durations, frequency of occurrence, or sequence of the classes of these microstates. Meanwhile, Merrin et al. (1990) reported that significantly more classes ("types") of microstates ("segments") in the theta frequency band occurred in schizophrenics than in normals and that medication reduced the number of classes of microstates.

Second, we tested the microstates in normals for possible behavioral correlates. In another study of eight normal subjects (Lehmann et al. 1987) we found that different classes of microstates (different maps) indeed corresponded to a measurable variable in behavior, selective motor reaction time to auditory stimuli. Between subjects there were similar differences in reaction time for the 26 microstate classes which occurred in all subjects (Friedman ANOVA $p < 0.025$). This shows that even in a subtle range of functional states, in terms of duration of state and range of state changes, the instantaneous microstate of the brain measurably influences the fate of incoming information.

If such gross measures as reaction time are affected by the momentarily existing microstate, more subtle phenomena such as conscious experience might be expected to be reflected by these states. Based on a series of experiments in humans, Libet (1982) suggested that there is a necessary minimal time of presence of information in the brain that qualifies the information to reach access to consciousness, and he estimated 500 ms for this. The question arises whether our microstates indeed can be the building blocks of consciousness, accepting Libet's conditions. As noted above, stable microstates of more than 508 ms covered only 25% of the time in our study. Of course, there are several methodological issues in the electric definition of a microstate, essentially related to the window/hysteresis problem of recognition. Accepting our results at face value for further speculation, it was interesting that some of the microstate landscapes in our study appeared to be much more "popular" than others: they reoccur frequently. On the average across the six subjects of the first study (Lehmann et al. 1987) the microstate class that was most "popular" covered about 20% of the total time, while it constituted 12% of all classes. May it be that reentering the same microstate repeatedly at some minimal interval can substitute for persistence, in order to qualify the microstate content for consciousness? It might also be that a brief repeated sequence of different microstates constitutes a higher unit that qualifies all participating states for consciousness – we have not yet systematically investigated possible rules of concatenations of microstates. It is also conceivable that, besides duration, the characteristic of intensity of the brain's electric condition – which is known to play a role in the access to consciousness (Libet 1982; Skrandies 1987) – might somehow be present in the microstate and not yet identified by us.

Recently, we performed a series of investigations that tested two hypotheses about the microstates: (1) that the putative brain functional microstates indeed are sufficiently characterized by one instantaneous brain electric map whose landscape may or may not be repeated at preceding or later times and thus belonging to a shorter or more extended state; determining a momentary map characterizes the momentary microstate. (2) that a given microstate reflects the type of momentary thought or emotion. The basis for this is, as stated above, that different types of thoughts or emotions are expected to involve different sets of activated neural elements in the brain, however subtle these differences might be in terms of activated sets or types of conscious experience.

In several earlier studies, lawful relations between mentations and extended EEG epochs were observed. In normal subjects, types of thoughts executed as tasks (e.g., visual imagery and numerical computations, Ehrlichmann and Wiener 1980; Makino et al. 1989) and types of spontaneous thoughts (e.g., visual imagery vs abstract thoughts during reverie, Lehmann et al. 1981) showed correlations with several frequency domain characteristics of the EEG time series during, say, 20 s after the command to perform a prespecified mentation or before the signal to report the preceding spontaneous thought. Since we suspect that execution of a particular type of thought might require powerful brain resources concerned with task execution with which the thought type might be confounded, so that thought type might be less prominent in the electric landscape, we prefer to study spontaneous unrestricted thoughts, classifying them post-hoc after elicited reporting. Encouraged by the studies of relations between fairly long EEG epochs and types of mentations, we decided to examine the hypothesis that the different microstates which we had recognized on formal grounds and which we had found to be associated with some information-processing differences in behavior might in fact represent different classes of subjective (private) experiences.

We have found support for this hypothesis in several studies (Lehmann et al. 1990; see also below) in which we collected the different types of freely varying spontaneous thoughts and investigated their relations to the momentary microstates defined by the brain electric maps. In general, the experimental design has been close to that of the latest study: the subjects were comfortably seated, and, at random intervals of about 3 min, were prompted by a gentle tone to briefly report what just had gone through their mind. The reports were tape recorded, transcribed, and each report was classed by two independent raters in various categories, for example, concerning the following classes in three categories: (1) as to visual imagery vs abstract thought; (2) as to content being related to past experience, present lab situation, or future planning; and (3) as to distinct emotions involved vs relaxed emotional condition (emotional load is considered as an inherent aspect of conscious experience, see Ciompi 1991), on the same level as strategy/type of thought (see Koukkou and Lehmann 1983). Typically in these studies, about 70% of the required classifications are unanimous between the two raters; these are then used for further analysis.

The continuously recorded multichannel EEG recordings were searched backwards from the prompt for the last moment of maximal strength of the brain electric map before the prompt signal (among other reasons, in order to use data with an optimal signal to noise ratio). Typically, this map was found within 50 ms preceding the prompt and was accepted as representing the putative momentary brain state during the thought/emotion reported a brief moment later after the prompt.

A map's landscape is described most parsimoniously by the locations of its most positive and most negative potential values, i.e., the locations of the two extreme values of the map. For each subject, the locations of these extremes of all maps associated with each class of thought and emotion were collected. For each subject, the median location of all extremes was computed for each class of thought and emotion. Finally, the grand median locations of the extremes across subjects were computed for each class of thought and emotion. The differences in location between classes of the same category were statistically compared using paired tests.

The locations of the extreme potentials are not only a primary formal descriptor and classifier of landscape. Adopting a single-generator model of brain electric state, the locations of the map's potential extremes led to an estimate of the location of the hypothetical brain generator: the first estimate is the center point between the two extremes (centroid or center of gravity). Since the momentary maps evidently contain an appreciable amount of noise, we computed the median location of the extremes collected from all maps belonging to the same class in a given thought/emotion category to achieve a robust estimate of the hypothetical generator location. Let me note here that the concept is not directly concerned with hypothetical generators. Rather, the location of the hypothetical generator is taken as a data reducing descriptor of the entire landscape of the map that characterizes a microstate: if the location of the extracted location differs, a different map and hence a different microstate must have been present (different microstates by definition are generated by at least partially different generators, see above).

With B. Henggeler, another study was done on the hypothesized relation between types of spontaneous conscious mentation and brain functional microstates defined by electric map landscapes. We examined 13 male volunteers who were prompted 30 times for reports of subjective experiences in three recording sessions each. Significant differences in the grand median locations of the map extreme values were observed in the anterior-posterior direction on the scalp between microstate maps associated with: (1) thoughts related to the past vs thoughts related to the present, (2) thoughts related to the past vs thoughts related to the future, and (3) reports rated as associated with emotions (positive or negative) vs reports associated with a relaxed emotional condition. Significant across the 13 subjects, microstates concerning "past" were more posterior than "present" and "future"; microstates concerning "emotional" conditions were more posterior than those associated with a relaxed emotion.

The evidence in the reported series of pilot studies suggests that it is possible to recognize short-lasting brain functional microstates in the subsecond range when utilizing the momentary spatial distribution of the brain electric field. Given microstates are stable for varying brief durations and show a rapid transition into the next state, not only in event-related potential studies (Brandeis and Lehmann 1989) but also in spontaneous EEGs, as discussed above. The data indicate that input during different microstates leads to different motor reaction times and that different types of spontaneous thoughts and emotions are associated with different microstates that existed immediately prior to the report of the private experience. This suggests that the microstates defined by brain electric map landscapes might qualify for the electric representation of conscious mentation, as building blocks or "atoms of thought and emotions."

It is hypothesized that normal and pathological brain mechanisms of mentation might differ in the vocabulary (repertoire), the concatenations (syntax), and the frequencies of occurrence (see Merrin et al. 1990) of these microstates.

References

Brandeis D, Lehmann D (1989) Segments of event-related potential map series reveal landscape changes with visual attention and subjective contours. Electroencephalogr Clin Neurophysiol 73:507–519

Ciompi L (1991) Affects as central organizing and integrating factors; a new psychosocial/biological model of the psyche. Br J Psychiatry 159:97–105

Ehrlichman H, Wiener MS (1980) EEG asymmetry during covert mental activity. Psychophysiology 17:228–235

Gath I, Lehmann D, Bar-On E (1983) Fuzzy clustering of EEG signal and vigilance performance. Int J Neurosci 20:303–312

Itil T, Itil KZ (1986) CEEG and dynamic brain mapping in the bioavailability and bioequivalence of psychotropic drugs. In: Shagass C, Josiassen RC, Roemer RA (eds) Brain electric potentials and psychopathology. Elsevier, Amsterdam, pp 345–358

John ER, Prichep LS, Fridman J, Easton P (1989) Neurometrics: computer-assisted differential diagnosis of brain dysfunctions. Science 239:162–169

Koukkou M, Lehmann D (1983) Dreaming: the functional state-shift hypothesis. Br J Psychiatry 142:221–231

Koukkou M, Manske W (1986) Functional states of the brain and schizophrenic states of behavior. In: Shagass C, Josiassen RC, Roemer RA (eds) Brain electric potentials and psychopathology. Elsevier, Amsterdam, pp 91–114

Lehmann D, Koukkou M, Andreae A (1981) Classes of day-dream mentation and EEG power spectra. Sleep Res 10:152

Lehmann D, Ozaki H, Pal I (1987) EEG alpha map series: brain micro-states by space oriented adaptive segmentation. Electroencephalogr Clin Neurophysiol 67:271–288

Lehmann D, Kofmel BA, Weiss Y (1990) The atoms of thought: momentary EEG state and classes of subjective experiences during "day dreaming." Brain Topography 2:247

Libet B (1982) Brain stimulation in the study of neuronal functions for conscious experience. Hum Neurobiol 1:235–242

Makino A, Horie S, Ebisutani D, Matsumoto K (1989) Topographical display of EEG change during mental task. In: Tsutsui J (ed) EEG Topography 1987. Neuron, Shinagawa, Tokyo, pp 47–56

Merrin EL, Meek P, Floyd TC, Callaway E (1990) Topographic segmentation of waking EEG in medication-free schizophrenic patients. Int J Psychophysiol 9:231–236

Pfurtscheller G, Klimesch W (1990) Topographical display and interpretation of event-related desynchronization during a visual-verbal task. Brain Topography 3:85–93

Saletu B (1989) EEG imaging of brain activity in clinical psychopharmacology. In: Maurer K (ed) Topographic brain mapping of EEG and evoked potentials. Springer, Berlin Heidelberg New York, pp 482–506

Skrandies W (1987) Visual persistence of stereoscopic stimuli: electric brain activity without perceptual correlate. Vision Res 27:2109–2118

Mapping of Scalp Potential Fields Elicited by Cortical Generators: The Use of Dynamic Random Dot Stereograms

W. SKRANDIES[1]

The mammalian visual system offers a unique possibility to study electrophysiologically cortical neuronal mechanisms without interference by subcortical activity. Since the input of the two eyes remains separated up to the level of the visual cortex, evoked potential components generated exclusively by cortical structures may be investigated when dynamic random dot stereograms (RDS; Julesz 1960, 1971) are presented binocularly. The perception of such stereograms depends on the fusion of two, nonidentical, horizontally disparate, monocular inputs in the visual cortex. Under monocular viewing conditions a given RDS stimulus cannot be perceived stereoscopically (see below and data in Fig. 1C).

This article will describe the topographical features of stereoscopically evoked responses in humans derived from multichannel recordings of electrical brain activity using an electrode array over the occipital brain areas. Evoked potentials were obtained from both healthy adults and from patients with reduced stereovision. Dynamic RDS stimuli were presented as stereoscopic checkerboard patterns in different parts of the visual field resulting in the perception of a checkerboard pattern standing in front of the display, and the stereoscopically elicited scalp potential distributions were compared to those evoked by conventional two-dimensional checkerboard reversal stimuli of the same mean luminance and retinal extension (for technical details see Skrandies and Vomberg 1985; Skrandies 1987, 1991). In all our experiments only local changes of horizontal disparity occur and the RDS stimulus can be perceived throughout the recording epoch; thus no attentional effects are introduced in the stereo condition. As a control, a comparable checkerboard pattern with contrast borders is presented in an identical fashion on the same monitor, and all stimulus parameters are as similar as possible to the RDS in order to produce a comparison stimulus in which only the contrast change triggers the visual evoked potential (VEP). In this way we are able to compare directly the effects of contrast inversion (contrast stimulus) and local disparity changes in selected parts of the display (stereo stimulus).

[1] Physiologisches Institut, Justus-Liebig-Universität, Aulweg 129, W-6300 Giessen, FRG.

Imaging of the Brain in Psychiatry and Related Fields
Edited by K. Maurer

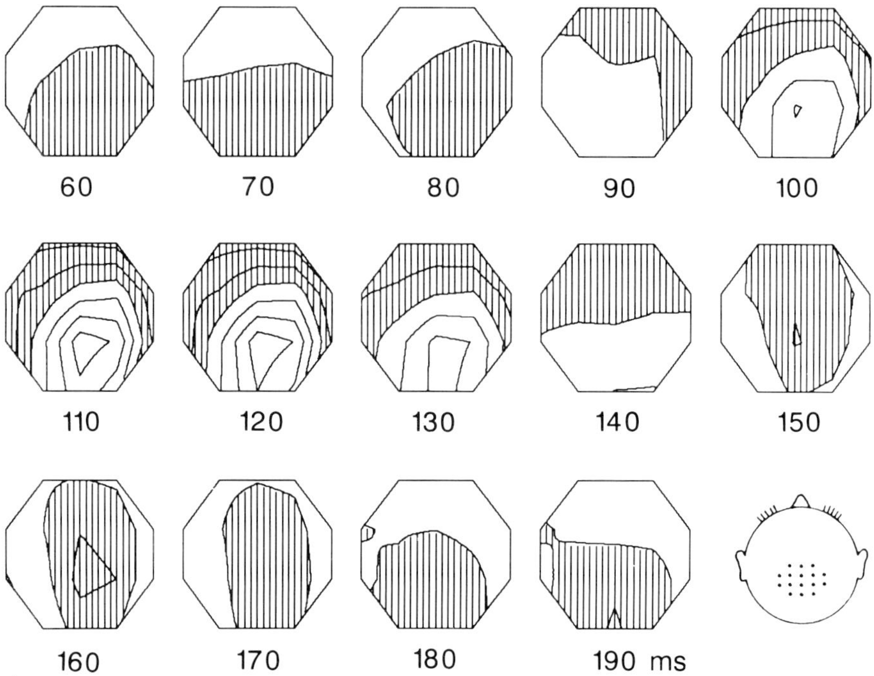
60
70
80
90
100
110
120
130
140
150
160
170
180
190 ms

A

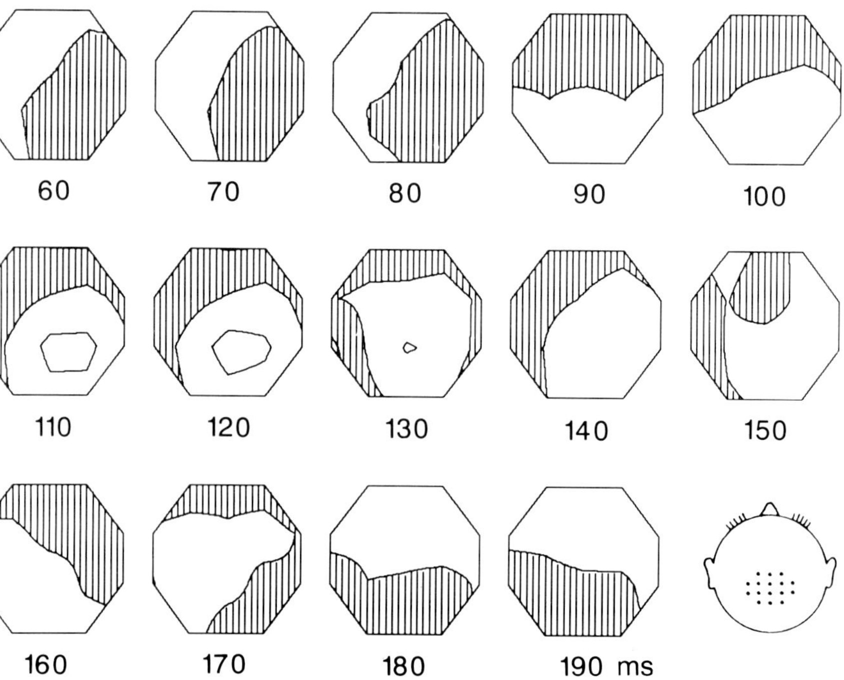
60
70
80
90
100
110
120
130
140
150
160
170
180
190 ms

B

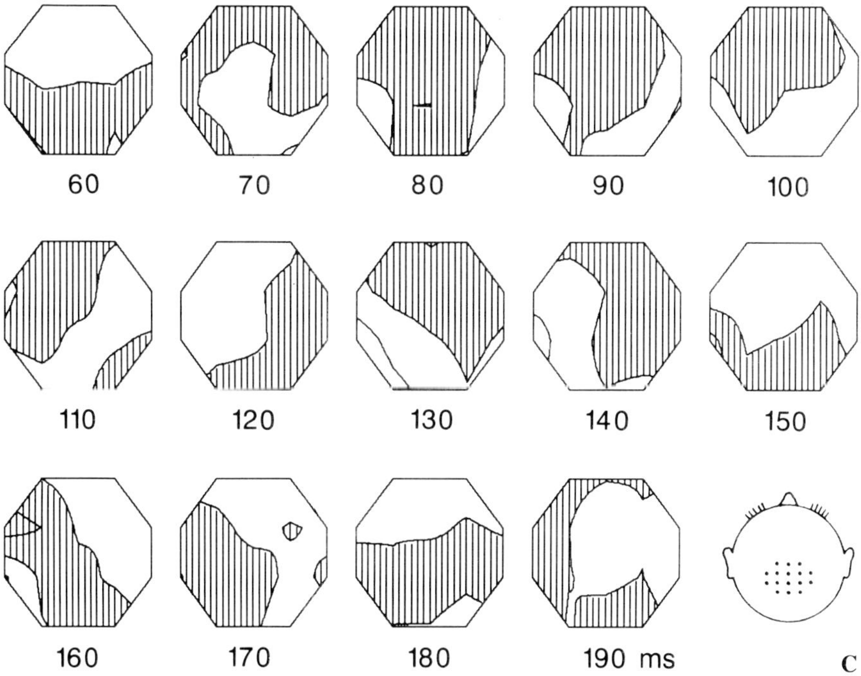

Fig. 1A–C. Potential map series between 60 and 190 ms evoked in different stimulus conditions. **A** Contrast reversal stimuli (65% contrast) presented with central fixation. **B** Dynamic random dot stimuli (disparity changes of 9.6 min of arc) presented binocularly as red-green anaglyphs with central fixation. **C** Control condition in which the same random dot stereogram (RDS) stimuli as in **B** were presented monocularly. Note that no stimulus locked activity may be seen. Numbers give poststimulus times in milliseconds; equipotential lines are in steps of 2 μV for **A** and 1 μV for **B** and **C**; electrode array with regular interelectrode distances between the inion and Pz (see *inset*); average reference data; *hatched areas* are negative.

The size of the test field (10.8° × 14.6°), mean luminance (16 cd/m^2), and spectral composition of the display were identical in all stimulus conditions

Major differences between stereoscopic and contrast evoked brain activity are found in the strength of the potential fields and in their topographic characteristics. However, the latencies of the major occipital components which correspond to the conventional P100 component are not influenced by stimulus mode (see also Skrandies and Vomberg 1985; Skrandies 1986, 1991), suggesting that the binocular information flow to the visual cortex has a similar time course for both the processing of contrast borders and dynamic RDS stimuli.

Potential distributions evoked by a contrast reversal stimulus characteristically display an occipital positivity about 120 ms following the stimulus (see Fig. 1A). Component latency was determined quantitatively by the computation of global field power (GFP, Lehmann and Skrandies 1980;

Skrandies 1989), and it was maximal for the contrast evoked activity shown in Fig. 1A at 116 ms.

Stereoscopically evoked brain activity has a very similar appearance with a concentrically organized positivity over the occiput in the latency range of the P100 component. Figure 1B shows the corresponding potential fields of the same subject evoked by a depth reversal (i.e., disparity change of 9.6 min arc) of a checkerboard pattern of the same mean luminance and retinal extension as the contrast stimulus used to generate the data in Fig. 1A. The occipital positivity coincides with maximal GFP at 120 ms indicating that there are similar component latencies for contrast and disparity evoked brain activity. This was repeatedly observed in various subject populations (Skrandies and Vomberg 1985; Skrandies 1986, 1987, 1991).

An important control in all RDS experiments consists in the proof that the observed activity is generated selectively by disparity-sensitive neurons and that there are no monocular cues. Figure 1C illustrates the results of monocular fixation of the display when RDS patterns are presented in the same way as for Fig. 1B. It is obvious that no stimulus related brain activity is elicited in this condition (compare Fig. 1B and 1C). Thus only binocular disparity-sensitive neurones are excited by the presentation of our dynamic RDS patterns.

The latencies of the evoked components are similar for contrast and stereoscopic stimuli, while significant differences occur with the strength of the evoked potential fields, as is evident from Fig. 1. The amplitudes of the fields are much higher for the contrast than the stereo condition (note that the fields in Fig. 1A and B are scaled differently). This is also reflected in the GFP values (4.14 μV for contrast stimuli; 0.73 μV for stereo stimuli) suggesting that RDS stimuli are less effective in exciting many neurones simultaneously. One possible interpretation of this finding is that there are fewer neurones in the visual cortex that are selectively sensitive to binocular disparate stimuli than there are neurones responding to contrast changes. It also appears conceivable that there are more contrast-sensitive neurones than there are disparity-sensitive neurones. This interpretation is in line with our previous data obtained from patients with reduced stereovision; in these patients the electrical brain activity evoked by dynamic RDS patterns displayed smaller amplitudes (and longer latencies) than in healthy controls. In such patients there occurs an inverse linear relationship between stereoscopically evoked potential amplitudes and psychophysical disparity thresholds ($r = 0.80$) while in stereoblind patients no such VEP activity may be obtained (Vomberg and Skrandies 1985).

It is also evident from Fig. 1B that stereoscopic stimuli elicit potential fields that are symmetrical with respect to the sagittal midline. The interhemispheric symmetry of the potential fields was quantitatively assessed in a larger subject population (Skrandies 1991), and the results support our earlier findings that no differences of electrical brain activity between the

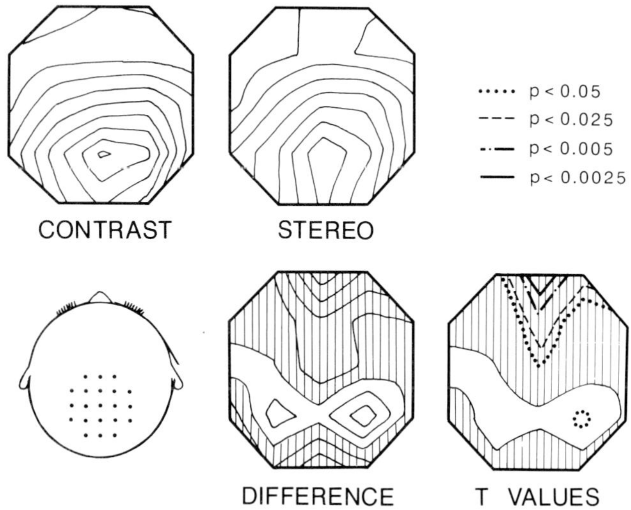

Fig. 2. *Top*: Grand mean potential distribution maps of 13 subjects at component latency scaled individually to an equal potential range (*lines* are in steps of 10% of the potential range). *Bottom*: Difference map (contrast-stereo) (*lines* in steps of 4%) and significance probability map illustrating direct comparisons of the complete potential field distributions at component latency by computations of paired *t* tests using the amplitude values of 13 subjects recorded from 21 occipital electrodes (individual data were scaled in order to remove extreme values). With stereoscopic stimuli significantly larger amplitudes are found over more anterior brain areas while significantly larger amplitudes are evoked by contrast over posterior areas. Negative areas are *hatched*; significance levels as indicated. Equal spacing between electrodes with an electrode array as in *inset*: the most anterior electrode is in the midline at Pz and the most posterior midline electrode is at the inion. (Data from Skrandies 1991)

left and the right hemisphere are observed when the subjects are presented dynamic RDS stimuli (Skrandies 1987). This suggests that the visual areas of both hemispheres of the human brain are able to process horizontally disparate information. Slightly larger differences are observed, however, over the right hemisphere when stereoscopic and contrast evoked field distributions are compared directly (Fig. 2).

Topographical differences between stereo and contrast evoked activity also become evident when the whole scalp field distributions are compared directly. Figure 2 illustrates the mean potential distributions computed from the data of 13 subjects at individual GFP latency of the P100 component. Differences in absolute field strength were removed by scaling the data of each subject to an equal potential range of the scalp field. Thus, Fig. 2 shows differences in the field characteristics independent of the amplitude differences described above. The results of the corresponding statistical comparison are also displayed in Fig. 2 as scalp distributions of *t* values as a significance probability map. With central retinal stimuli, the difference map shows a topographic pattern roughly symmetrical with respect to the midline. Stereoscopic evoked activity is significantly larger mainly over more frontal regions within the electrode array (corresponding to Pz) while contrast evoked activity is more pronounced posteriorly at Oz (Fig. 2, lower half). This is in line with our finding of a more anterior component location for stereoscopically evoked brain activity (Skrandies and Vomberg 1985; Skrandies 1986, 1991). We also note that significant lateral topographic differences between stereoscopic and contrast evoked brain activity have been found when lateralized stimuli were investigated (Skrandies 1991). All these data indicate that stereoscopic perception in humans relies on the activation of different cortical structures than the perception of contrast stimuli.

In summary, the cortical processing of both contrast and stereoscopic stimuli revealed by multichannel evoked potential recordings has a similar time course, while there appear to be fewer neurones activated by dynamic RDS stimuli. Our findings suggest that stereoscopic stimuli activate neuronal populations outside area 17. This interpretation is consistent with data derived from animal experiments which have shown that area 18 contains more neurones that are sensitive to binocular disparate stimuli than area 17 (Hubel and Wiesel 1970, 1973; von der Heydt et al. 1981). In addition, stereoscopic and contrast stimuli appear to be processed in a different way, as our earlier findings on the electrophysiological and perceptual persistence of visual stimuli have demonstrated (Skrandies 1987).

Acknowledgement. Dr. Ch. Michel, Department of Neurology, University Hospital Zürich, helped with programming.

References

Hubel DH, Wiesel TN (1970) Cells sensitive to binocular depth in area 18 of the macaque monkey cortex. Nature 225:41–42

Hubel DH, Wiesel TN (1973) A re-examination of stereoscopic mechanisms in area 17 of the cat. J Physiol (Lond) 232:29P–30P

Julesz B (1960) Binocular depth perception of computer-generated patterns. Bell Syst Tech J 39:1125–1162

Julesz B (1971) Foundations of cyclopean perception. University of Chicago Press, Chicago, p 406

Lehmann D, Skrandies W (1980) Reference-free identification of components of checkerboard-evoked multichannel potential fields. Electroencephalogr Clin Neurophysiol 48:609–621

Skrandies W (1986) Visual evoked potential topography: methods and results. In: Duffy FH (ed) Topographic mapping of brain electrical activity. Butterworths, Boston, pp 7–28

Skrandies W (1987) Visual persistence of stereoscopic stimuli: electric brain activity without perceptual correlate. Vision Res 27:2109–2118

Skrandies W (1989) Data reduction of multichannel fields: global field power and principal components. Brain Topography 2:73–80

Skrandies W (1991) Contrast and stereoscopic visual stimuli yield lateralized scalp potential fields associated with different neural generators. Electroencephalogr Clin Neurophysiol 78:274–283

Skrandies W, Vomberg HE (1985) Stereoscopic stimuli activate different cortical neurones in man: electrophysiological evidence. Int J Psychophysiol 2:293–296

Vomberg HE, Skrandies W (1985) Untersuchung des Stereosehens im Zufallspunktmuster-VECP: Normbefunde und klinische Anwendung. Klin Monatsbl Augenheilkd 187:205–208

von der Heydt R, Hänni P, Dürsteler M, Peterhans E (1981) Neuronal responses to stereoscopic stimuli in the alert monkey – a comparison between striate and prestriate cortex. Pfügers Arch 391:R34

EEG Characteristics of Aggression with Respect to Sorrow and Joy

S. Debus[1], W. Machleidt, and H. Hinrichs

Introduction

The goal of psychophysiological research of basic emotion is an answer to the question: Is there an apparent relationship between the phenomenological characterization of emotion and physiological patterns? The process involves a detailed description of different emotional dispositions, observable variables of behavior, and physiological measurements.

Based on extensive empirical studies, the latest concept of basic emotion (Machleidt et al. 1989) in psychophysiological electroencephalogram (EEG) research is that the spontaneous activity of the EEG is specifically modulated by emotional disposition. Both phenomenological and EEG analytical differentiation increase with the intensity of emotion. The identification of five basic emotions, intention, anxiety, aggression, sorrow, and joy, resulted in a psychological understanding of emotion (Izard 1977; Lungwitz 1947). Six dynamic EEG parameters (Machleidt 1982, 1987; Machleidt et al. 1989) could be analyzed. These are summarized in Table 1. The θ, α, and β powers increase with aggression, while α peak frequency and α bandwidth remain unchanged. The aim of a follow-up study was to validate these results by replication (Debus 1990). For instance, according to Machleidt (1987), contrasting aggression with sorrow should result in differences in the θ, α and β bands; contrasting aggression with joy should lead to differences primarily in the θ and β bands. Here, we present two case reports from this follow-up study.

Methods

Based on the different emotional dispositions of the volunteers, as described in their biographies, we devised an imagination exercise. The volunteers sit or lie down on a comfortable couch and describe a positive and negative event from their lives. The volunteers close their eyes and EEG recording begins. They are then requested to allow uncontrolled flow of their ideas

[1] Neurologische Klinik, Med. Hochschule Hannover, Konstanty-Gutschow-Str. 8, W-3000 Hannover, FRG.

Imaging of the Brain in Psychiatry
and Related Fields
Edited by K. Maurer

Table 1. Differentiation of five basic emotions by six spectral EEG parameters

EEG parameter	Intention	Anxiety	Aggression	Sorrow	Joy
α Power	Increase	Decrease	Increase	Decrease	Increase
α Modus	Increase	Increase	Unchanged	Decrease	Unchanged
α Bandwidth	Decrease	Increase	Unchanged	Increase	Decreased
θ Power	Unchanged	Increase	Increase	Decrease	Decrease
β Power	Unchanged	Increase	Increase	Decrease	Decrease
Complexity	Decrease	Increase	Decrease	Increase	Decrease

Dynamic with increasing intensity of emotion. Anxiety, joy, aggression, and sorrow are characterized by opposite changes of EEG parameters. Intention shows typical changes in α parameters. Complexity behaves analogous to α power. Differentiation of the various emotions is possible by means of multivariate discriminant analysis of the six EEG parameters.

and imagination. We subsequently offer keywords during the free association phase, thereby reactivating life event memories. At the end of the exercise a catamnestic interview follows. Later, while viewing a videorecording of the exercise, the volunteers are asked to comment and to rate their own psychodynamic. The emotional epochs are registered (Künkel 1972) on a 13-channel EEG recorder and video-tape (electrode montage: Fp1, Fp2, F7, F8, F3, F4, Fz, T3, T4, C3, C4, Cz unipolar vs A2 according to the 10–20 system).

The psychophysiological information is analyzed according to the following scheme: After EEG recording the intensity and quality of emotions are rated by means of anamnesis, videorecording, catamnesis, and self-rating. Independent rating is performed synchronously with the EEG every 12 s by two psychologically trained raters. Only those segments in which the raters agreed in their assessment of the basic emotion are statistically analyzed. The EEG signals are evaluated by means of spectral analysis resulting in one spectrum every 12 s. The ratings of emotion (quality and average intensity) are correlated with the EEG spectra (Fig. 1). Finally, the data are interpreted in three stages: Stage 1 describes the psychic context; notice is taken of, e.g., physical sensations in special psychodynamic constellations and regression. Stage 2 involves testing nonparametrically (Mann-Whitney) the spectral parameters of all basic emotions against each other including hemispheric asymmetries. Topographic maps of spectral parameters are computed by two-dimensional interpolating splines (programs in Engeln-Müllges and Reutter 1988). With respect to the limited number of EEG channels, mapping is restrained to the frontal cortex region. In stage 3, correlation of spectral parameters with the rated emotional intensity scale is estimated along with testing of the regression line against a zero slope.

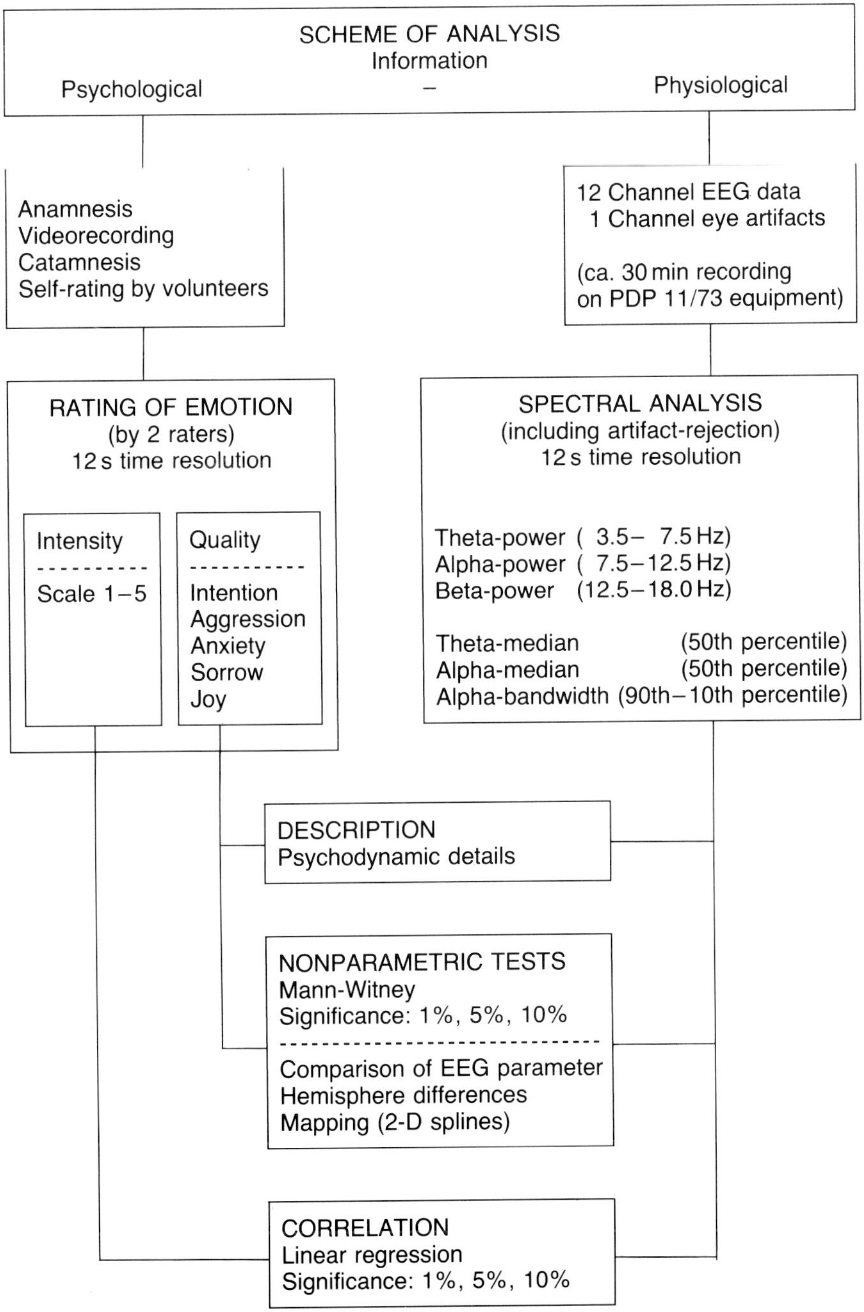

Fig. 1. Three stages of analyzing psychophysiological information. The choice of spectral parameters differs slightly from those given in Table 1. Since complexity did not supply any new information, it was replaced by the θ median; instead of α modus we chose the α median, which proved to be more stable

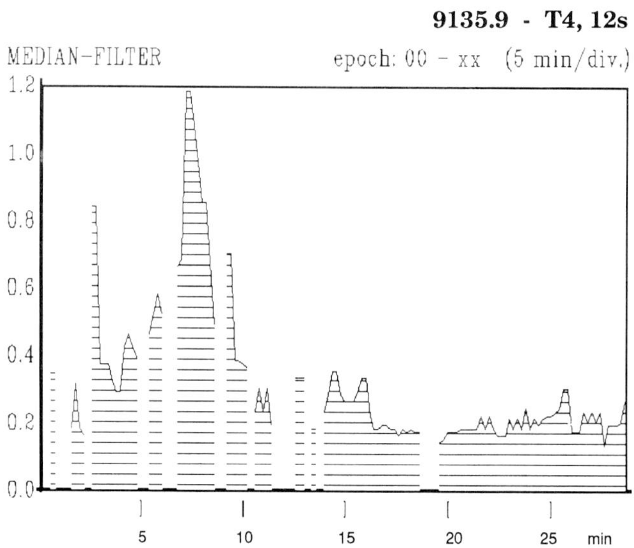

Fig. 2. Increase of α power with aggression, decrease with sorrow. α EEG derived at location F4. The 12 s intervals that were completely contaminated by artifacts are left as blank areas. ⊟, Alpha-Power

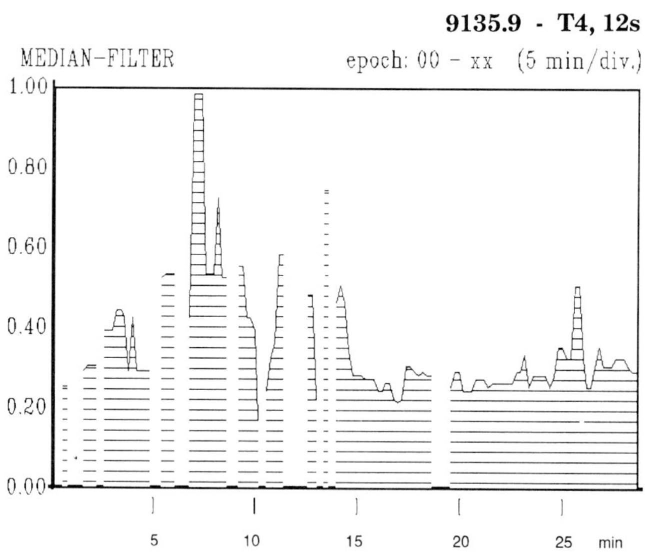

Fig. 3. The θ power dynamic. See legend to Fig. 2 for details. ⊟, Theta-Power

Table 2. EEG 9135: correlation of spectral parameters with rated intensity of aggression

Topography	Fp1	Fp2	F7	F8	F3	F4	Fz	T3	T4	C3	C4	Cz
θ Power			NS	+++	+	+++	+++		+++	++	+++	+++
α Power			++	NS	+++	+++	++		+++	+++	+++	+++
β Power			NS	NS	++	++	NS		+++	++	++	+
α Bandwidth			NS	NS	NS	+	NS		++	NS	NS	NS
θ Median			NS	++	NS	NS	NS		NS	NS	NS	NS
α Median			NS	NS	NS	NS	NS		NS	NS	NS	NS

There is a significant increase of θ, α, and β, power with aggression. Channels Fp1, Fp2, and T3 are excluded from analysis because of contamination by artifacts. Significance levels increase: +, 10%; ++, 5%; +++, 1%; NS, not significant.

Results

Case report; EEG 9135. In the imagination exercise, the female volunteer relives the aggression towards her reproachful and discriminating mother. With increasing α power (minute 4–9, see Fig. 2) she tries aggressively to defend herself against these reproaches. At minute 9, despair, a mixed emotion comprised of aggression and sorrow, occurs and slowly transforms the aggression into deeply depressed sorrow. From minute 17 to the end of the exercise, the epoch of pure sorrow is accompanied by low levels of α power. Until the climax of aggression (minute 9), the dynamic θ power (Fig. 3) increases parallel to α power. The power of the θ, α, and β bands decreases with increasing sorrow. This typical dynamic of aggression and sorrow is not restrained to one channel and can be shown throughout the topography.

Table 2 summarizes the significance of six spectral parameters: with aggression the power of the θ, α, and β bands increases. The α bandwidth and θ and α medians remain unchanged.

Case report; EEG 9015. The volunteer, a practitioner of Zen meditation, relives a LSD trip he had 10 years ago. His destructive fantasies are imagined in pictures of aggressive cars and very large attacking eagles. With increasing aggression the β power increases up to the climax in minute 15. Then the aggression slackens until minute 25 when the volunteer becomes more quiet. He reports feelings of euphoria at the end of the session (Fig. 4). Comparing Tables 2 and 3 there is a remarkable parallelism between the spectral dynamic and aggression.

Looking for lateralization effects of emotion, we tested the hemispheric differences (difference: mean of all channels on the left side − mean of all channels on the right side) with respect to the different emotions. The result

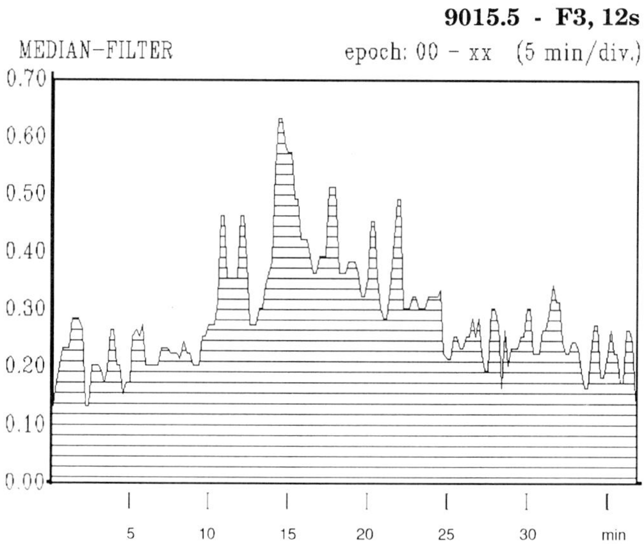

Fig. 4. Modulation of β power with varying intensity of highest level of aggression at minute 15. β EEG obtained at location F3. The EEG is almost free of artifacts. ⊟, Beta-Power

Table 3. EEG 9015: correlation of spectral parameters with rated intensity of aggression

Topography	Fp1	Fp2	F7	F8	F3	F4	Fz	T3	T4	C3	C4	Cz
θ Power	NS	++	+	NS	++	++	+++	+	NS	++	+	++
α Power	+++	+++	+++	+++	++	+++	++	+++	NS	++	++	++
β Power	+++	+++	+++	++	++	NS	+	+++	NS	+++	+	+++
α Bandwidth	NS	NS	NS	NS	NS	NS	NS	NS	NS	NS	NS	NS
θ Median	NS	NS	NS	NS	NS	NS	NS	NS	NS	NS	NS	NS
α Median	NS	NS	NS	NS	NS	NS	NS	+++	NS	NS	NS	NS

There is a significant increase of θ, α, and β, power with aggression. Significance levels increase: +, 10%; ++, 5%; +++, 1%; NS, not significant.

was that, although we could find some significant changes of side differences in the α and β powers, these effects were not systematic and were only of intraindividual relevance. To illustrate the topographic side effects, maps of the α power with respect to aggression and joy are shown in Fig. 5a and 5b respectively.

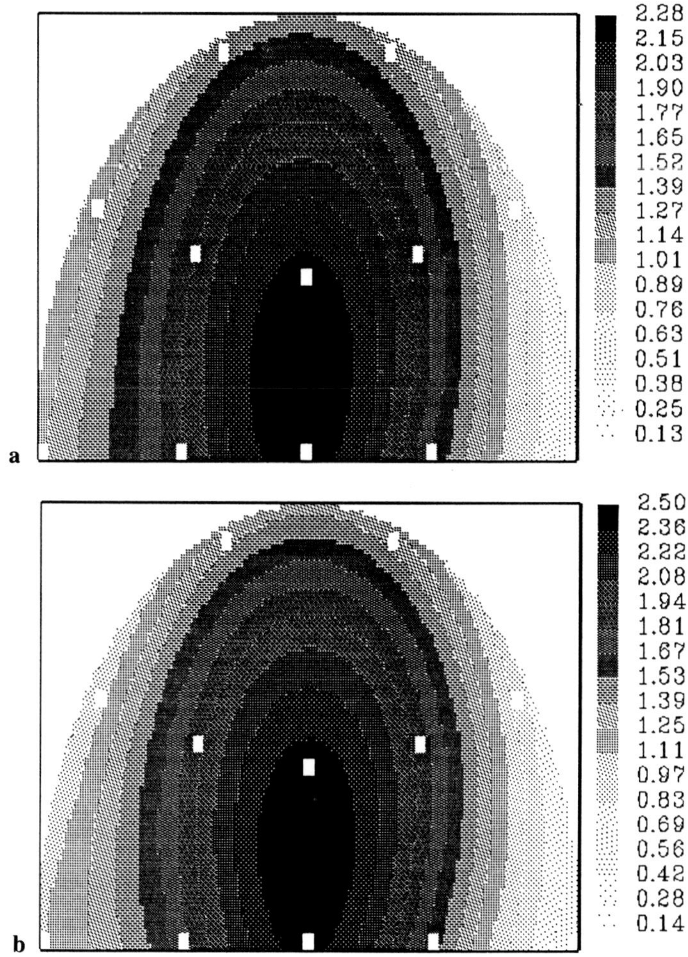

Fig. 5a,b. Mappings of α power with respect to aggression (**a**) and joy (**b**) in both frontal hemispheres (position of electrodes marked with *white squares*). There is no systematic indication of "affective split brain"

Conclusions

Two single case studies are presented which support the hypothesis that aggression, as a basic emotion, may be specifically identified by EEG spectral parameters, as predicted by the basic emotion model (Table 1). The same result is found within the entire collective. The absence of systematic side effects confirms the holistic point of view, that basic emotions are not lateralized.

References

Debus S (1990) EEG-dynamic in basic emotion and regression. Clin Neurophysiol 20:47

Engeln-Müllges G, Reutter F (1988) Formelsammlung zur numerischen Mathematik mit Standard-Fortran 77 Programmen. BI Wissenschaftsverlag, Mannheim

Izard CE (1977) Human emotions. Plenum, New York

Künkel H (1972) Simultane Vielkanal-Online-EEG-Analyse in Echtzeit. Z EEG-EMG 3:30

Lungwitz H (1947) Die Entdeckung der Seele. de Gruyter, Berlin

Machleidt W (1982) Emotionelles Erleben im EEG. Ein Beitrag zur biologischen und sozialen Fundierung psychodynamischer Abläufe. Thesis, Medical School Hanover

Machleidt W (1987) Systematisierung affektiver Verläufe mit der EEG-Spektralanalyse In: Weinmann H (ed) Zugang zum Verständnis höherer Hirnfunktionen. Zuckschwerdt, Munich

Machleidt W, Gutjahr L, Mügge A (1989) Grundgefühle. Springer, Berlin Heidelberg New York

The Quantification of Variability in Event-Related Potentials and Its Application to Schizophrenia*

J. ANDERSON[1], C. RENNIE, E. GORDON, and R. MEARES

Introduction

Schizophrenics are more variable than normals on almost any psychophysiological measure (Callaway 1975). One of these variable measures is the event-related potential (ERP), which is the brain's transient electrical response to discrete events. Previous investigations of ERP variability in schizophrenia have employed curve fitting techniques, peak picking, or principal component analysis to determine amplitude or latency variability of individual ERP components, particularly the P300 component (Michalewski 1986; Thomas et al. 1989). Such approaches are, however, made difficult by the presence of the ongoing EEG.

In this study we avoid the problem of peak identification in the presence of superimposed EEG by instead examining the variability throughout the epoch – without any attempt to determine a priori the variability of any single component. The method involves taking a set of single-trial evoked potentials and calculating the variance for each of the 256 (in our case) points within the sampling window. We refer to the result as a response variance curve (RVC). Consisting as it does of variances, one for each sampled point, the RVC directly complements the traditional average ERP.

Both ERPs and RVCs are examined in this study to determine whether schizophrenics show greater target ERP variability than normal controls, at what latency this variability is maximal, and the topographical distribution of this enhanced variability.

Patients and Methods

Ten unmedicated male schizophrenics, with mean age 23.8 yrs (SD = 5.3), were sex and age matched (within 4 years) to ten medicated schizophrenic subjects (mean age of 24.7 years) and with 10 normal control subjects (mean

* The financial support of the Rebecca Cooper Foundation of NSW and IBM Australia is gratefully acknowledged.

[1] Neuroscience Unit, Department of Psychiatry, Westmead Hospital, Westmead, NSW 2145, Australia.

Imaging of the Brain in Psychiatry
and Related Fields
Edited by K. Maurer

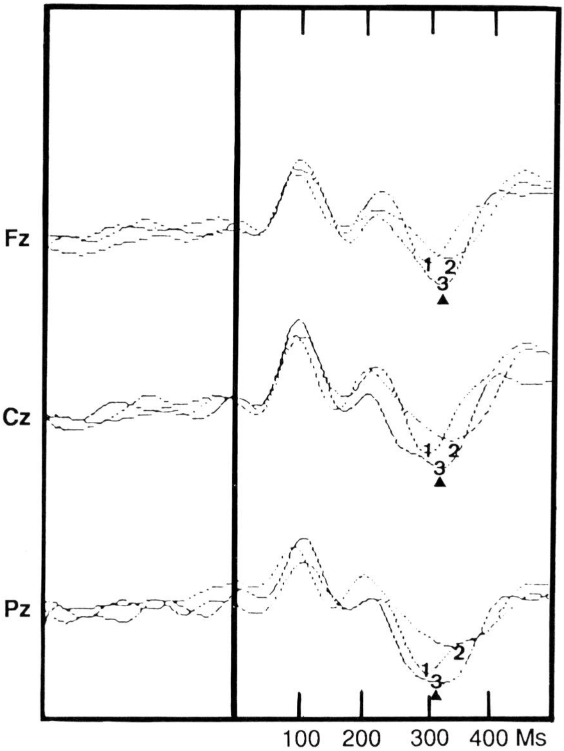

Fig. 1. Group results for conventional averaged event-related potential (ERP) target responses at *Cz*. Amplitude of P300 of unmedicated schizophrenics (n = 10) (*1*), medicated schizophrenics (n = 10) (*2*) is compared to normals (n = 10) (*3*). Each curve is the result of 234 single-trial ERPs

age 23.3 years). Patients were interviewed using the Composite International Diagnostic Interview (Robins et al. 1987) from which RDC (Endicott and Spitzer 1979) and DSM III-R diagnoses of schizophrenic disorder were derived. Normal control subjects with any history of neurological or psychiatric disorder were excluded.

The auditory "oddball" paradigm was used. Tone bursts were presented at a rate of 1/1.3 s: 85% of the tones were of 1000 Hz (background tones) and the remaining 15% were of 1500 Hz (target tones). The stimulus responses were recorded from 15 sites of the international 10–20 system, while linked earlobes served as reference. In addition, two electrodes were used to record potentials arising from eye movements. Participants were instructed to press a response button "as fast as possible" to the target tones. Acquisition continued until 30 target responses were obtained. In order to control for fatigue and habituation effects only the first 30 target responses of each subject were analyzed, and artifact-free responses were included for further analysis only if both the experimental and the control subjects correctly identified the target. Using this procedure, 234 target responses (out of a maximum possible of 300) were extracted to represent each of the three groups.

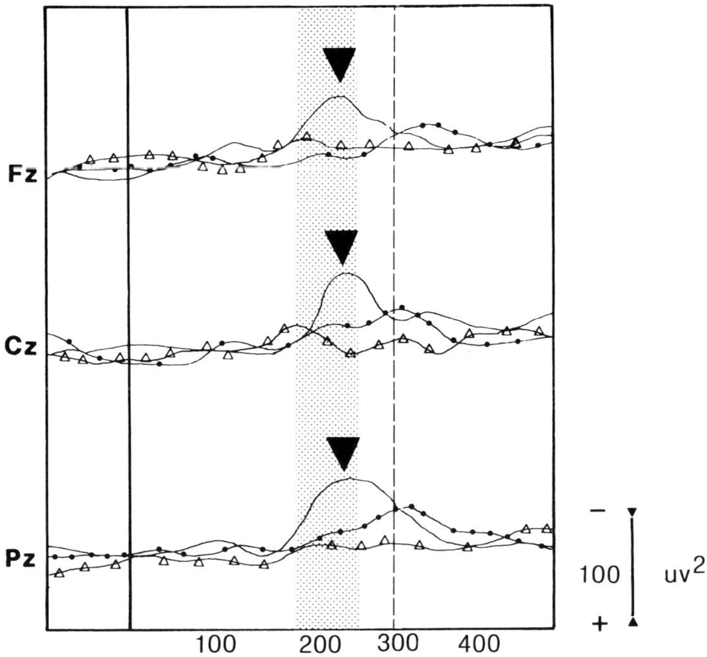

Fig. 2. Group results for response variance curves (RVCs) at *Fz*, *Cz*, and *Pz* electrode sites: —, unmedicated schizophrenic group (n = 10); -△-△-△-, medicated schizophrenic groups (n = 10); -●-●-●-, normals (n = 10)

First, individual and group average ERP waveforms were determined from the selected subset of single-trial epochs. The corresponding variance curves were subsequently determined by calculating the variance at each of the 256 points in the sampling window. This procedure was carried out for each subject and for each group. Finally, topographic ERP and RVC maps were obtained on a 64 × 64 grid using a nearest neighbor interpolation routine.

Results

Group Differences

Figure 1 shows the conventional average target ERPs for the three groups. Using a repeated measure one way analysis of variance there were no significant between-group differences in the amplitude or latency of any of the major components (N100, P200, N200, P300). This is in contrast to the group average RVCs, shown in Fig. 2, in which a difference is particularly evident at about the N200 latency. The distribution of variance at this latency is shown in Fig. 3.

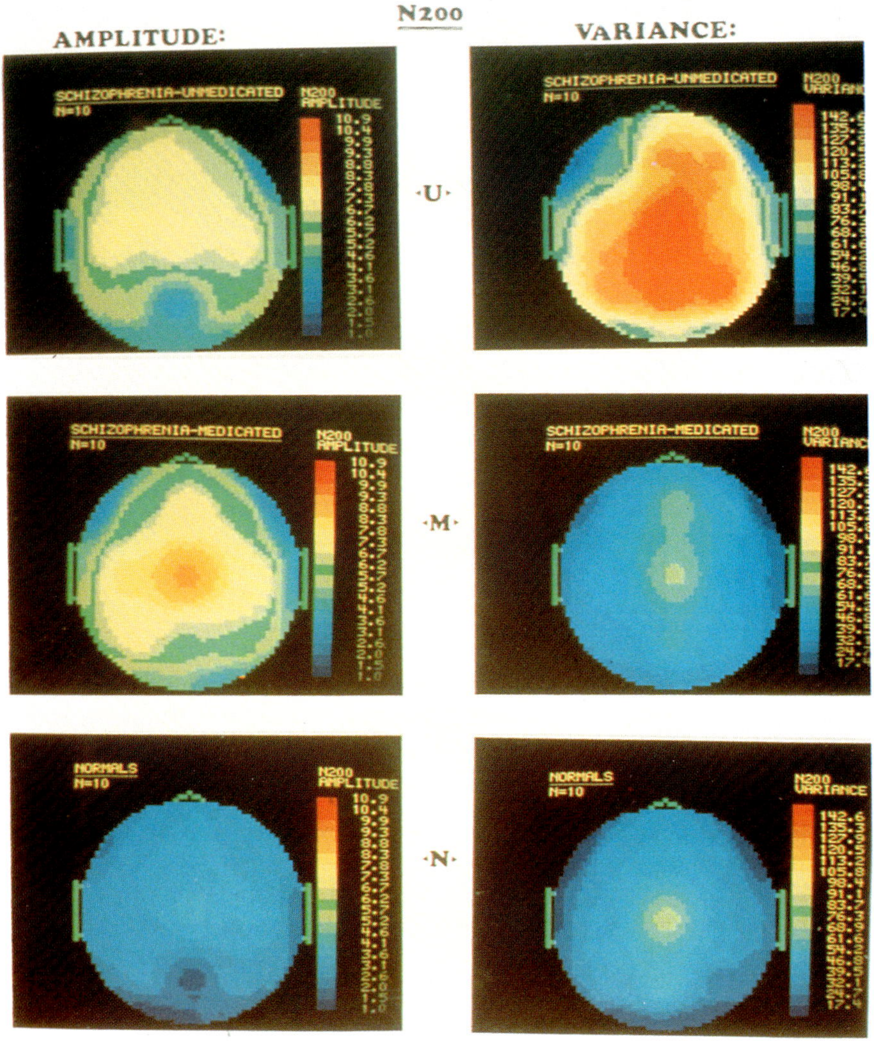

Fig. 3. Topographic distribution of group results for conventional amplitude measures (*left*) and response variance curves (RVCs) (*right*) of the N200 component at Cz: unmedicated schizophrenic group (*U*); medicated schizophrenic group (*M*); normals (*N*)

Individual Differences

The RVCs at Cz for each of the subjects are shown in Fig. 4. There was an increase in variance evident within the latency range of 190–250 ms in eight of the ten schizophrenics. Only two unmedicated schizophrenic subjects

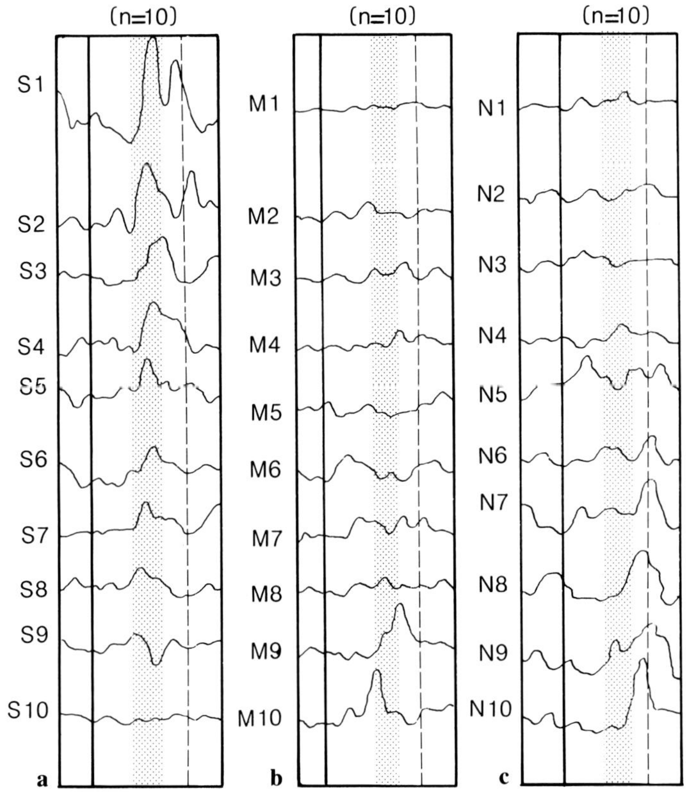

Fig. 4a–c. Individual response variance curve (RVC) results for unmedicated schizophrenics (**a**), medicated schizophrenics (**b**) and normals (**c**). Each curve is the result of between 17 and 30 single trial waveforms and has been arranged to demonstrate more clearly the range of responses. The site is Cz; the *solid line* marks stimulus onset

(subjects S9 and S10) were considered as not exhibiting a maximum variance peak within this latency range. In contrast to the unmedicated schizophrenics, perhaps two of the ten medicated schizophrenics (subjects M9 and M10), and two of the normals (subjects N1 and N4) had a variance peak at the N200 latency. If there was a peak in either of these groups, it tended to occur later, at about the P300 latency.

Discussion

In this study, the traditional average ERP technique showed only insignificant P300 amplitude differences between both schizophrenic groups and controls. However, when, instead of the mean, we look at the variance of all the responses, we found that in the unmedicated schizophrenic group eight of the ten subjects showed a clear increase in variance occurring at or near the latency of the N200 component. This was in contrast to the medicated and normal groups in which only two subjects were considered to have a comparable increase in variability around the N200 component latency. The complementary nature of average waveforms and RVCs is well exemplified in the comparison of medicated and unmedicated schizophrenics. The average showed no significant differences, in clear contrast to the RVCs in which there were significant differences between the variance curves. As a result it appears that medication has normalized the variability of response. This suggestion needs to be verified by examining the same patient before and after medication.

The topographical distribution of variance at the N200 latency was examined in each group. As can be seen in Fig. 3, there are extensive differences in the variance scores, particularly in the centroparietal regions. Topographic distribution of the RVC measure clearly demonstrates significant differences that were not evident using the conventional averaging technique. This was borne out by statistical analysis using repeated measure analysis of variance which determined that there were only three sites where significant differences in N200 ERP amplitude (F3, F7, and C3) and the RVC (190–250 ms) of the three groups (F8, C3, C4, Pz, P3, P4, O2) occurred.

The finding of increased ERP variability within a defined latency window may provide a useful measure for the examination of the stages of information processing (as reflected by late component ERPs) that are postulated to be dysfunctional in schizophrenia.

References

Callaway E (1975) Evoked potential variability and cognitive variability. In: Callaway E (ed) Brain electrical potentials and individual psychological differences. Grune and Stratton, New York, pp 63–79

Endicott J, Spitzer RL (1979) Use of the research diagnostic criteria and the schedule for affective disorders and schizophrenia. J Nerv Ment Dis 171:34–39

Michalewski HJ, Prasher DK, Starr A (1986) Latency variability and temporal interrelationships of the auditory event-related potentials (N1, P2, N2, and P3) in normal subjects. Electroencephalogr Clin Neurophysiol 65:59–71

Robins LN, Wing J, Helzer J (1987) Composite International Diagnostic Interview. World Health Organization, Geneva

Thomas DG, Neer CM, Price JM (1989) Analyses of single-trial N1 amplitude and latency variability and their influence on the average evoked potential. Electroencephalogr Clin Neurophysiol 74:228–235

Haloperidol-Induced Changes of Computerized Electroencephalogram Topography in Drug-Free Schizophrenic Patients

S. Galderisi[1], A. Mucci, M.L. Mignone, M. Maj, and D. Kemali

Introduction

An increase in slow activity in the electroencephalogram (EEG) of schizophrenic patients, as compared to healthy subjects, has been rather consistently reported in quantitative EEG studies (Itil et al. 1972; Karson et al. 1987; Miyauchi et al. 1990). Since neuroleptic administration in normal subjects induces an increase of slow activities (Fink 1974), a possible role of drug treatment in producing these findings has been hypothesized. In this connection, it should be pointed out that most of the studies reporting δ increase in schizophrenia involved unmedicated patients (Itil et al. 1972; Karson et al. 1987), and a decrease of δ activity following neuroleptic administration in schizophrenics has been reported in studies based on a test-retest design (Saletu et al. 1986).

As to the topography of this abnormality, it is still unclear whether it involves different cortical regions or is confined to frontal areas. Computerized EEG (CEEG) topography studies have so far reported contradictory results (Morihisa et al. 1983; Karson et al. 1987). Investigations addressing more specifically the problem of eye movement contribution to frontal slowing did not find a frontal localization and reported a widespread increase of δ (Karson et al. 1987).

In the present study, the topography of δ activity and its relationship to neuroleptic treatment have been investigated in 20 DSM III-R drug-free schizophrenics.

Subjects and Methods

Schizophrenic patients included in the experimental sample had an age range of 19–37 years (mean ± SD, 25.6 ± 4.8) and a mean length of illness of 0.6–17 years (mean ± SD, 6.01 ± 4.8). 18 patients had to complete a washout period of at least 15 days (45 days for long-acting neuroleptics)

[1]Department of Psychiatry, First Medical School, University of Naples, Largo Madonna delle Grazie, 80138 Naples, Italy.

Imaging of the Brain in Psychiatry
and Related Fields
Edited by K. Maurer

Table 1. Differences in relative power between drug-free schizophrenics and healthy controls

Frequency bands	Leads											
	F3	F4	T3	T4	T5	T6	C3	C4	P3	P4	O1	O2
δ												
Schizophrenics[a]	23 ± 8	23 ± 7	23 ± 9	22 ± 6	17 ± 7	16 ± 7	22 ± 7	22 ± 6	18 ± 7	18 ± 7	14 ± 7	14 ± 7
Controls	16 ± 7	17 ± 8	16 ± 6	19 ± 8	13 ± 6	11 ± 6	16 ± 8	16 ± 9	14 ± 9	14 ± 9	12 ± 9	11 ± 8
α_2												
Schizophrenics[b]	17 ± 11	17 ± 11	18 ± 10	17 ± 11	30 ± 16	30 ± 17	20 ± 13	21 ± 12	31 ± 16	31 ± 18	34 ± 21	35 ± 21
Controls	28 ± 12	29 ± 12	29 ± 11	31 ± 9	37 ± 16	40 ± 16	33 ± 11	33 ± 11	41 ± 14	43 ± 14	48 ± 21	50 ± 18

[a] Significant increase of δ in schizophrenics: $p < 0.05$.
[b] Significant reduction of α_2 in schizophrenics: $p < 0.02$.

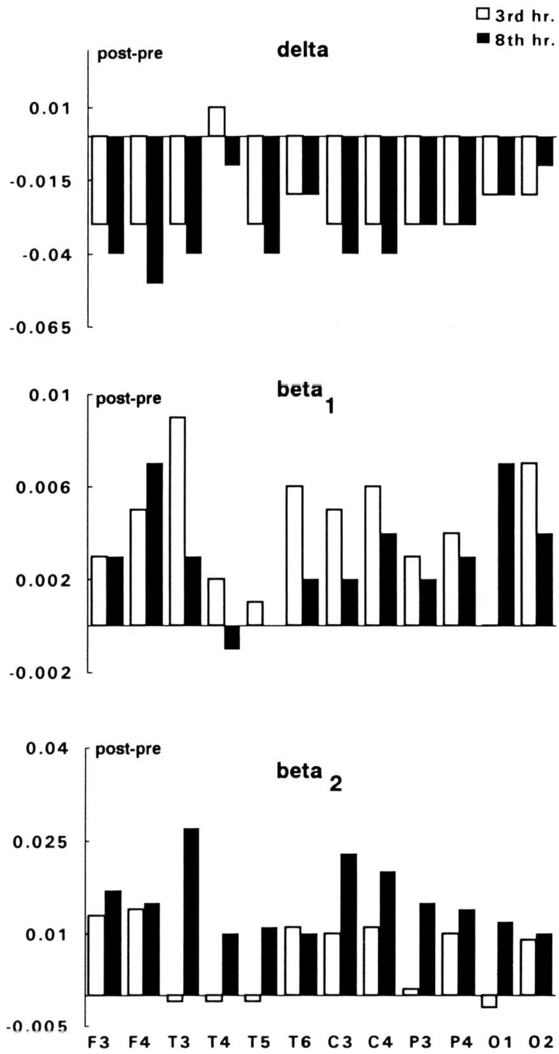

Fig. 1. Changes in relative power observed in schizophrenics after haloperidol acute treatment. Reduction of δ: 3rd hour, $p < 0.006$; 8th hour, $p < 0.0001$. Increase of β_1: 3rd hour, $p < 0.03$. Increase of β_2: 8th hour, $p < 0.006$

before entering the study; the remaining two were drug-naive. A total of 11 healthy volunteers, comparable with patients for age, sex, and handedness, were used as the control group.

10 min of resting, eyes closed, EEG were recorded at the end of the washout period, and these baseline recordings were compared to baseline EEGs of the control group; further recordings were obtained 1, 3, 6, and 8 h after a single oral dose of haloperidol (3 mg) and after 7, 14, and 28 days of chronic treatment. The EEG was recorded from 16 unipolar leads of the international 10–20 system, each referred to the ipsilateral ear lobe. Eight frequency bands were considered (δ, 1.3–3.5 Hz; θ_1, 3.75–5.5 Hz; θ_2,

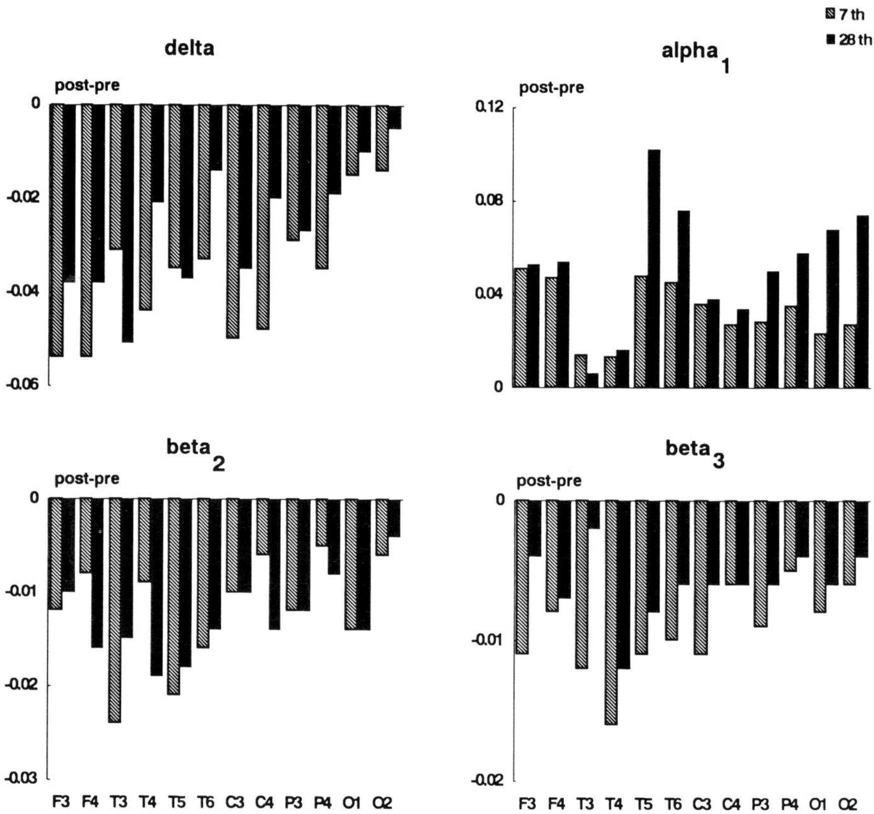

Fig. 2. Changes in relative power observed in schizophrenics after haloperidol chronic treatment. Reduction of δ: 7th day, $p < 0.001$; 28th day, $p < 0.02$. Increase of α_1, 7th day, $p < 0.01$; 28th day, $p < 0.04$. Decrease of β_2, 7th day, $p < 0.03$; 28th day, $p < 0.04$. Decrease of β_3, 7th day, $p < 0.01$

5.75–7.5 Hz; α_1, 7.75–9.5 Hz; α_2, 9.75–12.5 Hz; β_1, 12.75–15 Hz; β_2, 15.25–26 Hz; β_3, 26.25–35 Hz). Differences between patients and controls and changes in relative power (RP) following acute and chronic neuroleptic treatment were evaluated by means of two-way ANOVAs (for further details about CEEG procedure and analysis, see Galderisi et al. 1990).

Results

A comparison between baseline CEEG recordings of patients and healthy controls revealed a widespread significant increase of δ and a significant reduction of α_2 in schizophrenics (Table 1).

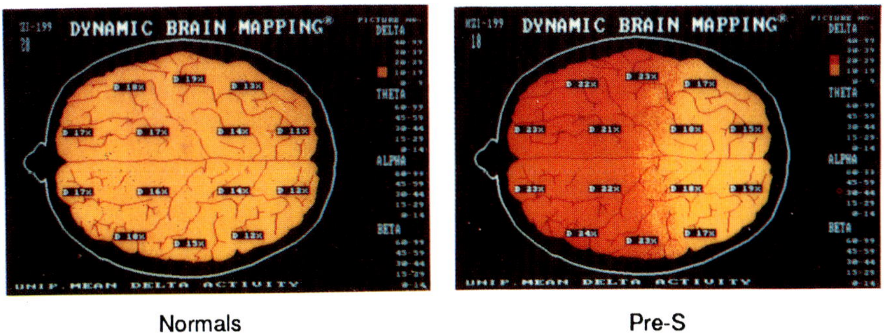

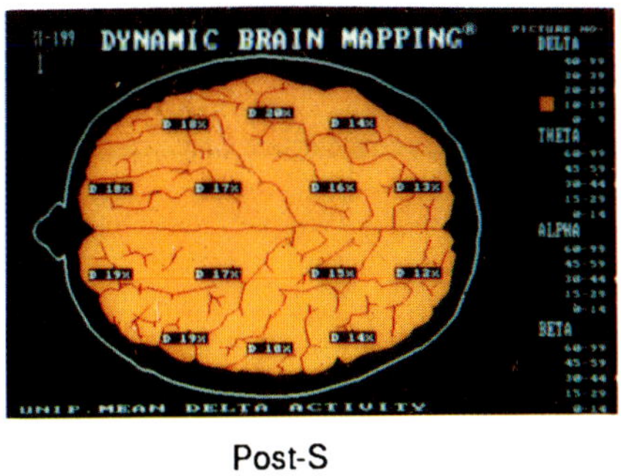

Fig. 3. Group maps showing the increase of δ relative power in drug-free schizophrenics (*Pre-S*) as compared with *Normals* and its decrease in schizophrenics after haloperidol treatment (*Post-S*)

No significant change was detected 1 h after drug administration. Since CEEG modifications were very similar after 6 and 8 h and after 14 and 28 days, only results observed after 3 and 8 h, for the acute treatment, and after 7 and 28 days, for the chronic treatment, will be reported.

Significant changes induced by acute treatment included a reduction of δ RP and an increase of β_1 and β_2 RP (Fig. 1). After chronic treatment, significant changes included a decrease of δ and fast β RP and an increase of α_1 RP (Fig. 2).

Discussion

In summary, an increase of δ RP was observed in a group of drug-free schizophrenics as compared to healthy controls. The δ increase observed in our patients was not localized to frontal areas, but involved all cortical regions, which argues against an electro-oculogram (EOG) contamination. Antipsychotic treatment cannot account for the increase of slow activity in schizophrenia. As a matter of fact, both acute and chronic haloperidol administration induced a significant decrease of δ activity (Fig. 3).

As to the pathophysiological meaning of increased δ in schizophrenia, two main hypotheses have been proposed. According to the first one, the increase in δ activity is an index of lowered arousal (Lifshitz and Gradijan 1974); this hypothesis does not provide much insight into the pathophysiological meaning of δ activity and does not fit with a large body of evidence supporting a hyperarousal hypothesis of schizophrenia (Spohn and Patterson 1979). The second hypothesis has been outlined on the basis of some studies showing decreased cortical metabolism in schizophrenic patients and a significant negative correlation between δ activity and cortical metabolism (Buchsbaum and Haier 1987). In this connection, it is worth mentioning that an association has also been found between reduced metabolism in cortical areas and hypermetabolism in subcortical regions (Early et al. 1987). Within this frame, the δ increase in schizophrenia might be considered as the result of an impaired cortical-subcortical integration, possibly based on a dysfunction of dopaminergic systems. This interpretation would also explain δ reduction following neuroleptic administration.

References

Buchsbaum MS, Haier RJ (1987) Functional and anatomical brain mapping: impact on schizophrenia research. Schizophr Bull 13:115–132

Early TS, Reiman EM, Reichle ME, Spitznagel EL (1987) Left globus pallidus abnormality in never-medicated patients with schizophrenia. Proc Natl Acad Sci USA 84:561–563

Fink M (1974) EEG profiles and bioavailability measures of psychoactive drugs. In: Itil TM (ed) Psychotropic drugs and the human EEG. Karger, Basel, pp 76–98 (Modern problems of pharmacopsychiatry, vol 8)

Galderisi S, Mucci A, Di Gregorio MR, Bucci P, Maj M, Kemali D (1990) C-EEG Brain mapping in DSM-III schizophrenics after acute and chronic haloperidol treatment. European Neuropsychopharmacology 1:51–54

Itil TM, Saletu B, Davis S (1972) EEG findings in chronic schizophrenics based on digital computer period analysis and analog power spectra. Biol Psychiatry 5:1–13

Karson CN, Coppola R, Morihisa JM, Weinberger DR (1987) Computed electroencephalographic activity mapping in schizophrenia: the resting state reconsidered. Arch Gen Psychiatry 44:514–517

Lifshitz K, Gradijan J (1974) Spectral evaluation of the electroencephalogram: power and variability in chronic schizophrenics and control subjects. Psychophysiology 11:479–490

Miyauchi T, Tanaka K, Hagimoto H, Miura T, Kishimoto H, Matsushita M (1990) Computerized EEG in schizophrenic patients. Biol Psychiatry 28:488–494

Morihisa JM, Duffy FH, Wyatt RJ (1983) Brain electrical activity mapping (BEAM) in schizophrenic patients. Arch Gen Psychiatry 40:719–728

Saletu B, Küfferle B, Grünberger J, Anderer P (1986) Quantitative EEG, SPEM, and psychometric studies in schizophrenics before and during differential neuroleptic therapy. Pharmacopsychiatry 19:434–437

Spohn HE, Patterson T (1979) Recent studies of psychophysiology in schizophrenia. Schizophr Bull 5:581–611

Changes and Clinical Correlations of P300 in Schizophrenia

G. Eikmeier[1], E. Lodemann, H.M. Olbrich, D. Zerbin, and M. Gastpar

Introduction

A significantly reduced amplitude of the P300 component of the event-related potential (ERP) in schizophrenic patients has frequently been reported and is considered to be characteristic of schizophrenia. However, there are several other questions that remain concerning other parameters of the ERP and the clinical relevance of the changes (Blackwood et al. 1987; Pfefferbaum et al. 1989; Pritchard 1986). The present study tries to clarify two questions in P300 research in schizophrenia: (1) Is P300 latency prolonged in schizophrenic patients? (2) Are there relationships between P300 amplitude/latency and clinical symptoms of schizophrenia?

Subjects and Methods

A total of 15, right-handed, schizophrenic patients (8 males, 7 females, mean age: 30 ± 6 years) were included in the study. Most of the patients were under neuroleptic medication (acute phase, T_0: $n = 9$; remission, T_1: $n = 10$). Different neuroleptics were used (mean chlorpromazine equivalents T_0, 1134 ± 1228; T_1, 556 ± 634). The group without neuroleptic treatment consisted of drug-free patients (T_0: $n = 2$, T_1: $n = 1$) and patients receiving the antidepressant trimipramine. Additionally, ten right-handed controls of the same age and educational level and without personal or family history of psychiatric illness were studied.

ERP were recorded during a two-tone auditory discrimination task (frequent tone: p = 0.85, 800 Hz, 20 ms duration; infrequent tone: p = 0.15, 1400 Hz, 20 ms duration; interstimulus interval: sequence quasirandom 1.1–4.1 s) from 13 leads of the 10–20 system. ERP recordings were done twice, the first time in the acute phase of schizophrenia (T_0, mean Brief Psychiatric Rating Scale score: 50 ± 7), the second time after remission (T_1, mean Brief Psychiatric Rating Scale score: 31 ± 7; mean Scale for Assess-

[1] Klinik für Allg. Psychiatrie, Universitätsklinikum Essen, Hufelandstr. 55, W-4300 Essen, FRG.

Imaging of the Brain in Psychiatry and Related Fields
Edited by K. Maurer

Table 1. P300 amplitude and latency at C_z

	Schizophrenics		Controls		Schizophrenics versus controls
	T_0	T_1	T_0	T_1	
Amplitude (μV)	4.8 ± 3.6	6.7 ± 3.6	13.4 ± 5.6	15.3 ± 7.5	**
Latency (ms)	354 ± 31	349 ± 37	320 ± 22	314 ± 22	*

ANOVA results for main factor "group"; $^*p < 0.05$; $^{**}p < 0.005$.
T_0, acute phase; T_1, remission.

ment of Negative Symptoms score: 31 ± 14; mean Intentionalitäts scale (INSKA) score: 14 ± 6). The control subjects were studied in the same manner with an interval between the two recordings comparable to that in the patient group.

Results

Two-way ANOVA (group by time) for repeated measurements (t) showed a prolonged P300 latency and a reduced P300 amplitude in the schizophrenic patients; the interaction between the main factors was not significant (Table 1). Except in age there were no differences in demographic data or ERP between patients with and without neuroleptic treatment (t test).

In the acute phase we found no significant correlation between P300 amplitude/latency and the brief psychiatric rating scale (BPRS) total score or one of the the BPRS subscores. In the remitted state P300 amplitude was correlated ($p < 0.05$) negatively with the scale for assessment of negative symptoms (SANS) ($\rho = -0.54$) and INSKA ($\rho = -0.56$) total scores. Looking at the SANS subscores there was a negative correlation between the subscore "anhedonia-asociality" and P300 amplitude ($\rho = -0.57$; $p < 0.05$) and a positive correlation between the subscore "attentional impairment" and P300 latency ($\rho = 0.56$, $p < 0.05$).

Discussion

Besides the expected reduction of P300 amplitude in schizophrenics, the main findings of our study are: (1) The schizophrenic patients showed a significantly prolonged P300 latency. (2) P300 changes seem to be independent of the presence/absence of florid symptoms and of neuroleptic treatment. (3) P300 amplitude was correlated negatively with the negative syndrome of schizophrenia.

In summary, our data again show that changes of P300 are robust psychobiological phenomena in schizophrenia. Furthermore our analysis showed a significant correlation between P300 amplitude and the negative syndrome evaluated by two different rating scales. This seems to be of interest, since the P300 amplitude – indicating altered information processing – and negative symptoms are regarded as basic disturbances in schizophrenia. The correlation between P300 amplitude and anhedonia supports the view that P300 is a marker of anhedonia, which in our opinion is a core feature of the negative syndrome.

References

Blackwood DH, Whalley LJ, Christie JE, Blackburn IM, St Clair DM, McInnes A (1987) Changes in auditory P3 event-related potential in schizophrenia and depression. Br J Psychiatry 150:154–160

Pfefferbaum A, Ford JM, White PM, Roth WT (1989) P3 in schizophrenia is affected by stimulus modality, response requierements, medication status, and negative symptoms. Arch Gen Psychiatry 46:1035–1044

Pritchard WS (1986) Cognitive event-related potential correlates of schizophrenia. Psychol Bull 100:43–66

Cognitive Components of Auditory Evoked Potentials in Schizophrenic Disorders: Topography and Clinical Correlations

W.K. Strik[1], T. Dierks, T. Müller, and K. Maurer

Introduction

The amplitude reduction of the P300 component of event related potentials in schizophrenics has been found to be a nonspecific, but sensible marker in schizophrenia (Roth and Cannon 1972; Levit et al. 1973; Roth et al. 1981). Neuroleptic medication seems rather to enhance than to reduce P300 amplitude (Pfefferbaum et al. 1989).

Topographical mapping might be able to discriminate schizophrenics from normals and from patients with dementia by the pattern of the spatial distribution of the maxima of the P300 amplitudes (Maurer et al. 1989).

Morstyn et al. (1983) found a diminished peak of auditory P300 in schizophrenic patients compared to controls. The topographical distribution of the P300 maxima was displaced anteriorly and to the right in contrast to the control group, who had a small asymmetry with maxima on the left.

Shenton et al. (1989) confirmed the P300 amplitude reduction in 11 schizophrenics. Within the schizophrenic group positive symptoms were associated with high P300 amplitude over the left temporal areas. The authors tried to explain these results with the presence of two factors, one responsible for the overall schizophrenic-normal difference and another operating within the schizophrenic group, reflecting secondary and compensatory processes.

Pfefferbaum et al. (1989) found an inverse correlation between P300 amplitude and negative symptoms in a group of 13 medicated and 18 drug-free schizophrenics. Like Shenton et al., these authors could not confirm the amplitude reduction over left temporal areas reported by Morstyn. They concluded that P300 amplitude reduction in schizophrenia is a clear psychobiological phenomenon that is present regardless of medication status.

The purpose of our study was to determine whether negative and psychotic symptoms in schizophrenics are associated with different P300 amplitudes, latencies, and topography.

[1] Psychiatrische Klinik der Universität Würzburg, Füchsleinstr. 15, W-8700 Würzburg, FRG.

Imaging of the Brain in Psychiatry and Related Fields
Edited by K. Maurer

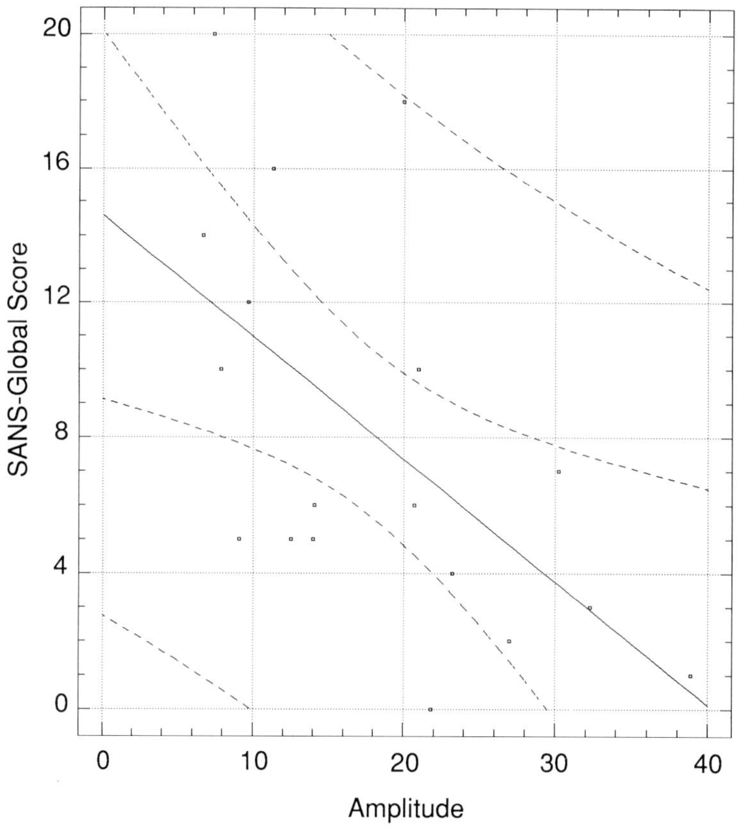

Fig. 1. Correlation between P300 amplitude and the global score of the Scale for Assessment of Negative Symptoms (SANS)

Subjects and Methods

We studied 20 schizophrenic patients (8 females, 12 males) with a mean age of 31 years. All of them met the criteria of DSM III-R. Evoked potentials (EPs) were elicited according to the method described by Maurer et al. (1987), based on the oddball paradigm. Recordings were realized from 19 electrodes, applied according to the international 10–20 system, and linked mastoid references. The data were processed into topographical maps of electric field distribution. Latencies of P300 were determined as a peak of the global field power (Lehmann 1987) in the 270–470 ms time window. Amplitudes were calculated as the difference between P300 maximum and minimum. For clinical ratings we applied the Scale for Assessment of Negative Symptoms (SANS; Andreasen and Olsen 1982) and the Brief Psychiatric Rating Scale (BPRS).

Table 1. Correlations between clinical ratings and P300 parameters

P300	SANS		BPRS		
	Total	Global	Anxiety	Emotional withdrawal	Affective flattening
Amplitude	−0.48*	−0.57**	0.34	−0.20	0.04
Latency	−0.45	−0.32	−0.49*	−0.53*	−0.56**

Pearson's correlation coefficient; * = $p < 0.05$; ** = $p < 0.02$.
SANS, Scale for Assessment of Negative Symptoms; BPRS, Brief Psychiatric Rating Scale.

Table 2. Clinical ratings of patients with the minimum of the equivalent dipole over the left and right hemispheres

	BPRS			
	Thought disorders* (av./σ)	Ideas of grandeur**	Depressive mood	Motor retardation
Left ($n = 7$)	3.57/2.07	2.43/2.50	0	0
Right ($n = 12$)	1.67/1.83	0.42/1.44	0.42/0.1	0.83/1.4

Students t test; $^{*}p = 0.039$, $^{**}p = 0.052$.
BPRS, Brief Psychiatric Rating Scale.

Results

A total of 18 patients could be reliably assessed for P300 amplitude. Low amplitudes correlated significantly with the total ($r = -0.48$, $p < 0.05$) and with the global score ($r = -0.58$, $p < 0.02$) (Fig. 1) of the SANS. Furthermore, short latencies of the P300 correlated with high total scores of the SANS ($r = -0.45$, n.s.) and with high scores on the BPRS items "anxiety" ($r = -0.49$, $p < 0.05$), "emotional withdrawal" ($r = -0.53$, $p < 0.05$), and "affective flattening" ($r = -56$, $p < 0.05$) (Table 1). Those patients who had the minimum of the equivalent dipole in the left hemisphere ($n = 7$) had higher scores of the BPRS itmes 4 ("thought disorders," $p = 0.05$) and 8 ("ideas of grandiosity," $p < 0.04$), and lower scores of the items 9 ("depressive mood," n.s.) and 13 ("motor retardation," n.s.) than those patients ($n = 11$) with the minimum in the right hemisphere (Table 2).

Discussion

Our results demonstrate the existence of relationships between clinical features and neurophysiological variables within the group of schizophrenic disorders. Negative symptoms, assessed with the SANS and the BPRS, are associated with shorter latencies of the P300 wave, and the sums of the SANS scores, especially the global score reflecting the severity of impairment by negative symptoms, were associated with low P300 amplitudes. No inverse relationships have been found with the positive symptoms assessed with the BPRS, indicating that positive and negative symptoms are independent and not located on one axis.

Some characteristic psychopathological features were associated with different topographical distributions of the P300. This might indicate that the state of mood and impulse depends on lateralized brain activities, but further investigation is necessary.

References

Andreasen BC, Olsen S (1982) Negative symptoms versus positive schizophrenia: Definition and validation. Arch Gen Psychiatry 39:789–794

Lehmann D (1987) Principles of spatial analysis. In: Gevins AS, Rémond A (eds) Methods of analysis of train electrical and magnetic signals. Handbook of electroencephalography and clinical neurophysiology (revised, vol I). Elsevier Amsterdam

Levit RA, Sutton S, Zubin J (1973) Evoked potential correlates of information processing in psychiatric patients. Psychol Med 3:487–494

Maurer K, Lowitsch K, Stöhr M (1987) Evozierte Potenziale, Einführung und Atlas. Enke, Stuttgart

Maurer K, Dierks T, Ihl R, Laux G (1989) Mapping of evoked potentials in normals and patients with psychiatric diseases. In: Maurer K (ed) Topographic brain mapping of EEG and evoked potentials. Springer Berlin Heidelberg New York

Morstyn R, Duffy FH, McCarley RW (1983) Altered P300 topography in schizophrenia. Arch Gen Psychiatry 40:729–734

Pfefferbaum A, Ford JM, White PM, Roth WT (1989) P3 in schizophrenia is affected by stimulus modality, response requirements, medication status, and negative symptoms. Arch Gen Psychiatry 46:1035–1044

Roth WT, Cannon EH (1972) Some features of the auditory evoked response in schizophrenics. Arch Gen Psychiatry 27:466–471

Roth WT, Pfefferbaum A, Kelly AF, Berger PA, Kopell BS (1981) Auditory event related potentials in schizophrenia and depression. Psychiatry Res 4:199–212

Shenton ME, Faux SF, McCarley RW, Ballinger R, Coleman M, Torello, Duffy FH (1989) Correlations between abnormal auditory P300 topography and positive symptoms in schizophrenia: a preliminary report. Biol Psychiatry 25:710–716

Electroencephalogram Mapping in Hemispheric Vascular Insults

I. Szirmai[1], Gy. Surek, and A. Kamondi

Introduction

Spectral analysis has extended the usefulness of the electroencephalogram (EEG) through the quantitation and extraction of more information than that obtainable from visual analysis (Cohen et al. 1976; Duffy 1989; Oken et al. 1989). The EEG is generally asymmetric in vascular diseases of the brain (Jonkman et al. 1985). The goal of this article is to demonstrate the relevance of EEG mapping in patients with hemispheric vascular diseases through the comparison of visual analysis, clinical, and computerized tomography (CT) scan findings.

Patients and Methods

A 16-channel routine and computerized EEG analysis was performed in 51 cerebrovascular patients in the first week after the stroke. All patients had focal signs and 30 out of 51 showed infarction on CT scans. The signals were A-D converted on an IBM PC with a digitizing frequency of 64 and 128 cps. CZ- or averaged-reference was used. After fast Fourier transformation, power and coherence spectra were computed in the frequency range of 0.25–30 HZ. Absolute, relative power mapping (RPM) and averaged power spectra were displayed in 2 and 4 s epochs, respectively (software work was done by E. Dologh (RKFT) Budapest). For closer analysis of α asymmetries, a 15-electrode α roster, placed on the posterior regions of the skull, was used. Paired Wilcoxon and student *t* tests for evaluation of side and field differences of resting power and photo reactivity were used.

Results

Visual analysis of slightly irregular EEGs are not of diagnostic value for the estimation of severity of hemispheric ischemia in the acute phase of the

[1] Clinic of Neurology, University Medical School Pecs, 7623 Pecs, Ret u.2., Hungary.

Imaging of the Brain in Psychiatry
and Related Fields
Edited by K. Maurer

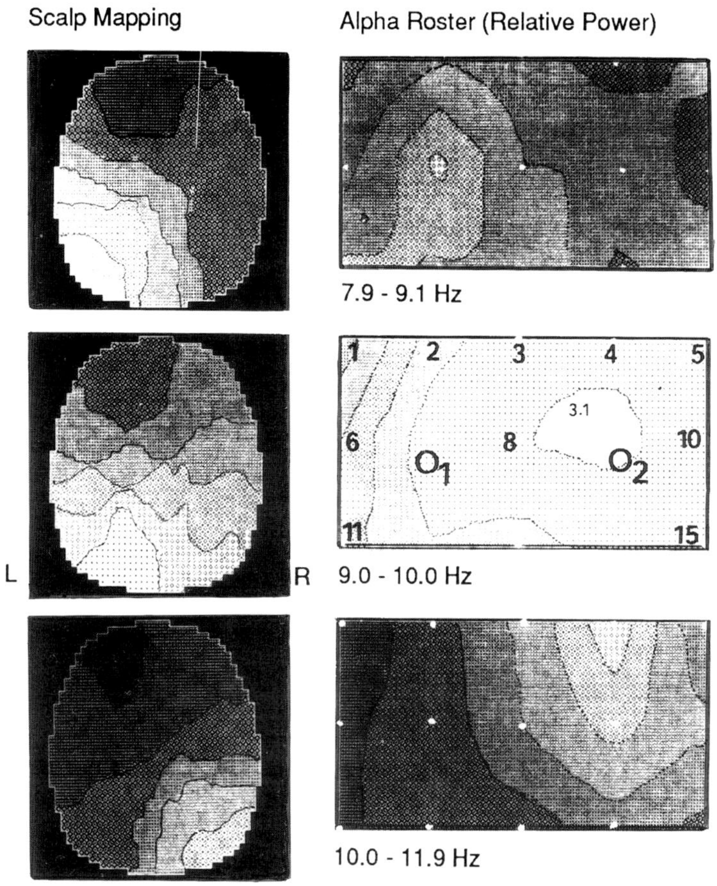

Fig. 1. 2 HZ reduction of α peak frequency on the left (*L*) parietooccipital region in comparison to the right (*R*) in a patient with left internal carotid artery (ICA) occlusion. Asymmetry of averaged power fields can be better visualized on the occipitally placed α roster. Placement of electrodes signalized by *O1* and *O2* points. Values of relative power: *brightest* = 3.1, *darkest* = 0.5. Scale divided in ten steps

disease. Recognition of θ and δ waves in the visual and computerized analysis of the EEG was approximately equal, but in the α domain, mapping revealed 20% more significant power asymmetries than found by descriptive analysis of the EEG. An optimally chosen frequency window using RPM can be helpful in finding significant asymmetries of close power ranges.

Original topograms of a 52 year old male patient with right hemisensory deficit and fluent aphasia caused by occlusion of the ICA are demonstrated in Fig. 1. The CT scan was negative. The significant occipital power asymmetry in the sub-α range suited the cortical type lesion. In three other patients with capsular infarction, EEG mapping demonstrated unexpectedly

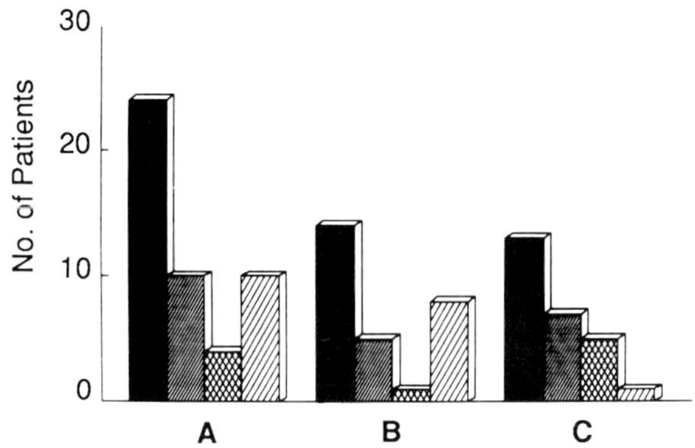

Fig. 2. Effect of photostimulation on α power asymmetry (n = 51). Group *A* = α power (AP) in rest higher on the intact side; *B* = AP higher on the infarct side; *C* = AP difference is not significant. In group *B*, in more than half of the patients the AP asymmetry decreased after photostimulation. In group *C*, photostimulation with the dominant (trigger) frequency induced significant AP differences in 40% of patients. ■, Values in rest; ▨, no photo drive; ▩, asymm higher; ▧, asymm lower

widespread power reduction. In evaluation of statistically significant α power differences, the strongest argument is the ipsilateral presence of slow waves or downward shifting of α frequency. The T values of α power asymmetries stand in significant negative correlation ($r = -0.59$) with the corresponding θ and δ waves. There is no correlation between neurological scores and T values of slow wave asymmetry ($r = 0.37$).

In some instances, photostimulation helped to judge the field of dampened electrogenesis (Fig. 2). When the lesion did not affect the α generators the probability of significant activation of one side was only 40%. This type of α power asymmetry can be better visualized using the splain fitting technique derived from multivariant analysis. The "mountain diagrams" facilitate the recognition of the effect of photodrive.

Discussion

In considering α asymmetries, the interpreter must be aware that in 50% of male adults the α activity is significantly higher on the right occipital region (Wienecke et al. 1980). Models of human α sources are rather inconsistent. Inouye et al. (1986) discussed endogenous (posteriorly) and exogenous (predominantly frontal-central localized) generators. Nunez and Katznelson (1981) found that a slower α component was generated in the anterior regions, while a faster α component was generated in the posterior regions. Our case analysis suggests that asymmetric α power can be either a consequence of cortical or subcortical lesions of the occipital segments. The hypothesis whether the effect of bilateral photostimulation could help in specifying the extent of the vascular lesion cannot be proved (nor rejected) by statistical argumentation.

In summary, EEG mapping provides fast and interpretable information in the acute stage of stroke. It helps to quantify minimal EEG asymmetries and facilitates the recognition of functional derangements of cortical tissue. Spectral analysis is a proper tool in the follow-up of infarcted territories after strokes. Nonetheless, the clinical usefulness of EEG topography depends exclusively on the interpreter.

References

Cohen BA, Bravo-Fernandez EJ, Sances A (1976) Quantification of computer analyzed serial EEGs from stroke patients. Electroencephalogr Clin Neurophysiol 41:379–386

Duffy FH (1989) Why mapping? In: Maurer K (ed) Topographic brain mapping of EEG and evoked potentials. Springer, Berlin Heidelberg New York, pp 19–52

Inouye T, Shinosaki K, Yagasaki A, Shimizu A (1986) Spatial distribution of generation of alpha activity. Electroencephalogr Clin Neurophysiol 63:353–360

Jonkman EJ, Poortvliet DJC, Veering MM et al. (1985) The use of neurometrics in the study of patients with cerebral ischemia. Electroencephalogr Clin Neurophysiol 61:333–341

Nunez PL, Katznelson RD (1981) Electric fields of the brain. Oxford University Press, New York, pp 214–280

Oken BS, Chiappa KH, Salinsky M (1989) Computerised EEG frequency analysis: sensitivity and specificity in patients with focal lesions. Neurology 39:1281–1287

Wienecke GH, Deinema CHA, Spoelstra P et al. (1980) Normative spectral data on alpha rhythm in male adults. Electroencephalogr Clin Neurophysiol 49:636–645

Correlation Maps: On the Relation of Electroencephalographic Slow Wave Activity to Computerized Tomography and Psychopathometric Measurements in Dementia

B. SALETU[1], E. PAULUS, P. ANDERER, J. GRÜNBERGER, and R. FREY

Topographic mapping of the electroencephalogram (EEG) has become an important method in the field of neuropsychiatry, specifically in geriatric medicine. In the latter, it is possible to relate functional EEG mapping to other imaging techniques such as computed tomography (CT) which shows structural and morphological changes. In addition, mapping data should be correlated to clinical psychopathological and psychometric data.

In 111 demented hospitalized patients (77 females, 34 males) ages 58–98 (mean 82) years, clinical and psychometric studies and morphological CT and functional EEG imaging were carried out, with patients being off psychopharmaceutical agents for at least 14 days. They were diagnosed according to DSM III criteria and subdiagnosed according to Hachinski score and CT in 54 senile dementia of Alzheimer type (SDAT) and 57 multi-infarct dementia (MID) patients.

CT measures included the following cerebrospinal fluid (CSF) space variables according to Meese et al. (1980): greatest distance between the anterior horns; distance between the caudate nuclei; width of third ventricle; distance between the choroid plexuses; greatest distance between the lateral ventricles at the level of cella media. In addition, cortical density was measured in 1.7 mm^3 cubes under 17 EEG electrodes in Hounsfield units.

Brain mapping was based on 3 min vigilance-controlled EEG (eyes closed). A total of 17 EEG leads were recorded vs averaged mastoids. After automatic artifact rejection and computing of the common average reference, spectral analysis was carried out and 36 target variables were quantified (Anderer et al. 1987).

Clinical and psychometric evaluations included Sandoz Clinical Assessment Geriatric (SCAG) scale, the Clinical Global Impression (CGI) scale, the Digit Symbol Substitution Test (DSST), the Trail Making Test (ZVT), and the Digit Span (DS) test.

Compared to normals, untreated SDAT and MID patients demonstrated an increased δ/θ activity. In addition, SDAT and MID patients showed decreased β activity and slowing of the dominant frequency and

[1] Universitätsklinik für Psychiatrie, Währinger Gürtel 18-20, 1090 Wien, Austria.

Imaging of the Brain in Psychiatry and Related Fields
Edited by K. Maurer

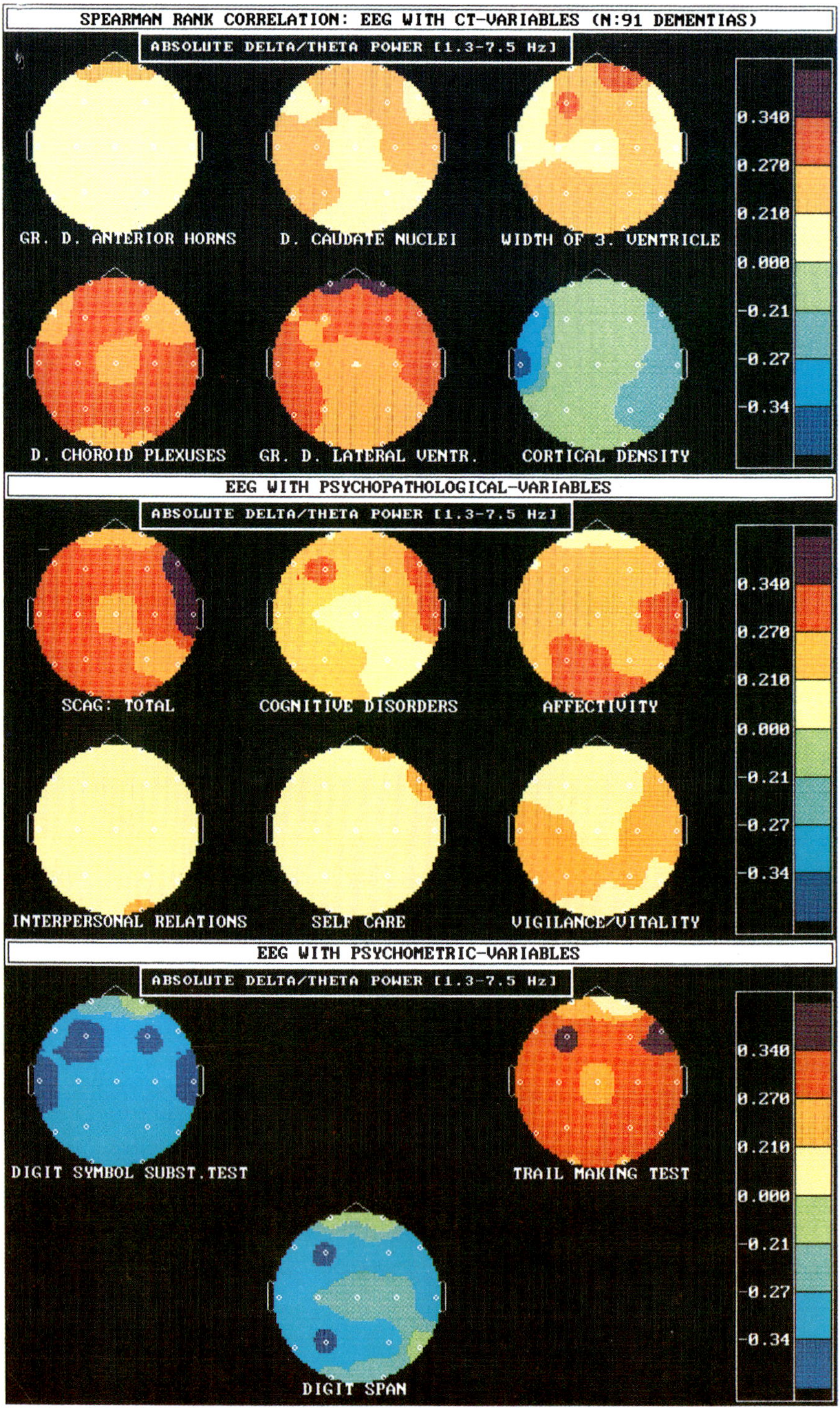

SPEARMAN RANK CORRELATION: EEG WITH CT-VARIABLES (N:91 DEMENTIAS)
ABSOLUTE DELTA/THETA POWER [1.3-7.5 Hz]
GR. D. ANTERIOR HORNS
D. CAUDATE NUCLEI
WIDTH OF 3. VENTRICLE
D. CHOROID PLEXUSES
GR. D. LATERAL VENTR.
CORTICAL DENSITY
0.340
0.270
0.210
0.000
-0.21
-0.27
-0.34
EEG WITH PSYCHOPATHOLOGICAL-VARIABLES
ABSOLUTE DELTA/THETA POWER [1.3-7.5 Hz]
SCAG: TOTAL
COGNITIVE DISORDERS
AFFECTIVITY
INTERPERSONAL RELATIONS
SELF CARE
VIGILANCE/VITALITY
EEG WITH PSYCHOMETRIC-VARIABLES
ABSOLUTE DELTA/THETA POWER [1.3-7.5 Hz]
DIGIT SYMBOL SUBST.TEST
TRAIL MAKING TEST
DIGIT SPAN

centroid of the total activity. While SDAT patients exhibited these differences specifically over the parietal and temporal regions, MID patients showed these differences over all brain regions (Saletu et al. 1988).

Correlation maps regarding the relationship between CT and EEG slow wave activity demonstrated that the lower the cortical density and the wider the CSF spaces, the higher the δ/θ power (Fig. 1, upper row). Furthermore, the more pronounced the slowing of brain function, the worse the psychopathology, as evaluated by the clinician utilizing the SCAG score (Fig. 1, middle row). Finally, the slower the brain activity, the worse the performance, with regard to recognition, and memory of the patient, as evaluated by means of the DSST, the ZVT, and the DS tests (Fig. 1, lower row).

References

Anderer P, Saletu B, Kinsperger K, Semlitsch H (1987) Topographic brain mapping of EEG in neuropsychopharmacology – part I: Methodological aspects. Methods Find Exp Clin Pharmacol 9:371–384

Meese W, Kluge W, Grumme T, Hopfenmüller W (1980) CT evaluation of the CSF spaces of healthy persons. Neuroradiology 19:131–136

Saletu B, Anderer P, Paulus E, Grünberger J, Wicke L, Neuhold A, Fischhof PK, Litschauer G, Wagner G, Hatzinger R, Dittrich R (1988) EEG brain mapping in SDAT and MID patients before and during placebo and xantinolnicotinate therapy: reference considerations. In: Samson-Dollfus D, Guieu JD, Gotman J, Etevenon P (eds) Statistics and topography in quantitative EEG. Elsevier, Paris, pp 251–275

←

Fig. 1. Significance probability maps based on Spearman rank correlation coefficients between absolute δ/θ power and CT measurements (*upper row*), SCAG scores (*middle row*), and psychometric scores (*lower row*) in demented patients (n = 91). *Hot colors* represent positive, *cold colors* negative correlation ($r > 0.21$: $p < 0.05$; $r > 0.27$: $p < 0.01$; $r > 0.34$: $p < 0.001$). The wider the CSF spaces and the less the cortical density (specifically over temporal regions), the higher the δ/θ power. The higher the δ/θ activity, the worse the psychopathology, as measured by the total SCAG score (SCAG factors "vigilance/vitality," "cognitive disorders," and "affectivity"). The higher the δ/θ power, the less symbols could be substituted within 90 s, the more time it took patients to finish the trail making test, and the fewer the number of digits that could be remembered

Electroencephalogram Mapping During Cognitive Effort in Normals and Neurotics

M. ROTHER[1], W. KRAUSE, C. SCHLEUSSNER, U. KRAUSE, and H. WITTE

Introduction

Simplification by effective structuring of information in order to reduce mental effort is one basic component of human problem solving. This simplification depends on the ability to find representative structures in the learning material. The more effective the structures, the more effectively can problems be solved. Similarly uneffective structuring should demand higher cognitive effort to solve problems. Cognitive effort may change the basic rhythm of the electroencephalogram (EEG) (Creutzfeld et al. 1969). These changes can be found at different locations depending on the brain structures involved during different kinds of activation. Topographical differences can be described by the EEG mapping method. Thus, in the first part of the study, we examined whether ineffective structuring by untrained persons is accompanied by more EEG desynchronization than effective structuring by trained persons.

We supposed that patients suffering from performance disabilities during daily work may not structure effectively. They need more cognitive effort to solve problems. The greater effort may lead to inadequate tiredness during long-lasting mental load. Thus, in the second part of the study, changes of EEG activity during a problem solving paradigm by patients with performance disabilities were compared to the results of the normal controls examined during the first part of the study.

Subjects and Methods

The control group consists of 21 healthy volunteers (11 trained and 10 untrained in problem solving). Nine patients suffering from performance disabilities during daily work (reason for consultation of the psychiatrist) were included in the study. None of the patients showed abnormalities during routine psychological testing (behavioral questionnaires). All subjects

[1] Klinische Forschung LFWK, Hoechst Aktiengesellschaft, Werk Kalle-Albert, Postfach 3540, W-6200 Wiesbaden, FRG.

Imaging of the Brain in Psychiatry
and Related Fields
Edited by K. Maurer

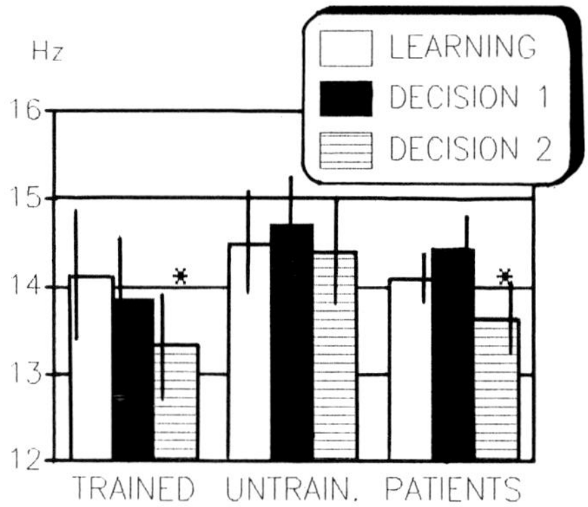

Fig. 1. Global mean frequency of the α/β frequency band during the test periods for trained controls, untrained controls, and patients. *Statistical differences ($p < 0.05$ level) between decision 1 and decision 2

were right-handed, free of medication, without neurological or psychiatric diseases in the case history, and well educated (graduated or students).

The paradigm consists of a learning and a decision period. The learning material is paired relational statements which had to be structured (for more details see Schleußner et al. 1991). The learning statements can be used as often as seems necessary for the subjects. During the decision part of the test the subjects had to use their internal structures to answer questions on the relation between two elements. "Yes" and "no" were the possible answers. The time interval between the presentation of the question and the answer was measured as reaction time; 444 questions were given to the subjects.

The EEG was recorded simultaneously with the presentation of the learning material during the learning period and the first 32 questions during decision parts 1 and 2. A 15-channel EEG (10–20 system, reference: $A_1 + A_2$; see Fig. 2) was used. The EEG was digitized with a sampling rate of 100 Hz for 256 data points for each interval. After fast Fourier transformation the mean frequency and the square root of summarized spectral power within the θ (4–8 Hz) and α/β (8–30 Hz) frequency bands were calculated. Only visually inspected artifact-free segments were considered for quantitative analysis. For artifact detection, the electrooculogram (EOG) was recorded simultaneously with the EEG.

The global mean frequency representing the grand average of all mean frequencies of all 15 EEG montages and the global spectral power representing the grand average of the square root of summarized spectral power of the θ and α/β frequency band for all channels were calculated. The global mean frequency and the global spectral power were averaged for all epochs of the learning period, the decision 1 period, and the decision 2 period (Fig. 1). Statistical comparisons between the global parameters of all epochs were made by the Wilcoxon test for paired data for the groups of interest. For the calculation of the topographical maps the four nearest neighbor method was used for interpolation. Statistical differences of EEG

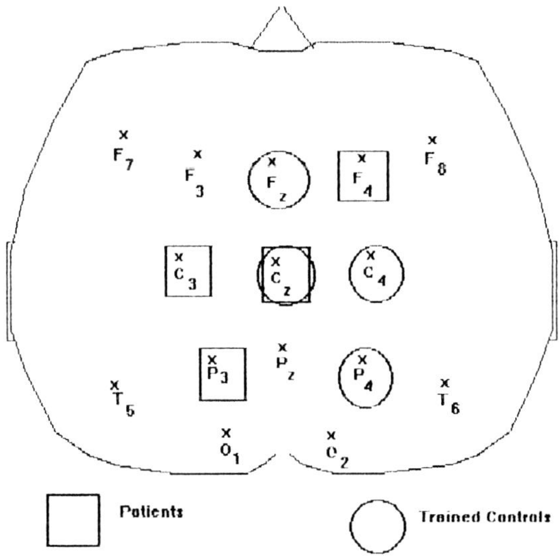

Fig. 2. Statistical differences ($p < 0.05$) of the mean frequency of the α/β frequency band for the trained controls and the patients between decision 1 and decision 2. Significant differences ($p < 0.05$) at the electrode positions are marked with *circles* or *rectangles*

topography during the different test epochs in all groups were verified by the Wilcoxon test statistic considering the parameters separately for every electrode montage (Fig. 2).

Results and Discussion

The mean frequency of the α/β frequency band in the trained controls shows the expected significant reduction during the decision part of the study (Fig. 1) indicating less cognitive effort than in the learning part. This mean frequency was not decreased or even higher during the decision part in untrained controls indicating high mental effort during the decision period too. This is probably due to ineffective structuring during the learning period. It corresponds to our previous results showing higher mean frequencies during an ineffective structuring paradigm in one and the same subject than during an effective structuring paradigm (Schleußner et al. 1991).

In neurotics we found an increase of mean frequency during the first part of decision indicating higher mental effort because of insufficient structuring during the learning period. In contrast to the untrained controls we found a significant decrease of mean frequency during decision 2. This phenomenon might be caused because better structuring was performed during decision 1 with subsequent effective problem solving, as in the trained controls. A second explanation could be that the frequency decrease is caused by inadequate tiredness. The latter explanation is supported by the long-lasting reaction time in the patients in comparison to the trained controls (patients 1900 ms, untrained controls 1550 ms, trained controls 900 ms). That different mechanisms are involved in the frequency decrease during the decision part 2 of the trained controls and the patients can be shown by the different EEG topography of these changes in both groups (Fig. 2).

No effect of global spectral power of the θ and α/β frequency range or of the global mean frequency of the θ band was found. This might be due to global averaging. The significant increase of the parameter at some electrodes might be covered by a decrease at other electrodes. Such contrary changes of the α rhythm of frontal and parietooccipital regions in psychophysiological studies were shown by Pfurtscheller and Klimesch (1990). These topographical phenomena should be evaluated in further processing of the data. The cognitive load during the learning period should be characterized in further studies by comparison to an unspecific reference (control) situation.

References

Creuzfeld O, Grünewald G, Simonova O, Schmitz H (1969) Changes of the basic rhythms of the EEG during the performance of mental and visuomotor tasks. In: Evans CR, Mulholland B (eds) Attention in neurophysiology. Butterworth, London, pp 148–168

Pfurtscheller G, Klimesch W (1990) Topographic display and interpretation of event-related desynchronization during a visual-verbal task. Brain Topography 3(1): 85–93

Schleußner C, Rother M, Krause W (1991) Die Psychophysiologische Messung des Kognitiven Aufwandes. Z.F. Psychol Suppl 11:415–421

Topographic Brain Mapping of Emotion-Related Hemisphere Activity and Susceptibility to Psychosomatic Disorders

W. Wittling[1], R. Roschmann, and E. Schweiger

Introduction

There is some evidence that the cerebral hemispheres markedly differ in their capability to regulate physiological processes during emotional situations. The right hemisphere plays an especially dominant role in the control of emotion-related cardiovascular and neuroendocrine responses (Hugdahl et al. 1983; Wittling 1990; Wittling and Pflüger 1990). Moreover, deviations from the normal pattern of functional hemisphere asymmetry may be associated with a heightened risk for developing psychosomatic and autoimmune disorders. Geschwind and Behan (1982, 1984) were the first to show that left-handedness is up to three times more frequent in psychosomatic disordered individuals. These findings have been widely confirmed in further studies (Lelong et al. 1986; Smith 1987; Searleman and Fugagli 1987; Betancur et al. 1990).

There are some problems, however, in interpreting this association between sinistrality and psychosomatic diseases because the findings are not based on direct measurements of cerebral dominance patterns. They only provide indirect evidence, as it must be taken into account that only about 50% of left handers show deviations from the normal pattern of functional hemisphere asymmetries. Therefore, the purpose of the present study was to examine whether individuals with a high or low degree of susceptibility to psychosomatic disorders differ in their emotion-related hemisphere activity as measured by topographic brain mapping of event-related potentials.

Method

A total of 42 subjects (20 males, 22 females) aged 21–30 years participated in the experiment. All subjects were students at the Catholic University of Eichstätt. Only right-handed subjects with normal speech lateralization were accepted for the experiment.

[1] Abt. für Physiologische und Klinische Psychologie, Kath. Universität Eichstätt, Ostenstr. 26-28, W-8078 Eichstätt, FRG.

Imaging of the Brain in Psychiatry
and Related Fields
Edited by K. Maurer

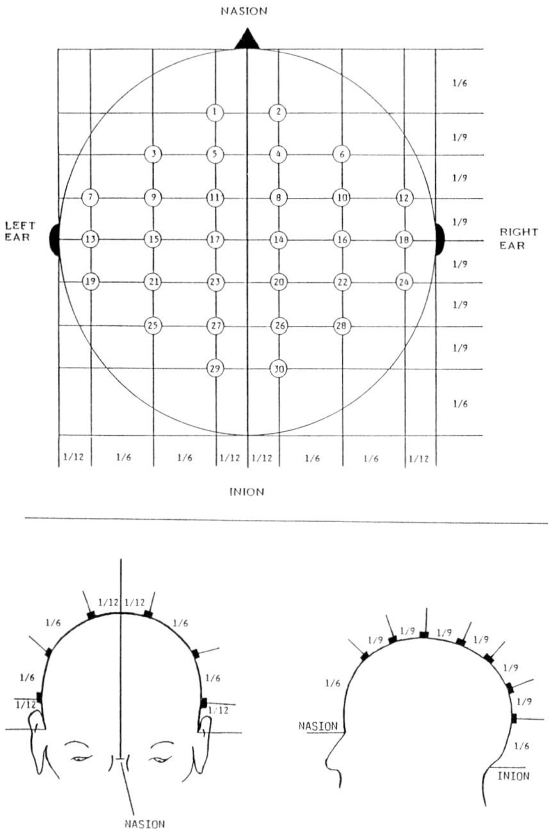

Fig. 1. Placement of electrodes

To establish two experimental groups differing in their degree of psychosomatic susceptibility, a well-known German personality inventory, the revised form of the *Freiburger Persönlichkeits-Inventar* (FPI-R), was used (Fahrenberg et al. 1984). Subjects were selected according to their score on the somatic complaints scale (scale 8) of the FPI-R. Subjects scoring extremely high on the somatic complaints scale (stanine 6–9) were classified as the group of psychosomatic disordered individuals, whereas the other group consisted of subjects showing an extremely low level of psychosomatic disorders (stanine 1–4). The two experimental groups were matched according to sex (10 males, 11 females each) and age. In an additionally administered questionnaire developed by ourselves the two groups also showed significant differences in the frequency of specific psychosomatic diseases.

Subjects were shown 130 color slides of human faces grouped into two emotion-related categories. Photographs of normal human faces served as neutral stimuli, while faces deformed by dermatologic diseases were used as emotional stimuli representing a clearly aversive emotional quality. The series of emotional and neutral stimuli each included 65 different slides. The pictures were presented tachistoscopically with a stimulus duration of 150 ms in central vision in a random order sequence.

The brain mapping system we used was constructed in accordance with the brain electrical activity mapping (BEAM) technique of Duffy et al. (1979, 1981). The electrical activity of the brain was recorded from 30 electrodes attached to the scalp with collodion. The electrodes were placed according to the system depicted in Fig. 1 and allowed a high electrode density with electrodes positioned systematically symmetric to the midline. Monopolar recordings with a time constant of 0.3 s and a upper cutoff of 32 Hz were made with linked earlobes as reference. In order to detect artifacts, horizontal and vertical eye movements were registered. Data acquisition and stimulus presentation were under the control of an Eltec 68K computer, which digitized the electroencephalogram (EEG) and electro-oculogram (EOG) at 1.79 ms intervals providing a sampling rate of more than 550 Hz. The recordings covered a 200 ms pre- and a 1600 ms post-stimulus period for each slide presentation. Recording was carried out in a sound-attenuated electrically shielded chamber.

The potentials obtained for each subject were averaged separately for emotional and neutral stimulus conditions. Grand means for the two experimental groups and the whole subject group were calculated for both conditions. For statistical analysis topographic *t* test comparisons were performed and depicted by means of significance probability mapping.

Results

At first we compare the potentials evoked by neutral versus emotional stimuli for the whole subject group. A typical example of grand means obtained for neutral and emotional stimuli is illustrated in Fig. 2. The waveforms are characterized primarily by a positive component at about 350 ms latency followed by a long-lasting negativity. This negativity is especially marked for the emotional stimulus condition and reaches its maximum at about 1000 ms after stimulus onset.

Statistical analysis by *t* test comparisons confirms that emotional stimuli evoke a significantly higher negativity in the period between 800 and 1200 ms over the whole posterior region. A typical example for the distribution of these significant differences is presented in Fig. 3.

As a second step we compare the two experimental groups with low versus high susceptibility to psychosomatic disorders in their responses to both neutral and emotional stimuli by means of topographic *t* test comparisons. Generally, there are marked differences between the two subject groups for the emotional stimulus condition but not for the neutral one. Group differences are significant between 560 ms and 1000 ms. The differences indicate that individuals with a low susceptibility to psychosomatic

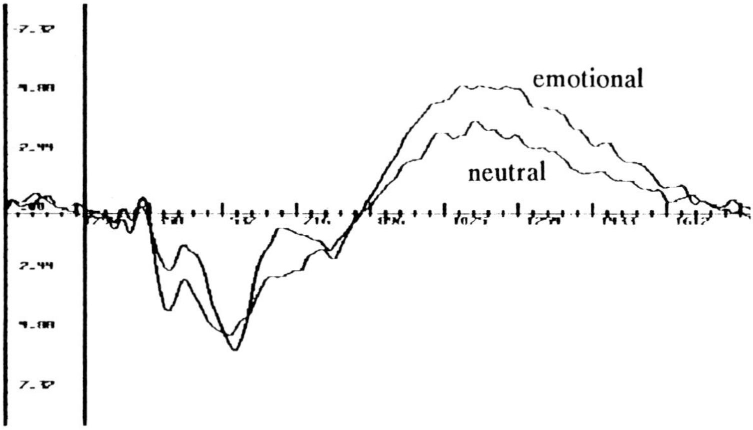

Fig. 2. Example of grand means obtained for neutral and emotional stimuli (electrode 22) for the whole subject group; the *vertical line* marks stimulus onset (prestimulus interval 200 ms); downward deflection indicates positivity

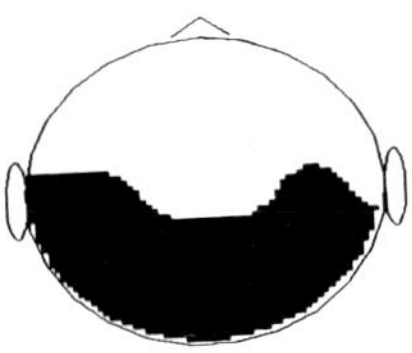

Fig. 3. Example of the *t* test probability maps for the comparison of neutral vs emotional stimulus conditions (913 ms latency); *black areas* indicate differences on a significance level of 5% representing a higher negativity in the emotional stimulus condition

disorders respond to emotional stimuli with a higher negative potential than subjects with a high susceptibility to such disorders. These differences are varying in their extent, but it becomes obvious that they are mainly restricted to the right hemisphere (Fig. 4).

Discussion

The findings indicate that individuals with a high susceptibility to psychosomatic disorders clearly differ from psychosomatically healthy individuals in the processing of emotionally laden material but not in the processing of neutral stimuli. In particular, they show a lower negativity in the late component of the potentials evoked by emotional stimuli. This late negativity has been found to be characteristic for the processing of emotionally laden material (Roschmann 1990; Roschmann and Wittling 1992). The observed group differences mainly occur over the right hemisphere.

It can be concluded that individuals with high levels of psychosomatic disorders show abnormal patterns of functional hemisphere asymmetry.

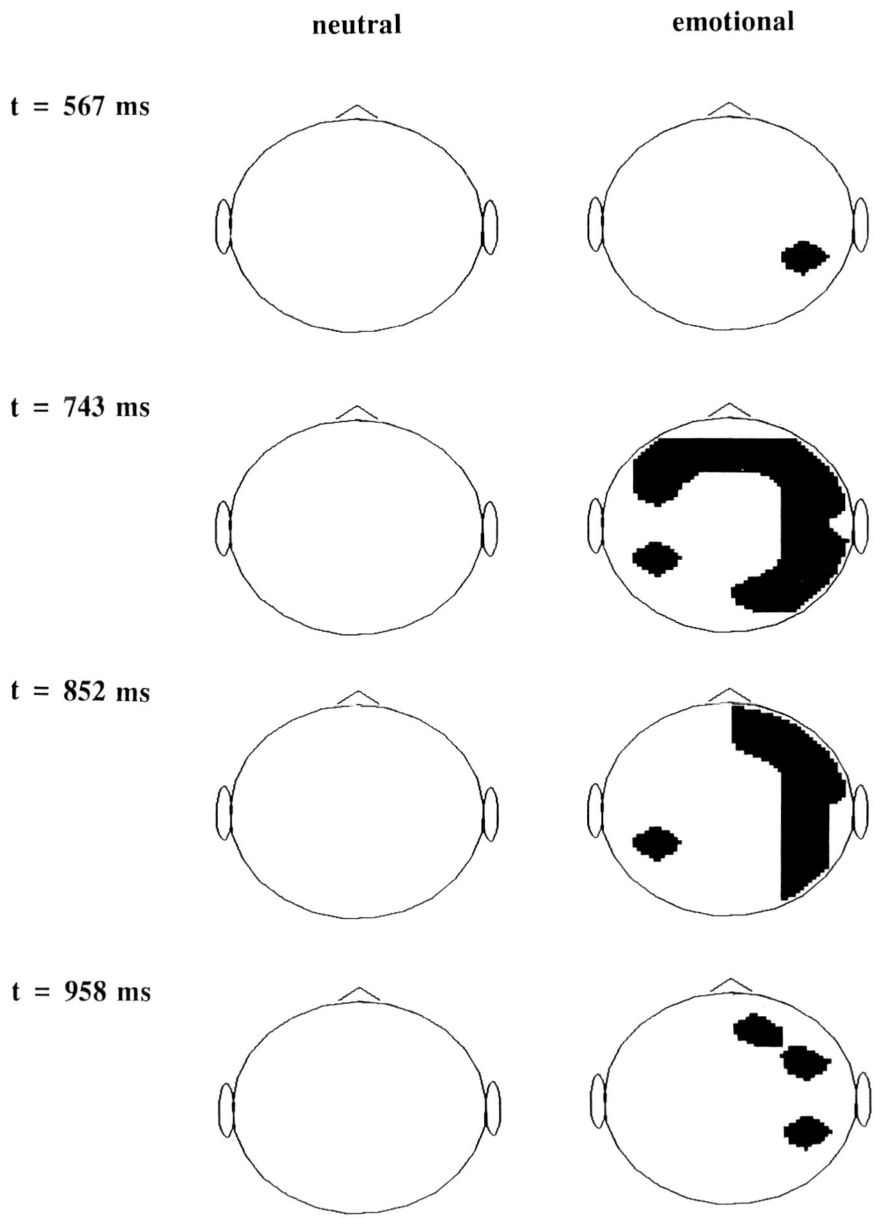

Fig. 4. Examples of the *t* test probability maps for the comparison between the two experimental groups for the neutral and emotional stimulus condition; black areas indicate differences on a significance level of 5% representing a lower negativity in the group of psychosomatically disordered subjects

They are characterized by a weakening of the normally leading role of the right hemisphere in the regulation of emotion-related responses. The results are in accordance with the findings of Geschwind and Behan (1982, 1984) in sinistrals and with our results of previous studies obtained with a technique of lateralized film presentation (Wittling et al. 1990).

References

Betancur C, Vélez A, Cabanieu G, LeMoal M, Neveu PJ (1990) Association between left-handedness and allergy: a reappraisal. Neuropsychologia 28: 223–227

Duffy FH, Burchfiel JL, Lombroso CT (1979) Brain electrical activity mapping (BEAM): A method for extending the clinical utility of EEG and evoked potential data. Ann Neurol 5:309–321

Duffy FH, Bartels PH, Burchfiel JL (1981) Significance probability mapping: an aid in the topographic analysis of brain electrical activity. Electroencephalogr Clin Neurophysiol 51:445–462

Fahrenberg J, Hampel R, Selg H (1984) Das Freiburger Persönlichkeitsinventar (FPI-R). Hogrefe, Göttingen

Geschwind N, Behan PO (1982) Left-handedness: association with immune disease, migraine and developmental learning disorder. Proc Natl Acad Sci USA 79: 5097–5100

Geschwind N, Behan PO (1984) Laterality, hormones, and immunity. In: Geschwind N, Galaburda A (eds) Cerebral dominance. The biological foundations. Harvard University Press, Cambridge

Hughdahl K, Franzon M, Andersson B, Walldebo G (1983) Heart rate responses (HRR) to lateralized visual stimuli. Pavlovian J Biol Sci 18:186–198

Lelong M, Thelliez F, Thelliez P (1986) Les gauchers sont-ils plus souvent des allergiques? Allerg Immunol 18:10–13

Roschmann R (1990) Emotionale Reizverarbeitung in den zerebralen Hemisphären. Untersuchung zur Topographie ereigniskorrelierter Potentiale bei emotionsbezogener visueller Stimulation. Pustet, Regensburg

Roschmann R, Wittling W (1992) Topographic brain mapping of emotion-related hemisphere asymmetries. Int J Neurosci 63:5–16

Searleman A, Fugagli AK (1987) Suspected autoimmune disorders and left-handedness: Evidence from individuals with diabetes, Crohn's disease and ulcerative colitis. Neuropsychologia 25:367–374

Smith J (1987) Left-handedness: its association with allergic disease. Neuropsychologia 25:665–674

Wittling W (1990) Psychophysiological correlates of human brain asymmetry: blood pressure changes during lateralized presentation of an emotionally laden film. Neuropsychologia 28:457–470

Wittling W, Pflüger M (1990) Neuroendocrine hemisphere asymmetries: salivary cortisol secretion during lateralized viewing of emotion-related and neutral films. Brain Cogn 14:243–265

Wittling W, Pflüger M, Schweiger E (1990) Zerebrale Hemisphären-Anomalien: Ein Risikofaktor für die Genese psychosomatischer Störungen. In: Frey D (ed) Bericht über den 37. Kongreß der Deutschen Gesellschaft für Psychologie in Kiel. Hogrefe, Göttingen, pp 696–697

Neurometric Quantitative Electroencephalogram Subtyping of Obsessive Compulsive Disorders

F. Mas[1], L.S. Prichep, E.R. John, and R. Levine

Introduction

Obsessive compulsive disorder (OCD) has been the subject of a growing body of biologically oriented psychiatric research. There is mounting evidence for a neurobiological basis for OCD. Early studies of the conventional electroencephalogram (EEG) generally showed a higher prevalence of abnormal records in obsessional patients (Pacella et al. 1944; Rockwell 1847). Using quantitative EEG (QEEG) in obsessional patients, Flor-Henry et al. (1979) noted abnormalties in the left temporal region.

In the present study, we evaluated the QEEG in OCD patients using the neurometric method. Neurometrics uses a standardized procedure in which 19 channels of data are collected using on-line artifact rejection. Quantitative features are extracted and log transformed to obtain Gaussianity, age-regressed, and Z-transformed relative to population norms (John et al. 1988a). Results of discriminant analyses, published elsewhere, demonstrate the differential diagnositic sensitivity and specificity of the neurometric method (John et al. 1988b; Prichep et al. 1990a).

The major objectives in this preliminary investigation were to identify features of the power spectrum that might identify subtypes within the OCD patient group and to correlate pretreatment subtype membership with subsequent pharmacologic response.

Patients and Methods

A total of 15 patients with DSM III-R diagnosis of OCD were studied in a drug-free state. The population consisted of 4 females and 11 males, with a mean age of 41.4 years. The patients were seated comfortably in a sound and light attenuated chamber. After 20 min of eyes closed, resting EEG data were collected from the 19 monopolar electrode sites of the international 10–20 system, referred to linked earlobes. A differential eye channel was

[1] Brain Research Laboratories New York, University Medical Center, 550 First Avenue, New York, NY 10016, USA.

Imaging of the Brain in Psychiatry
and Related Fields
Edited by K. Maurer

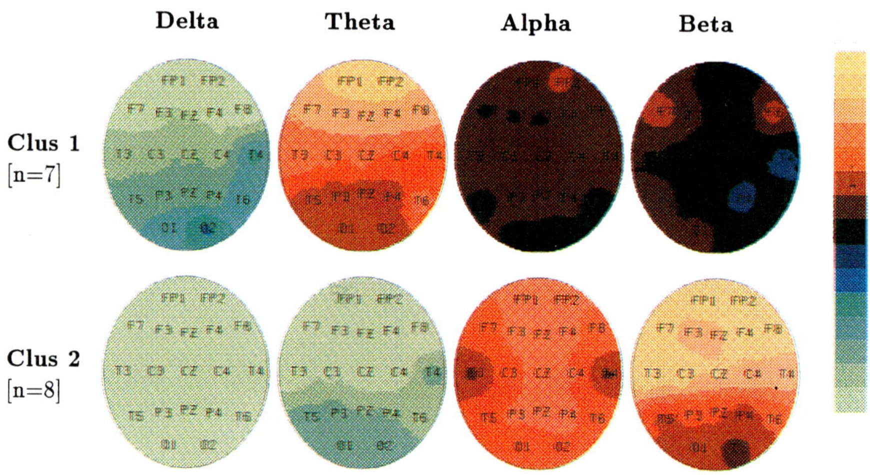

Fig. 1. Group average topographic maps (nose up) for Z relative power in the δ, θ, α, and β frequency bands for the two neurometric clusters of obsessive compulsive disorder OCD patients. Color coding is proportional to the mean Z score for each cluster in steps corresponding to those shown in the Z scale (range is ±1.64z). Note that in estimating the significance of the Z scale value for group data, the standard deviation (Z score) must be multiplied by the square root of the sample size; *clus*, cluster

used for the detection of eye movement. The EEG amplifiers had a bandpass from 0.5 to 30 Hz, with a 60 Hz notch filter; 2 min of artifact-free data were extracted from the EEG record for quantitative analysis.

After their baseline neurometric evaluations were obtained, the patients began treatment with a specific anti-OCD compound, such as chlomipramine or fluoxetine, together with supportive therapy. Treatment response was evaluated after 3 months utilizing the Clinical Global Improvement (CGI) rating system (Conners 1985). Responders were defined as markedly or moderately improved and nonresponders as those who showed minimal or no positive response.

In a previous evaluation of this data we studied the neurometric profiles of the responders and the nonresponders and reported clear differences in the group average topographic maps (Prichep et al. 1990b). In this analysis we used multivariate cluster analysis of the baseline (off medication) evaluations to identify subtypes in the population. Further, since we did not have enough patients in this preliminary study for a split-half replication, and since review of the data revealed no clear hemispheric findings, we did our initial cluster analysis of the baseline evaluations using a small subset of left hemispheric neurometric relative power variables and then repeated the cluster analysis with the right hemispheric homologous measures. The relationship between cluster membership and response to treatment was evaluated.

Results

Cluster analysis resulted in the identification of two subgroups of OCD patients, one containing seven and the other eight patients. The exact same cluster structure was obtained using the left and right hemispheric relative power variables, suggesting the strength of cluster structure. The variables contributing most to the cluster solution were frontotemporal θ central β, and posterior δ.

Group average topographic maps for Z relative power are shown in Fig. 1. Both clusters show a diffuse deficit of δ especially in the anterior regions. However, the members of cluster 1 show a slight anterior increase in θ, while the members of cluster 2 show a tendency toward increased α and a notable increase in β in the anterior and central regions.

Similar results were found for absolute power. Cluster 1 shows a tendency toward decreased power in δ, a tendency toward increased anterior power in θ with normal α and β distributions. Cluster 2 shows normal δ and θ distributions, but diffuse increased α and widespread increases in β, largest in the anterior and central regions.

It was found that 71% of the members of cluster 1 were considered to be nonresponders while 88% of the members of cluster 2 were found to be responders.

Conclusions

At baseline two clusters of OCD patients were identified: one containing the majority of those patients who later are identified as responders and the other containing most of the nonresponders. Responders show excess absolute and relative power in α and β, particularly in anterior leads, while nonresponders show less differences relative to norms, with a tendency towards anterior excess θ. The fact that the same clusters were obtained with either left or right hemisphere variables suggests the diffuse nature of the abnormalities.

While these findings need to be confirmed by larger studies (now in progress) which include additional quantitative clinical measurements, they suggest that OCD includes pathophysiological subtypes sharing a common clinical expression. The subtype involving the more β abnormalities appear more likely to respond to serotonin uptake blockades (alone or in combination with psychotherapy). However, the subtype with θ abnormalities do not appear to respond to the well known anti-OCD specific compounds used in this study but many respond more selectively to different psychopharmacologic and/or psycotherapeutic modalities not explored here.

References

Conners C (1985) Rating scales and checklists for child psychopharmacology. Psychopharmacol Bull 21:809–843

Flor-Henry P, Yeudall L, Koles Z, Howarth B (1979) Neuropsychological and power spectral EEG investigations of the obsessive-compulsive syndrome. Biol Psychiatry 14(1):119–130

John E, Prichep L, Friedman J, Essig-Peppard T (1988a) Neurometric classification of patients with different psychiatric disorders. In: Samson-Dollfus D (ed) Statistics and topography in quantitative EEG. Elsevier, Paris, pp 88–95

John E, Prichep L, Easton P (1988b) Neurometrics: computer assisted differential diagnosis of brain dysfunctions. Science 293:162–169

Pacella B, Polatin P, Nagler S (1944) Clinical and EEG studies in obsessive-compulsive states. Am J Psychiatry 100:830

Prichep L, John E, Essig-Peppard T, Alper K (1990a) Neurometric subtyping of depressive disorders. In: Cazzullo C, Invernizzi G, Sacchetti E, Vita A (eds) Plasticity and morphology of the central nervous system. MTP, London

Prichep L, Mas F, John E, Levine R (1990b) Neurometric subtyping of obsessive compulsive disorders. In: Stefanis CN, Rabavilas AD, Soldatos CR (eds) Psychiatry: a world perspective, vol. 1. Excerpta Medica, Amsterdam Elsevier, pp 557–562

Rockwell F (1947) The electroencephalogram and personality organization in the obsessive-compulsive reactions. Arch Neurol Psychiatry 57:71

Electroencephalogram Mapping in Sodium Lactate-Induced Panic Attacks: Preliminary Results

S. Pallanti[1], L. Rossi, G. de Palma, M, Checchi, C. Muscas, and C. Faravelli

Introduction

Response to sodium lactate infusion has been proposed as a laboratory model for evoking and studying panic attacks and as a possible biological marker for panic disorder (Liebowitz et al. 1984). However, electroencephalogram (EEG) recordings performed during this test yielded contrasting results. Fink et al. (1969) first reported that in five "anxious patients" EEG recording during lactate infusion showed increased β and decreased α bands compared to four healthy controls. Knott et al. (1981) reported α reduction and paradoxical increase of slow waves in six patients with DSM III panic disorder (PD). Lapierre et al. (1984), studying a larger sample of 23 patients with PD and 16 with generalized anxiety disorder (GAD), confirmed the increase of slow waves in the former but failed to find significant differences in the rate of lactate response between the two groups. However these authors did not use a control group of healthy subjects.

In an attempt to clarify EEG modifications we report our initial experience with EEG mapping in panic patients recorded during lactate infusion.

Patients and Methods

Five never-treated and presently drug-free patients (three females and two males; mean age 31, range 21–32) suffering from PD with agoraphobia according to DSM III-R were studied. The onset of the illness was datable to within 4 months of the recording.

The control group (four females and two males; mean age 25, age range 17–31) was drawn from hospital staff members; none had current or preceding psychopathological disorders or a family history of PD or major depression.

Informed consent was obtained from each subject. Lactate challenge was performed according to the procedure described by Liebowitz et al.

[1] Dept. of Neurological and Psychiatric Sciences, University of Florence, Viale Morgagni, 85 Florence, Italy.

Imaging of the Brain in Psychiatry and Related Fields
Edited by K. Maurer

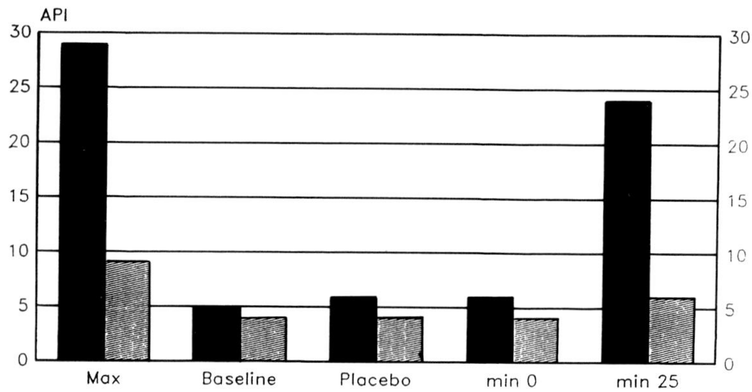

Fig. 1. Panic symptoms rating based on a modified version of the acute panic inventory. ■, P.D. patients; ▨, controls. (Adapted from Dillon et al. 1987)

(1984). A 16-channel EEG was performed on resting subjects while they received the infusion and Ag-AgCl electrodes were applied to the scalp according to the international 10–20 standard, in Fp1, Fp2, F3, F4, F7, F8, C3, C4, T3, T4, P3, P4, T5, T6, O1, and O2, and referred to linked ears. Electrode impedance was always <5 KΩ; high frequency cutoff was 70 Hz and CT 0.3 s. Artifact-free tracings were carefully selected and used as input to the analogue-to-digital converters of a brain surveyor computer for fast Fourier analysis and brain mapping. Brain mapping of absolute power spectrum in four frequency bands (θ 5.0–7.0 Hz, α 8.0–12.0 Hz, β1 13.0–20.0 Hz, β2 21.0–31.0 Hz) was compared from each brain electrode during placebo and lactate infusion. Variations in percentage of power spectrum from the left (F7, F3, C3, T3) and right (F8, F4, C4, T4) frontotemporooccipital and from the left (T5, P3, O1) and right (T6, P4, O2) parietotemporal areas were also compared. Symptoms of typical panic attack during infusion were rated by means of a modified version of the Acute Panic Inventory (API) (Dillon et al. 1987) and the occurrence of panic was established on the basis of both subjective and objective signs (increase of ventilation and heart rate – measured by ECG – of more than 30%).

Results

All the patients panicked during lactate infusion within a time ranging from 11 to 17 min of the infusion (mean time 15 min), while two control subjects reported light subjective discomfort without meeting the criteria for panic attack (Fig. 1).

Compared to the prelactate parameters, left and right frontotemporal and left parietooccipital significant increases of both the β bands were

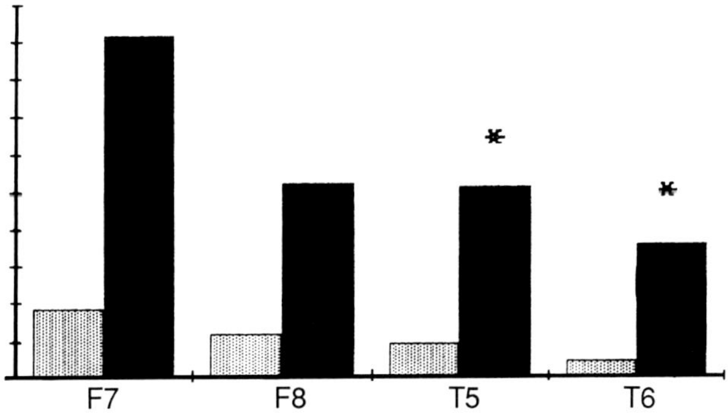

Fig. 2. Increased β1 band. *F7*, electrode pool F7, F3, T3; *F8*, electrode pool F8, F4, T4, C4; *T5*, electrode pool T5, P3, O1; *T6*, electrode pool T4, P4, O2. $^*p < 0.05$. ▨, controls; ■, patients

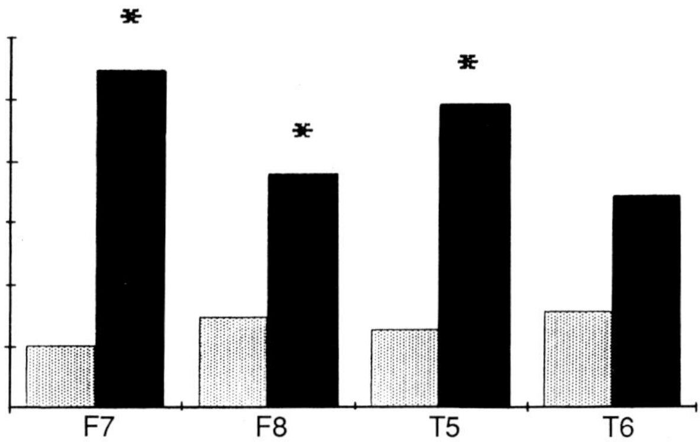

Fig. 3. Increased β2 band. *F7*, electrode pool F7, F3, T3; *F8*, electrode pool F8, F4, T4, C4; *T5*, electrode pool T5, P3, O1; *T6*, electrode pool T4, P4, O2. $^*p < 0.05$. ▨, controls; ■, patients

recorded in panic patients, while controls did not show any substantial modifications of their EEG parameters.

Statistical *t* maps showed a significant increase of β1 and β2 power spectrums during lactate-induced attacks. The main β1 increase was observed in the left parietooccipital area; a diffuse β2 increase was also observed (Figs. 2, 3).

Comments

EEG mapping could be used to improve the sensitivity of the diagnostic validity of lactate challenge for PD. The finding of an increase in fast frequencies (β1 and β2) is consistent with EEG changes usually seen in anxiety states (Lader 1975). The same EEG modification has been documented in GAD patients subjected to photostimulation (Grillon and Buchsbaum 1987).

References

Dillon DJ, Gorman JM, Liebowitz MR et al. (1987) The measurement of lactate induced panic and anxiety. Psychiatry Res 20:97–105

Fink M, Taylor M, Volavka J (1969) Anxiety precipitated by lactate. N Engl J Med 281:1429

Grillon C, Buchsbaum MS (1987) EEG topography of response to visual stimuli in generalized anxiety disorder. Electroencephalogr Clin Neurophysiol 66:337–348

Knott V, Chaudhry R, Lapierre YD (1981) Panic induced by sodium lactate: electrophysiological correlates. Prog Neuropsychopharmacol 5:511–514

Lader M (1975) The psychophysiology of anxious and depressed patients. In: Fowles D (ed) Clinical application of psychophysiology. Columbia University Press, New York

Lapierre YD, Knott V, Gray R (1984) Psychophysiological correlates of sodium lactate. Psychopharmacol Bull 20 n 1:50–57

Liebowitz MR, Fyer JA, Goram JM et al. (1984) Lactate provocation of panic attacks. Clinical and behavioral finding. Arch Gen Psychiatry 41:764–770

Hallucinations – Changes in Functional Brain Imaging (Electroencephalogram Mapping): Preliminary Data

T. MÜLLER[1], T. DIERKS, J. FRITZE, and K. MAURER

Introduction

Computerized tomography (CT) and magnetic resonance imaging (MRI) are excellent techniques for studying structural brain anatomy. Positron emission tomography, regional cerebral blood flow, and single photon emission CT (PET, RCBF, and SPECT) reveal brain function but suffer from the disadvantage of being invasive and requiring the subject to maintain a particular position for a relatively long period of time. These latter disadvantages are problematic when dealing with hallucinatory patients. In contrast, the electroencephalogram (EEG) has an extremely short analysis time and is not invasive. Our investigations involve EEG mapping, which allows display of the topographic distribution of functional states of brain electrical activity. The aim was to demonstrate topographic changes in the EEG caused by hallucinations.

Methods

EEG recordings, using a Brain Atlas III (Bio-logic System Corp.), of three, male, drug-free, schizophrenic patients diagnosed according to DSM III-R were made during a period of acute psychotic symptoms with auditory and visual hallucinations. A total of 19 electrodes were placed on the scalp according to the 10–20 system, linked mastoids were used as reference. Spectral analysis was performed on 20 s of artifact-free EEG (visually evaluated) using a fast Fourier transformation. Of special concern was to exclude fast segments suspected of containing muscle activity. The frequency spectra were analyzed in frequency bands according to the δ, θ, β, and α range.

[1] St. Josef-Hospital, Universitätsklinik, Neurologische Klinik, Gudrun-Str. 56, W-4630 Bochum 1, FRG.

Imaging of the Brain in Psychiatry
and Related Fields
Edited by K. Maurer

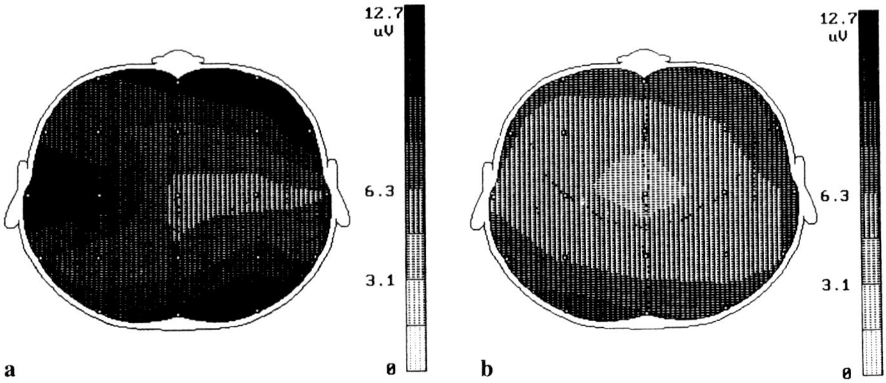

Fig. 1a,b. Mapping of EEG. **a** Hallucinatory symptoms: increased β activity on the left temporocentral and right occipital electrodes. **b** No hallucinatory symptoms: normal topographic distribution in the β range

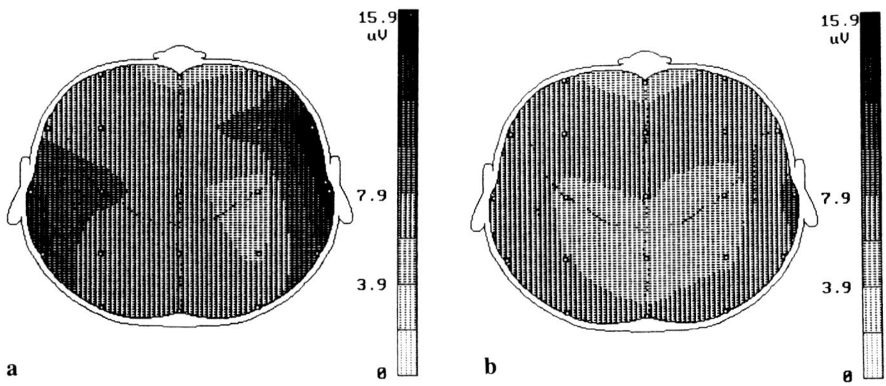

Fig. 2a,b. Mapping of EEG. **a** Hallucinatory symptoms: increased β activity on both temporal electrodes. **b** No hallucinatory symptoms: normal topographic distribution in the β range

Results

The β activity (15–23.50 Hz) showed an elevated activity over temporal (Fig. 2a, Fig. 3a) and temporocentral electrodes (Fig. 1a, Fig. 3a). Recordings taken after hallucinating psychotic states and after remission showed a normal topographic distribution (Fig. 1b, Fig. 2b, Fig. 3b). These changes had a high statistical significance level: the Z statistic on the β range over the C3 electrode was 3.7 SD (Fig. 4a) compared to healthy controls (Fig. 4b). In patients reporting delusions, thought disorder, and ideas of grandeur, these regions of increased β activity were not found.

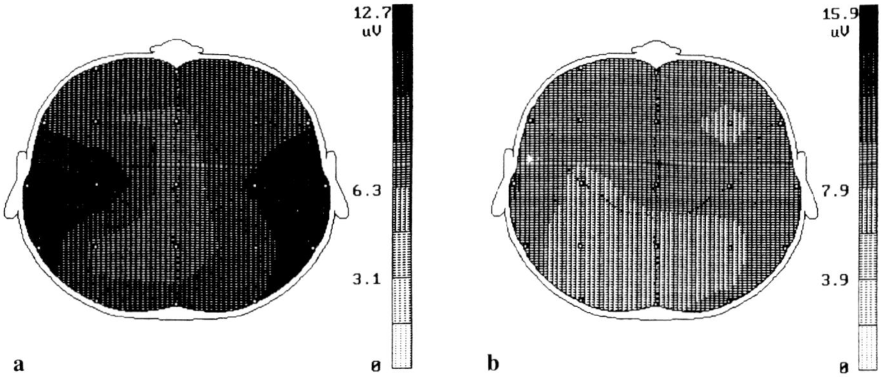

Fig. 3a,b. Mapping of EEG. **a** Hallucinatory symptoms: increased β activity on left temporocentral and right temporal electrodes. **b** No hallucinatory symptoms: normal topographic distribution in the β range

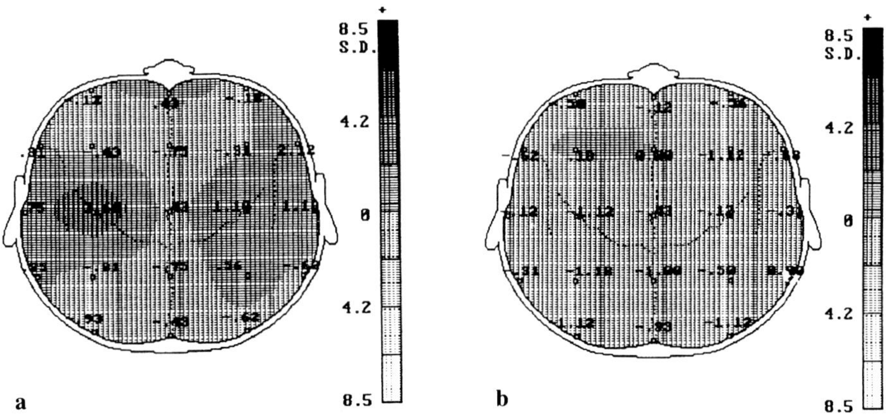

Fig. 4a,b. Z statistics in the β range **a** over the C3 electrode during hallucinatory symptoms: SD 3.7 compared to electrical activity in age-matched controls. **b** No hallucinatory symtoms

Discussion

Changes in neural activity in relation to different states of psychopathology has already been demonstrated by functional brain imaging using EEG mapping (Müller et al. 1989). Conventional multi-lead EEG recordings do not detect this localized increased β activity in acute hallucinatory patients. In drug-free schizophrenics with paranoid symptoms, these areas of increased β activity were not found. A positive correlation between electrical brain activity and cerebral blood flow has been noted (Günther et al. 1988);

therefore areas of elevated β activity could indicate increased regional brain perfusion in patients with hallucinatory symptoms. Highly significant correlations between blood flow measurements and the degree of psychoses were reported recently (Warkentin et al. 1990). Our findings are consistent with the hypothesis that positive symptoms in schizophrenia increase cerebral blood flow.

References

Günther W, Davous P, Godet JL, Guillibert E, Breitling D, Rondot P (1988) Bilateral brain dysfunction during motor activation in type II schizophrenia measured by EEG mapping. Biol Psychiatry 23:295–311

Müller T, Dierks T, Fritze J, Maurer K (1989) Functional brain imaging (mapping of EEG) in relation to psychopathologic changes in schizophrenia. Psychiatry Res 29:419–420

Warkentin S, Nilsson A, Risberg J, Karlson S, Flekköy K, Franzen G, Gustafson L, Rodriguez G (1990) Regional cerebral blood flow in schizophrenia: repeated studies during a psychotic episode. Psychiatry Res: Neuroimaging 35:27–38

Crack Cocaine Dependence: Discrimination from Major Depression Using Quantitative Electroencephalogram Variables

K.R. Alper[1], R.J. Chabot, A.H. Kim, L.S. Prichep, and E.R. John

The recognition of a syndrome of dependence associated with cocaine use is a relatively recent development. The statement that "Since only transitory withdrawal symptoms occur after cessation of or reduction in prolonged use, a separate category of dependence on cocaine is not included," quoted from DSM III (American Psychiatric Association 1980), has taken on an ironic significance in view of the present epidemic of crack cocaine use. Phenomenologic evidence for a syndrome of cocaine dependence indicates the existence of a characteristic progression of abstinence symptoms in withdrawing addicts which include anhedonia persisting for weeks after the last use (Gawin 1986). Evidence for biological correlates of the anhedonia of cocaine withdrawal includes the observation of decreased cerebral blood flow in abstinent cocaine abusers (Volkow et al. 1988) and reports of efficacy of pharmacological agents such as flupenthixol (Gawin et al. 1989a), desipramine (Gawin et al. 1989b), and bromocriptine (Giannini et al. 1989) in treating the anhedonia and craving associated with cocaine withdrawal. Collectively, the available behavioral, neurophysiological, and pharmacological evidence appears to support the concept of neuroadaptation in cocaine dependence (World Health Organization 1981).

In a poster presented at the meeting of the International Society for Neuroimaging in Psychiatry held in Wuerzburg in June 1990 our group presented pilot data from a quantitative electroencephalogram (QEEG) study of seven subjects with crack cocaine dependence who had been drug-free for 1–68 days. The major finding was an increase in absolute and relative α power. The contents of that poster have subsequently been published and are available elsewhere (Alper et al. 1990). Here, we wish to report on the evaluation of the above series of patients by a discriminant analysis using QEEG variables. The objective of this study was to determine if the profile features of the crack-dependent subjects resembled the profile of QEEG features we have previously reported for depression.

Our interest in the use of the depression QEEG discriminant arises from several lines of evidence indicating that there may be shared features of

[1] Brain Research Laboratories, New York University Medical Center, 550 First Avenue, New York, NY 10016, USA.

Imaging of the Brain in Psychiatry and Related Fields
Edited by K. Maurer

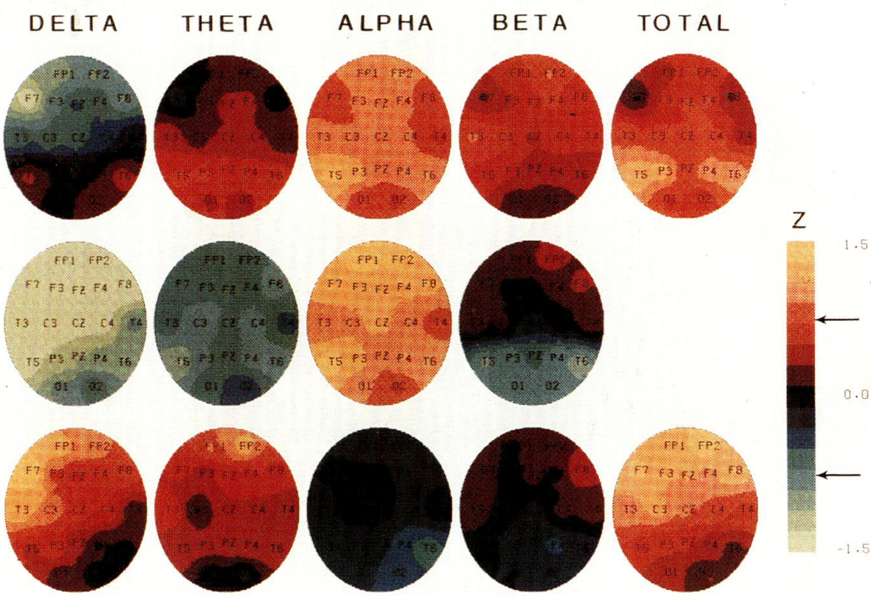

Fig. 1. Topographic head maps for group mean Z-scores for absolute power (*top row*), relative power (*middle row*), and mean frequency (*bottom row*). Color coding denotes the value of the group mean Z-score, which is proportional to the probability that the data obtained from the seven index subjects differ from the reference population of 150 normal adults. In estimates of the significance of a group mean Z-score, it is necessary to take the number of index subjects in the group into account. In the above figure, for example, the estimate of the critical value denoting significance at the level of $p = 0.05$ is $\pm 1.96/\sqrt{7} = \pm 0.74$ and is designated by the *horizontal arrows* to the right of the vertical color scale

depression and crack withdrawal. In the seven crack-dependent subjects we noted a mean Beck depression scale score of 18.9, a value that is in the range reported for subjects with major depression. In addition, four of these seven subjects had made suicide attempts, all subsequent to having begun the use of crack. A family history of affective disorder has been suggested to predispose to cocaine dependence (Nunes et al. 1988). Drugs with antidepressant activity such as desipramine and flupenthixol have been reported to facilitate abstinence for cocaine and to reduce the craving and anhedonia associated with cocaine withdrawal.

The QEEG profile of this group of crack cocaine-dependent subjects also supports the relevance of the comparison of cocaine withdrawal to depression. Figure 1 presents topographic maps of group mean Z-scores for absolute and relative power and mean frequency for each of the four frequency bands. It should be recalled that the color-coded values displayed designate the probability of a given value being within the confidence limits of EEG measurements obtained from normal individuals. The values are age-regressed and take into account the topographic variations of normative EEG data.

The major trend is an absolute and relative increase in α power. Values for excess α are significant at the 0.05 level at 17 of 19 leads for absolute power and 18 of 19 leads for relative power. Inspection of the data of individual subjects reveals that the relative α excess is present in each subject and is apparently consistent in each member of the group.

Absolute δ power is significantly decreased in five of the six frontal leads. A relative but not absolute "hyperfrontal" distribution of α power is due to decreased δ rather than significant topographic variability of increased α. There appears to a be a weak trend for increased absolute β power, which reaches significance in 4 of 19 leads. Relative power in all frequencies except α is decreased as a result of the widespread α excess. There is a trend for increased mean EEG frequency greater in the anterior leads for δ and θ but not α and β.

The apparent excess of α seen in these subjects bears an interesting relationship to the existing QEEG literature. Pollock and Schneider (1990), in a review of waking QEEG studies of depression, concluded that excess α was the most consistently reported QEEG correlate of depression. Itil (1983), in a review of pharmaco-EEG studies on depression, has suggested that the diminution of α typically seen with antidepressant drugs may serve a "corrective function," and that the similar QEEG profiles seen with multiple types of antidepressant drugs are determined by an underlying common pharmacological mechanism.

In the present investigation a two-way discriminant function, previously shown to discriminate depressed patients from normals, was used to classify the crack-dependent subjects. It was hypothesized that if the crack-dependent subjects were forced into this two-way discriminant they would tend to be classified as depressed. The development of this discriminant is described elsewhere (John et al. 1988a,b; Prichep et al. 1986).

It is possible to define cutoff levels for discriminant probability scores that correspond to confidence levels of classification accuracy (John et al. 1988b). In the present study we selected a cutoff score for classification as depressed corresponding to a false positive rate of less than or equal to 10%. Alternatively stated, a classification probability was used to categorize the crack cocaine-dependent patients as depressed such that the discriminant, if used to classify normal individuals, would falsely identify normals as depressed in less than 10% of cases. Table 1 displays the probability scores for depression in the discriminant for depression vs normal for each of the seven subjects. Three of the subjects have probabilities of being classified as depressed, significant at the 0.1 level and a fourth subject is above the frequently used 50% cutoff, which corresponds to a confidence level of approximately 0.2. By the criterion of discriminant classification in this

Table 1. Discriminant probability scores for depression in seven subjects with crack cocaine dependence: normal vs major depression discriminant

Subject	Major depression probability score
1	10.5
2	23.8
3	60.0[a]
4	56.8
5	93.6[a]
6	61.0[a]
7	45.8

[a] Discriminant scores exceeding the classification cutoff level $p \leqslant 0.10$, that is, the level at which the probability of a false positive classification is less than 10%.

small series of patients, crack dependence appears to share some common features with depression. Interestingly, all of the three patients classified as depressed at the 0.1 level had histories of suicide attempts, which were present in only one of the four individuals not classified as depressed at the 0.1 level.

The QEEG features that this laboratory has identified as having contributed most strongly to the discrimination of depressed from normal subjects are reduced anterior slow wave coherence, increased absolute power, and increased asymmetry of power values from the two cerebral hemispheres (John et al., 1988a,b; Prichep et al. 1986). Inspection of the individual QEEG results of each cocaine-dependent subject does not reveal a striking trend towards either anterior incoherence or power asymmetries. Increased absolute power, chiefly as a consequence of increased α power is present in the records of each of the seven subjects and likely contributes to the trend for classification of these cocaine-dependent individuals as depressed when forced into the two-way normal depression discriminant.

This apparent similarity of EEG states of crack withdrawal and depression might be explained by reduced neurotransmission of dopamine and serotonin systems in both states. The release of brain dopamine appears to underly cocaine's effects on reward mediated behavior. A consequence of exposure to pulsatile elevations of dopamine transmission may be a downregulation of dopamine receptors (Gawin 1986). Brain dopamine and serotonin systems are highly interdependent; there is a strong correlation reported for homovanillic acid and 5-hydroxyindoleacetic acid in cerebrospinal fluid (Agren 1983), and tricyclic antidepressants increase both dopaminergic and serotonergic neurotransmission (Jimerson 1987; Willner 1985). It is possible that the anhedonia of crack withdrawal and depression might involve a common abnormality in systems subserving reward mediated behavior. It is likely that, although some electrophysiological features may be shared, other features might differentiate the two disorders. Further studies of withdrawing cocaine addicts are presently underway and will hopefully clarify the relationship of cocaine dependence to mood disorders.

References

Agren H (1983) Depression and altered neurotransmission – states, traits and interactions. In: Angst J (ed) The origins of depression: current concepts and approaches. Springer, Berlin Heidelberg New York, pp 297–311

Alper K, Chabot R, Kim A, Prichep L, John E (1990) Quantitative EEG correlates of crack cocaine dependence. Psychiatry Res 35:95–106

American Psychiatric Association (1980) DSM-III: diagnostic and statistical manual, 3rd edn. American Psychiatric Association, Washington

Gawin F (1986) Abstinence symptomatology and psychiatric diagnosis in cocaine abusers. Arch Gen Psychiatry 43:107–113

Gawin F, Allen D, Humblestone B (1989a) Outpatient treatment of "crack" cocaine smoking with flupenthixol decanoate. Arch Gen Psychiatry 46:322–325

Gawin FH, Kleber H, Byck R, Rounsaville B, Kosten T, Jatlow P, Morgan C (1989b) Desipramine facilitation of initial cocaine abstinence. Arch Gen Psychiatry 46:117–121

Giannini AJ, Folts DJ, Feather J, Sullivan B (1989) Bromocriptine and amantadine in cocaine detoxification. Psychiatry Res 29:11–16

Itil T (1983) The discovery of antidepressant drugs by computer-analyzed human cerebral bio-electrical potentials (CEEG). Prog Neurobiol 20:185–249.

Jimerson D (1987) Role of dopamine mechanisms in the affective disorders. In: Meltzer H (ed) Psychopharmacology: the third generation of progress. Raven, New York, pp 505–511

John E, Prichep L, Fridman J, Easton P (1988a) Neurometrics: computer assisted differential diagnosis of brain dysfunctions. Science 293:162–169

John E, Prichep L, Friedman J, Essig-Peppard T (1988b) Neurometric classification of patients with different psychiatric disorders. In: Samson-Dollfus D (ed) Statistics and topography in quantitative EEG. Elsevier, Paris, pp 88–95

Nunes E, Quitkin F, Klein D (1988) Psychiatric diagnosis in cocaine abuse. Psychiatry Res 28:105–114

Pollock V, Schneider LS (1990) Quantitative, waking EEG research on depression. Biol Psychiatry 27:757–780

Prichep L, Lieber A, John E, Alper K, Gomez-Mont F, Essig-Peppard T, Flitter M (1986) Quantitative EEG in depressive disorders. In: Shagass C, Josiassen R, Roemer R (eds) Brain electrical potentials and psychopathology. Elsevier, Amsterdam, pp 223–244

Volkow N, Mullani N, Gould KL, Adler S, Krajewski K (1988) Cerebral blood flow in chronic cocaine users: a study with positron emission tomography. Br J Psychiatry 152:641–648

Willner P (1985) Antidepressants and serotonergic neurotransmission: an integrative review. Psychopharmacology (Berl) 85:387–404

World Health Organization (1981) Nomenclature and classification of drug and alcohol-related problems: a WHO memorandum. Bull WHO 59(2):225–242

Adrenergic-Cholinergic Balances: Interaction of Physostigmine and Clonidine in Behavior and Topographic Electrical Brain Activity

J. FRITZE[1], T. DIERKS, L. FRÖLICH, M. LANCZIK, T. MÜLLER, and K. MAURER

Introduction

Physostigmine in healthy volunteers induces a behavioral syndrome reminiscent of depression and characterized by anergia and anhedonia. Affectively ill subjects react supersensitively and possibly experience a transient but full-blown depression even in the euthymic interval (Janowsky et al. 1980). The electroencephalogram (EEG) is desynchronized by physostigmine (Domino 1968). The behavioral effects of physostigmine are accompanied by cardiovascular and endocrine stress phenomena (Janowsky et al. 1986). These effects might be due to a muscarinic-cholinergic stimulation of noradrenergic neuronal systems (Janowsky and Risch 1984). Indeed, in the rat, locus coeruleus neurons are cholinergically stimulated (Engberg and Svensson 1980). Therefore, the present study investigated, whether the α2-adrenergic agonist clonidine (Kobinger 1978), by stimulating presynaptic autoreceptors of noradrenergic neurons, might antagonize physostigmine.

Methods

Five healthy male volunteers (age 31–39 years) participated after giving their informed consent. The study had a double-blind crossover design with counterbalanced randomized order. EEG electrodes were placed according to the 10–20 system and electrical brain activity was recorded by 20 channels using the Brain Atlas III (Bio-Logic Systems, Mundelein, Illinois, USA). The EEG was recorded at rest (1:50 P.M.) and at 2:30 P.M., 2:55 P.M., 3:10 P.M., and 3:40 P.M. At 1:30 P.M., 0.2 mg glycopyrrolate were injected intramuscularly. Starting at 2 P.M. either 1 μg/kg clonidine in saline or placebo was infused via an intravenous tube over 10 min followed by 22 μg/kg physostigmine over 10 min at 2:40 P.M. EDTA-blood was drawn every 10 min for 2 h starting at 2 P.M. Heart and respiration rate were recorded continuously via electrocardiogram (ECG) electrodes, blood pressure was measured every 2 min. Mood and behavior were rated at 2:20

[1] Troponwerke, Berlinerstr. 156, W-5000 Köln 80, FRG.

Imaging of the Brain in Psychiatry and Related Fields
Edited by K. Maurer

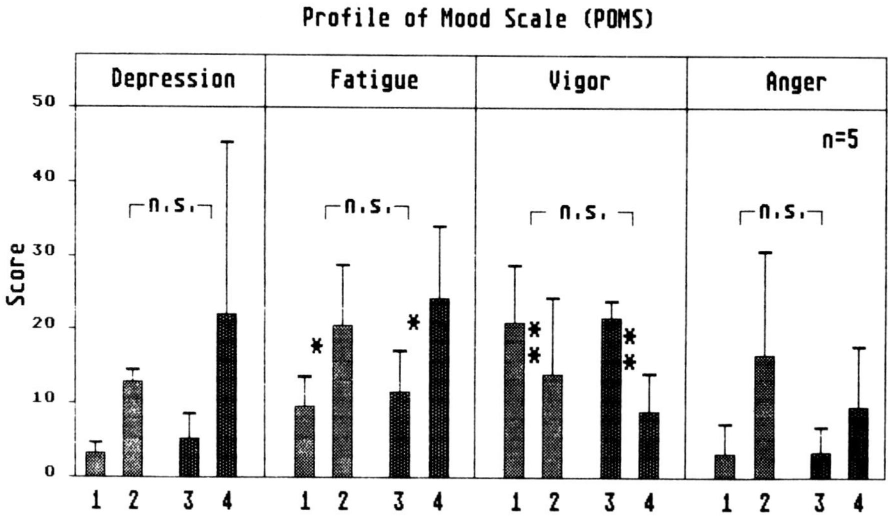

Fig. 1. Self-ratings (POMS) following placebo (*1*) → physostigmine (*2*) and clonidine (*3*) → physostigmine (*4*) demonstrating anergia and anhedonia uninfluenced by clonidine (ANOVA with repeated measures)

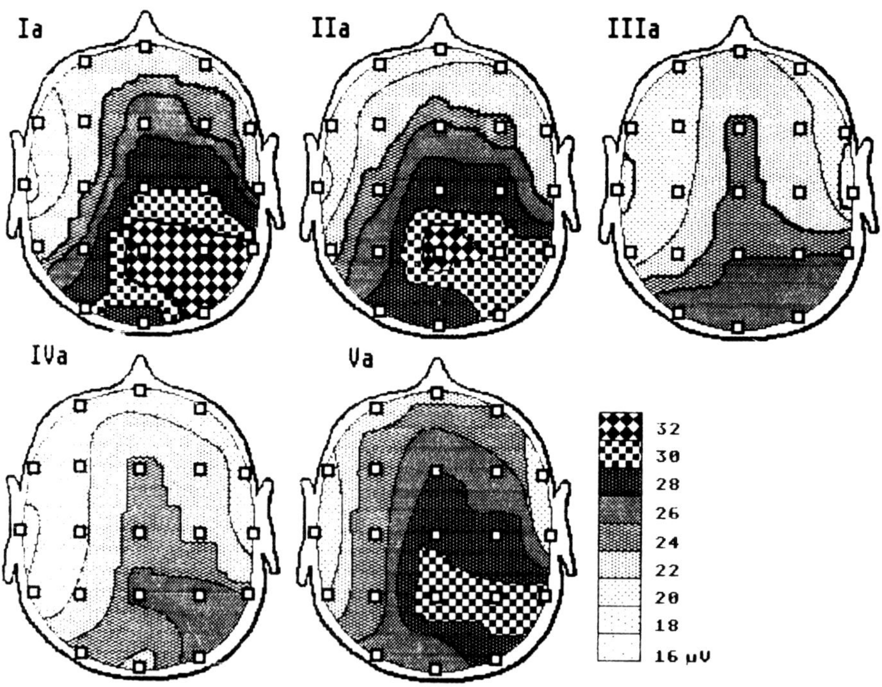

Fig. 2. Brain electric activity map: amplitude of 8–11.5 Hz activity at baseline (*I*), 30 min after placebo (*II*), and 15 min (*III*), 30 min (*IV*), and 60 min (*V*) after 22 μg/kg physostigmine following placebo ($n = 5$)

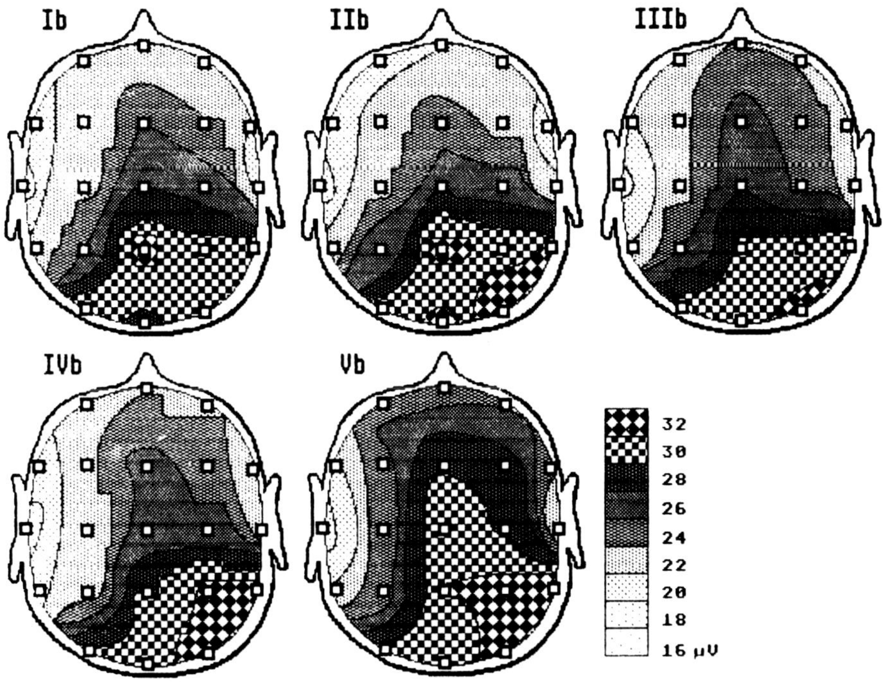

Fig. 3. Brain electric activity map: amplitude of 8–11.5 Hz activity at baseline (*I*), 30 min after 1 μg/kg clonidine (*II*), and 15 min (*III*), 30 min (*IV*), and 60 min (*V*) after 22 μg/kg physostigmine following clonidine ($n = 5$)

P.M. and 3:20 P.M. using the observer's version of the Activation Inhibition Scale (AIS; Janowsky et al. 1973) and the Profile of Mood Scale (POMS; McNair et al. 1971) for self-ratings.

Results

Physostigmine induced increases of heart rate, blood pressure, and plasma adrenaline, cortisol, and glucose (data not shown). These were behaviorally accompanied by anergia and anhedonia. All these effects were unaffected by clonidine (Fig. 1).

In contrast (Figs. 2 and 3), the time-dependent decrease of α-amplitude following physostigmine was antagonized by clonidine. This antagonism reached a trend towards significance ($p < 0.1$) over posterior brain regions, while the difference between both conditions was significant for 12–15.5 Hz activity ($p < 0.05$) (Fig. 4).

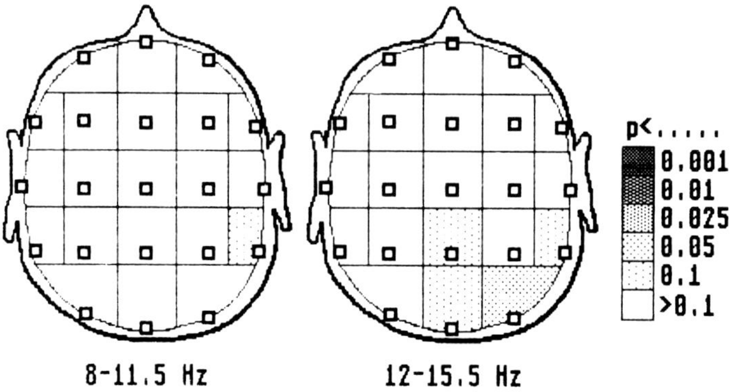

Fig. 4. Probability map. Student's paired *t* tests for the differences of the EEG amplitudes between both conditions 30 min after physostigmine, i.e., 60 min after placebo/clonidine (see IV in Figs. 2 and 3). The variances did not differ significantly from normality (Kolmogoroff-Smirnoff test)

Discussion

The effects of physostigmine on mood and drive and electrical brain activity as well as the accompanying stress phenomena correspond to previous findings. As they were unaffected by clonidine, they cannot simply be attributed to a noradrenergic overdrive secondary to cholinergic stimulation. This argument is strengthened by the antagonism by clonidine of the effects of physostigmine on the EEG. This dissociating effect of clonidine is most interesting in that it questions the relationship of cortical neuronal activity to limbic functions such as mood and drive. The present knowledge, however, does not allow an interpretation in terms of the neuronal circuits and synaptic processes involved.

References

Domino EF (1968) Cholinergic mechanisms and the EEG. Electroencephalogr Clin Neurophysiol 24:292–293

Engberg G, Svensson TH (1980) Pharmacological analysis of a cholinergic receptor mediated regulation of brain norepinephrine neurons. J Neural Transm 4:137–150

Janowsky DS, Risch SC (1984) Cholinomimetic and anticholinergic drugs used to investigate an acetylcholine hypothesis of affective disorders and stress. Drug Dev Res 4:125–142

Janowsky DS, El-Yousef MK, Davis JM, Sekerke HJ (1973) Antagonistic effects of physostigmine and methylphenidate in man. Am J Psychiatry 130:1370–1376

Janowsky DS, Risch SC, Parker DC, Huey LY, Judd LL (1980) Increased vulnerability to cholinergic stimulation in affective disorder patients. Psychopharmacol Bull 16:29–31

Janowsky DS, Risch SC, Kennedy B, Ziegler M, Huey LY (1986) Central muscarinic effects of physostigmine on mood, cardiovascular function, pituitary and adrenal neuroendocrine release. Psychopharmacology 89:150–154

Kobinger W (1978) Central alpha-adrenergic systems as targets for hypotensive drugs. Rev Physiol Biochem Pharmacol 81:40–100

McNair DM, Lorr M, Droppleman LF (1971) Profile of mood scale. Educational testing service, San Diego

Increased Reactivity in the Electroencephalogram During Voluntary Movements of Normal Volunteers Medicated with Haloperidol

K.P. Westphal[1], B. Grözinger, J. Reess, V. Diekmann, and H.H. Kornhuber

Introduction

Since applying power spectral analysis of the EEG in schizophrenia, higher δ, θ, and β activities have been described (Itil et al. 1974; Itil 1977). Itil demonstrated less and slower α activity in schizophrenics, which had also been reported by Giannitrapani and Kayton (1974). The latter group showed a lower dominant α frequency and greater α spread. EEG mapping studies carried out mainly during cortical activation led to the contradictory results of more frontal activity in the δ and θ bands (Morihisa et al. 1983; Morstyn et al. 1983; Günther and Breitling 1985; Karson et al. 1987; Williamson and Mamelak 1987). Depending on the various cognitive tasks and the different samples of schizophrenic patients, investigators were able to describe various dysfunctions in the activated EEG (Kemali et al. 1980; Kornhuber 1983; Saletu et al. 1986; Koukkou-Lehmann 1987; Schellenberg et al. 1988; Günther et al. 1989; Colombo et al. 1989; Gruzelier et al. 1990). The validity of EEG findings in schizophrenia during activation tasks had been under discussion (Karson et al. 1987; Kahn et al. 1988), since it seemed difficult to exclude components of eye movements and movement artifacts. Moreover, the influence of various neuroleptics on the EEG in the different groups of schizophrenics might be difficult to exclude, especially since differences in the EEGs of treated patients were calculated between responders and nonresponders (Ulrich et al. 1988). In particular, an increased δ and θ power over the frontal areas might partly be due to neuroleptic medication. A recent study (Miyauchi et al. 1990) showed slower activity only over the parietooccipital regions in acute untreated patients. Moreover, there was no difference in the topographical distribution of δ or θ power between untreated schizophrenics and controls (Westphal et al. 1989, 1990b).

To investigate whether the reported findings, especially those in treated patients with a known increase of power in the δ and θ bands and in the lower α band range (Itil et al. 1974; Westphal et al. 1990a) during rest,

[1] Abt. für Neurologie, RKU, Oberer Eselsberg 45, W-7900 Ulm, FRG.

Imaging of the Brain in Psychiatry
and Related Fields
Edited by K. Maurer

might be due to an EEG effect of the neuroleptic drug, normal volunteers who received neuroleptic medication were studied. The results will be presented here. Of particular interest was the change in reactivity during cortical activation in the treated normal volunteers, since most EEG findings (see above) in schizophrenic patients were found during various cognitive tasks. We hypothesized that normal volunteers should demonstrate similar abnormalities between untreated and treated conditions, as has been described in normal controls and treated schizophrenics.

In normal controls the influence of neuroleptic drugs on the EEG spectra is described usually after a single dose (Pfeiffer et al. 1968; Wieneke et al. 1981; Herrmann 1982; Herrmann and Kubicki 1981; Herrmann and Schärer 1986). Since patients are treated over a longer period of time with neuroleptics, the question arises whether the EEG effects following long-term administration of neuroleptics are similar to those after a single dose. Therefore, the normal volunteers received medication for 21 days.

Due to neuroleptic side effects (parkinsonoid), many treated schizophrenic patients receive anticholinergics, e.g., biperiden. Since the studies of Wickler (1952), a dissociation between EEG slowing and behavior has been known and was also described in humans (Itil and Fink 1966). The anticholinergic biperiden caused a loss of functional topography in the activated EEG during a voluntary motor task (Westphal et al. 1987). This was important, because most patients in our study of treated schizophrenics (Grözinger et al. 1984, 1986; Westphal et al. 1990a) received this anticholinergic. Other studies with treated patients seem to underestimate the influence of additionally administered anticholinergics during neuroleptic treatment. Activation patterns in the EEG might be modulated by cholinergic mechanisms (Buzsaki et al. 1988). Thus, the volunteers in the study reported here received biperiden during the last 7 days of haloperidol medication.

Voluntary movements (Bereitschaftspotential paradigm; Kornhuber and Deecke 1965) have been used for cortical activation, especially since disturbances of voluntary movements in schizophrenics are known (Marsden et al. 1975; Rogers 1985; Manschreck 1986). Moreover EEG analysis over a short time period (Diekmann 1985), about 1 s at rest, during preparation for voluntary movement in the *Bereitschaftspotential* (BP) period and during the voluntary movement phase itself, allows comparison of three different functional states (rest, preparation, movement) with a relatively high time resolution. In addition, cortical activation patterns before and during voluntary movements are well known from the literature (Jasper and Penfield 1949; Gastaut et al. 1952; Chatrian et al. 1959; Kornhuber and Deecke 1965); these changes can be described quantitatively (Pfurtscheller and Aranibar 1979; Pfurtscheller and Berghold 1989).

Methods

A total of 15, right-handed, male students (mean age 25.9 ± 6.6 years) were medicated for 14 days with haloperidol (HA) (about 0.04 mg/kg per day) and an additional 7 days with HA + biperiden (BI) (6 mg/day). EEGs were recorded on the 14th and 21st day; pretreatment and posttreatment sessions were also carried out. The posttreatment control took place at least 4 weeks after final administration of the drug. EEGs (Ag-AgCl electrodes) were recorded from F3, Fz, F4, C3′, Cz, C4′, P3, Pz, and P4, referred to linked earlobes. Electrode resistance was less than 5 kΩ. Eyes were closed. Electro-oculograms (EOGs) were recorded from the outer canthus and from the middle of the orbit. The galvanic skin response (GSR) was recorded from the hand (palmar-dorsal). EOGs and GSRs were used for artifact elimination only. The EEG was recorded with a bandpass filter from 0.13 Hz to 30 Hz. The sampling rate was 200 Hz, the sampling epoch 4000 ms. Trials contaminated with artifacts such as eye blinks, eye and head movements, or incorrect finger movements were excluded. The beginning of voluntary movement (flexion of the right index finger) in the electromyogram (EMG) started the EEG analysis. From 50–80 movement trial EEG spectra were calculated by fast Fourier transformation (FFT) for three EEG periods: (1) a resting period, starting 2.5 s before movement onset; (2) a BP period, beginning 1 s prior to the movement, and (3) a movement period. The intertrial interval was about 8 s. Non parametric Friedman and Wilcoxon-Wilcox tests (WWT) were used to compare normalized medians of the mean power density (MPD) and center frequency (CF) for each frequency band under different medications and for different movement related EEG periods (formulas and normalization procedure, see Diekmann 1985; Reinke and Diekmann 1987; Westphal et al. 1990a).

"Grand spectra," i.e., the spectra of all subjects, were computed for each electrode position, for each period, and for all four experimental conditions. Interindividual differences were eliminated by a normalization procedure (Westphal et al. 1990a). For statistical analysis of HA serum levels and for all psychometric tests the Wilcoxon matched pairs signed rank test was performed. For the reaction time test, analysis of variance was used.

Results

Comparison of the Four Medicated States

The δ MPD was higher under the HA and HA + BI conditions than in the untreated conditions at nearly all electrode positions during the rest period ($p < 0.05$ or 0.01, WWT). Moreover the θ MPD was higher under these conditions over the midline and the electrodes of the right hemisphere

($p < 0.05$, WWT). The α MPD tended to be higher in the HA state. HA + BI caused a significant decrease of α MPD at all parietal positions ($p < 0.05$, WWT). The β band MPD had significantly higher values in the HA condition than in all other states at nearly all electrode positions ($p < 0.05$, WWT).

The shift of power distribution within the α band towards a slower frequency range is reflected by a lower α CF at all electrode postions in the HA condition ($p < 0.05$, WWT) than in untreated states and a shift of θ CF in the HA condition towards a higher frequency range. The θ CF was also significantly higher at central and parietal areas ($p < 0.05$, WWT).

Comparison of the Three EEG Periods in Each State of Medication

The δ MPD increased steadily during the rest, BP, and movement periods and was significantly higher during the movement period than at rest. This was most pronounced in the HA + BI condition over the frontal-central areas (significant difference between rest and movement period, $p < 0.05$ or 0.01, WWT).

In contrast, the θ MPDs decreased during the movement period compared to rest in both the untreated state and the HA + BI condition. In these, there was an enhancement of θ power during the BP period. This was less prominent in the HA condition. The θ CF showed a steady decrease during the rest, BP, and movement periods and significant values were obtained when comparing rest and movement periods over motor-relevant areas in the region of the supplementary motor area (Cz) and over the motor cortex (C3′) contralateral to the movement ($p < 0.05$, WWT). This functional topographical sign during movement became more widespread in the HA condition and a significant reduction of θ CF between rest and movement appeared at all electrode positions except F4 and P4 ($p < 0.05$, WWT). In the HA + BI condition this effect was antagonized.

The α MPD was reduced (attenuated) between rest and movement at central and parietal regions. In the HA condition this attenuation was extended to the frontal areas. Additional administration of BI caused the disappearance of the attenuation effects during movement compared to rest. In the HA + BI condition there was even a tendency of higher α MPD during movement than during rest (paradoxical activation). The MPD of the β band demonstrated changes similar to those for the α MPD. These results between rest and movement periods in the different frequency bands are also demonstrated in the grand spectra (Fig. 1).

Psychometric Tests

Significant differences were calculated in the "adjective mood scale" and in the "complaint list" (von Zerssen 1982) between the HA condition (ad-

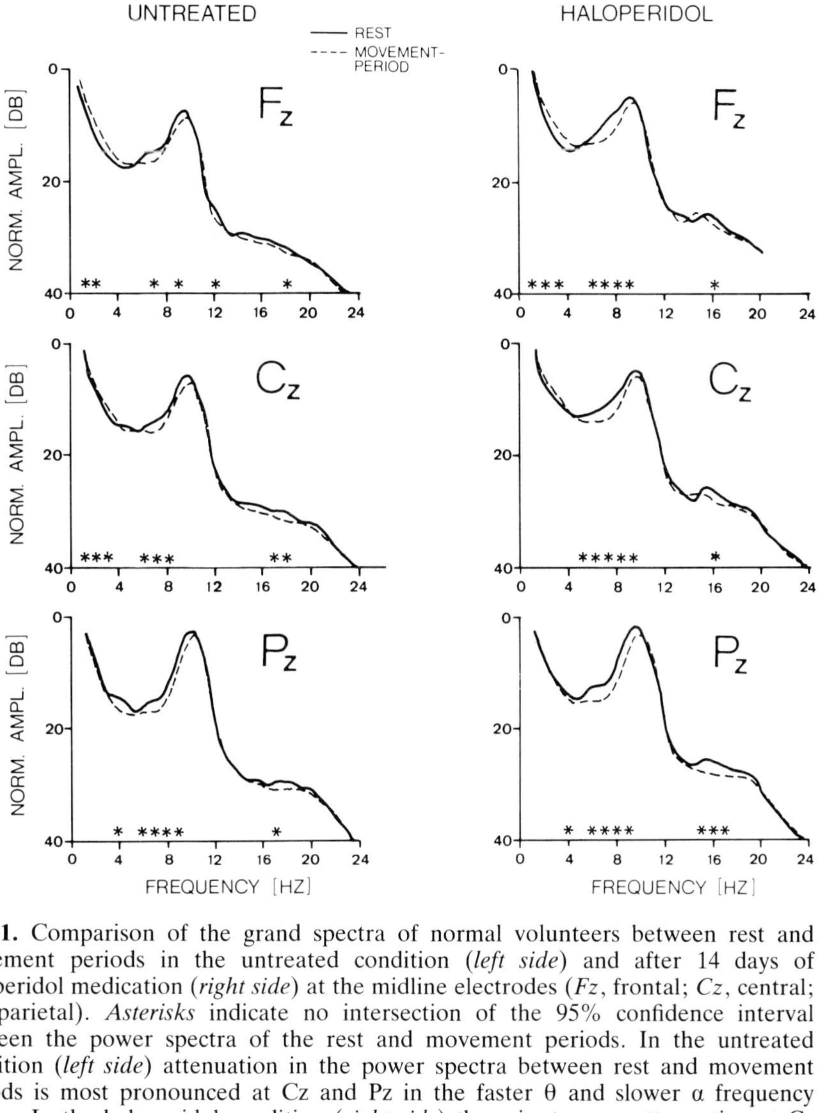

Fig. 1. Comparison of the grand spectra of normal volunteers between rest and movement periods in the untreated condition (*left side*) and after 14 days of haloperidol medication (*right side*) at the midline electrodes (*Fz*, frontal; *Cz*, central; *Pz*, parietal). *Asterisks* indicate no intersection of the 95% confidence interval between the power spectra of the rest and movement periods. In the untreated condition (*left side*) attenuation in the power spectra between rest and movement periods is most pronounced at Cz and Pz in the faster θ and slower α frequency ranges. In the haloperidol condition (*right side*) there is stronger attenuation at Cz and Fz than in the untreated condition (*left side*)

jective mood scale, 14.07 ± 8.18; complaint list, 25.57 ± 14.61; mean score ± SD), the HA + BI condition (adjective mood scale, 9.92 ± 8.96; complaint list, 16.43 ± 10.62; mean score ± SD), and the experiments without medication (adjective mood scale, 5.57 ± 4.73; complaint list, 12.29 ± 8.50).

Longer reaction times were obtained in the HA condition with interstimulus intervals of 5 s and 10 s than in the condition with presentation of constant interstimulus intervals. With randomized interstimulus intervals, significant differences, with longer reaction times in the HA condition, were found compared to the HA + BI condition with an interstimulus interval of 1 s ($p < 0.05$). Significantly higher HA plasma levels ($p < 0.001$) were found in the HA and in the HA + BI conditions (mean ± 1.30 ng/ml ± 0.08, 1.20 ng/ml ± 0.57 respectively).

Discussion

The results demonstrate that, when comparing the different states of medication, HA caused an increase of δ and θ powers. Additional administration of BI did not greatly change this increase. This effect was not found in the α and β bands; instead, HA caused a slowing of α power and a tendency towards a higher α power. However, in contrast to the δ and θ bands these phenomena were antagonized by the anticholinergic BI.

The results in the HA condition confirm the findings reported in the literature (Herrmann 1982; Herrmann and Kubicki 1981; Herrmann and Schärer 1986) obtained with a single dose of HA. Moreover, a lower α CF in the HA condition is in agreement with a lower α centroid in normal volunteers after application of chlorprothixene (Saletu 1989). Thus there seems to be similar EEG effects when comparing a single dose with administration over a 14 day period.

These results indicate that higher θ and δ powers and a slower α power in treated schizophrenics (see Introduction) should be assessed very carefully, since they might be due to neuroleptics.

The same holds true for the cortical activation pattern. Motor activation caused a decrease (attenuation) of θ, α, and β powers during the movement period compared to the rest period. These attenuation effects were mostly obtained over the central midline and the parietal midline electrode positions but also over the motor cortex and the parietal association cortex contralateral to the movement (Grözinger et al. 1990). This is in accordance with early findings reported in the literature (see Introduction) and the more recent data of Pfurtscheller and Berghold (1989). The functional topography is demonstrated by a multivariate, nonparametric, statistical method (Reinke and Diekmann 1987) and described elsewhere in detail (Diekmann et al. 1990).

Movement related attenuation became more extended in the HA condition. The HA effect, with more widespread functional topographical patterns, indicates that functional topography during cognitive tasks in treated schizophrenics may be changed by neuroleptic medication. The stronger and more extended attenuation effects during movement may be interpreted as an increase of reactivity during HA medication in normals.

Thus, higher reactivity during functional activation in treated schizophrenic patients than in an untreated state with low reactivity does not automatically mean that the increase is due to a therapeutic effect of the neuroleptic, i.e., a less psychotic state. Even normal volunteers demonstrated this increased reactivity under neuroleptic medication; therefore the same effect in medicated schizophrenics might simply be an EEG effect of the neuroleptic.

BI caused the disappearance of movement related attenuation effects, especially in the α band. This is in agreement with the literature. Buzsaki et al. (1988) described a cholinergic influence on EEG oscillations. According to their model of EEG modulation, the anticholinergic BI should interfere with cholinergically modulated activation patterns. Anticholinergic influences on the EEG effects of HA are discussed elsewhere (Westphal et al. 1992).

Acknowledgements. We thank Janssen in Neuss, Ratiopharm in Ulm, and Gry-Pharma in Kirchzarten, FRG for support. We are grateful to L. Frey for expert secretarial assistance.

References

Buzsaki G, Bickford RG, Pnomareff G, Thal LJ, Mandel R, Gage FH (1988) Nucleus basalis and thalamic control of neocortical activity in the freely moving rat. J Neurosci 8(11):4007–4026

Chatrian GE, Petersen MC, Lazarete JA (1959) The blocking of the rolandic wicket rhythm and some central changes related to movement. Electroencephalogr Clin Neurophysiol 11:497–510

Colombo C, Gambini O, Macciardi F, Bellodi L, Sacchetti E, Vita A, Cattaneo R, Scarone S (1989) Alpha reactivity in schizophrenia and in schizophrenic spectrum disorders: demographic, clinical and hemispheric assessment. Int J Psychophysiol 7:47–54

Diekmann V (1985) Kurzzeit-Spektral-Analyse von ereignisbezogenen EEG Abschnitten. In: Gänshirt H, Berlit P, Haack G (eds) Kardiovaskuläre Erkrankungen und Nervensystem. Neurotoxikologie. Probleme des Hirntodes. Springer, Berlin Heidelberg New York, pp 881–885 (Verhandlungen der Deutschen Gesellschaft für Neurologie, vol 3)

Diekmann V, Grözinger B, Westphal KP, Reinke W, Kornhuber HH (1990) The order of EEG activity of schizophrenic patients and the influence of haloperidol and biperidene on the EEG order of healthy subjects. In: Deecke L, Eccles JC, Mountcastle VB (eds) From neuron to action. An appraisal of fundamental and clinical research. Springer, Berlin Heidelberg New York

Gastaut H, Terzian H, Gastaut Y (1952) Etude d'une actvité électroencéphalographique méconnue: "le rhythme rolandique en arceau." Marseille Méd 89: 296–310

Giannitrapani D, Kayton L (1974) Schizophrenia and EEG spectral analysis. Electroencephalogr Clin Neurophysiol 36:377–386

Grözinger B, Neher KD, Westphal KP, Diekmann V, Kornhuber HH (1984) The EEG in schizophrenia. Changes in relation to voluntary movement in the theta and delta band. Naturwissenschaften 71:320

Grözinger B, Westphal KP, Diekmann V, Frech MM, Nitsch J, Andersen C, Scherb W, Neher KD, Kornhuber HH (1986) Schizophrene Patienten und Gesunde: EEG-Unterschiede bei Willkürbewegungen. In: Keup W (ed) Biologische Psychiatrie. Springer, Berlin Heidelberg New York, pp 181–196

Grözinger B, Westphal KP, Reess J, Leibing U, Kornhuber HH (1990) Changes in movement related EEG spectra in normal subjects on haloperidol and biperidene. In: Brunia C, Gaillard A, Kok A (eds) Psychophysiological brain research. Tilburg University Press, Tilburg

Gruzelier J, Liddiard D, Davis L, Wilson L (1990) Topographical EEG differences between schizophrenic patients and controls during neuropsychological functional activation. Int J Psychophysiol 8:275–282

Günther W, Breitling D (1985) Predominant sensorimotor area in left hemisphere dysfunction in schizophrenia measured by brain electrical activity mapping. Biol Psychiatry 20:515–535

Günther W, Steinberg R, Petsch R, Streck P, Kugler J (1989) EEG mapping in psychiatry: Studies on type I/II schizophrenia using motor activation. In: Maurer K (ed) Topographic brain mapping of EEG and evoked potentials. Springer, Berlin Heidelberg New York, pp 438–450

Herrmann WM (1982) Development and critical evaluation of objective procedure for electroencephalographic classification of psychotropic drugs. In: Herrmann WM (ed) EEG in drug research. Fischer, Stuttgart, pp 249–351

Herrmann WM, Kubicki S (1981) Beispiele für die Projektion von Substanzwirkungen typischer Psychopharmaka auf eine elektrophysiologische Messebene. Z EEG-EMG 12:21–32

Herrmann WM, Schärer E (1986) Pharmaco-EEG: computer EEG-analysis to describe the projection of drug effects on a functional cerebral level in humans. In: Lopes da Silva FH, Storm Leeuwen W, Rémond W (eds) Handbook of Electroencephalography and clinical neurophysiology: clinical applications of computer analysis of EEG and other neurophysiological signals, vol 2. Elsevier, Amsterdam, pp 385–445

Itil TM (1977) Qualitative and quantitative EEG findings in schizophrenia. Schizophr Bull 3:61–79

Itil TM, Fink M (1966) Anticholinergic drug-induced delirium: experimental modification, quantitative EEG and behavioral correlations. J Nerv Ment Dis 143:492–507

Itil TM, Saletu B, Davis S, Allen M (1974) Stability studies in schizophrenics and normals using computer-analyzed EEG. Biol Psychiatry 8:321–335

Jasper H, Penfield W (1949) Electrocorticogams in man: effect of voluntary movement upon the electrical activity of the precentral gyrus. Arch Psychiatr Nervenkr 183:163–174

Kahn EM, Weiner RD, Brenner RP, Coppola R (1988) Topographic maps of brain electrical activity – pitfalls and precautions. Biol Psychiatry 23:628–636

Karson CN, Coppola R, Morihisa JM, Weinberger DR (1987) Computed electroencephalographic activity mapping in schizophrenia. Arch Gen Psychiatry 44:514–517

Kemali D, Vacca L, Marciano F, Celani T, Nolfe G, Iorio G (1980) Computerized EEG in schizophrenics. Neuropsychobiology 6:260–267

Kornhuber HH (1983) Chemistry, physiology and neurophysiology of schizophrenia: towards an earlier diagnosis of schizophrenia I. Arch Psychiatr Nervenkr 233:415–422

Kornhuber HH, Deecke L (1965) Hirnpotentialänderungen bei Willkürbewegungen und passiven Bewegungen des Menschen: Bereitschaftspotential und reafferente Potentiale. Pflügers Arch 284:1–17

Koukkou-Lehmann M (1987) Hirnmechanismen normalen und schizophrenen Denkens. Springer, Berlin Heidelberg New York, pp XI-161

Manschreck TC (1986) Motor abnormalities in schizophrenia. In: Nasrallah HA, Weinberger DR (eds) Handbook of schizophrenia, vol 1. Elsevier, Amsterdam, pp 65–96

Marsden CD, Tarsy D, Baldessarine RJ (1975) Spontaneous and drug-induced movement disorders in psychotic patients. In: Benson DF, Blümer D (eds) Psychiatric aspects of neurological disease. Grune and Stratton, New York, pp 219–266

Miyauchi T, Tanaka K, Hagimoto H, Kishimoto H, Matsushita M (1990) Computerized EEG in schizophrenic patients. Biol Psychiatry 28:488–494

Morihisa JM, Duffy FH, Wyatt RJ (1983) Brain electrical activity mapping (BEAM) in schizophrenic patients. Arch Gen Psychiatry 40:719–728

Morstyn R, Duffy FH, McCarley RW (1983) Altered topography of EEG spectra content in schizophrenia. Electroencephalogr Clin Neurophysiol 1:262–271

Pfeiffer CC, Goldstein L, Murphree HB (1968) Effects of parenteral administration of haloperidol and chlorpromazine in man. I. Normal subjects: quantitative EEG and subjective response. J Clin Pharmacol 8:79–88

Pfurtscheller G, Aranibar A (1979) Evaluation of event related desynchronization (ERD) preceding and following self-paced movement. Electroencephalogr Clin Neurophysiol 46:138–147

Pfurtscheller G, Berghold A (1989) Patterns of cortical activation during planning of voluntary movement. Electroencephalogr Clin Neurophysiol 72:250–258

Reinke W, Diekmann V (1987) Uncertainty analysis of human EEG spectra: a multivariate information theoretical method for the analysis of brain activity. Biol Cybern 57:379–387

Rogers D (1985) The motor disturbance of severe psychiatric illness: a conflict of paradigms. Br J Psychiatry 147:221–232

Saletu B (1989) EEG imaging of brain activity in clinical psychopharmacology. In: Maurer K (ed) Topographic brain mapping of EEG and evoked potentials. Springer, Berlin Heidelberg New York, pp 482–506

Saletu B, Küfferle B, Anderer P (1986) On the orienting response in schizophrenics: quantitative EEG studies before and during therapy. In: Shagass C, Josiassen RC, Roemer RA (eds) Brain electrical potentials and psychopathology. Elsevier, Amsterdam, pp 59–81

Schellenberg R, Christoph B, Kluba J, Knorr W, Siewert B, Schindler M, Linsel A (1988) Nasopharyngeal EEG recordings in schizophrenic patients – preliminary remarks on the method and some first results. J Psychophysiol 2:283–289

Ulrich G, Gaebel W, Gaebel W, Pietzcker A, Müller-Örlinghausen B, Stieglitz RD (1988) Prediction of neuroleptic on-drug response in schizophrenic in-patients by EEG. Eur Arch Psychiatr Neurol Sci 237:144–155

von Zerssen D (1982) Clinical self rating scales (CSRS) of the Munich Psychiatric Information System (Psychis München) In: Sartorius N, Ben TA (eds) Assessment of depression. Springer, Berlin Heidelberg New York

Westphal KP, Grözinger B, Haag C, Scherb W, Diekmann V, Kornhuber HH (1987) The influence of biperidene on the EEG power spectra during the Bereitschaftspotential paradigm. In: Johnson R, Rohrbaugh JW, Parasuraman R (eds) Current trends in event-related research. Elsevier, Amsterdam, pp 556–561 (EEG Suppl 40)

Westphal KP, Grözinger B, Diekmann V, Scherb W, Reess J, Leibing U, Kornhuber HH (1989) Comparison of untreated and treated schizophrenic patients, normals and neuroleptic treated normals: "hypofrontalitiy" and different EEG spectra before and during voluntary movement. Psychiatry Res 9:395–398

Westphal KP, Grözinger B, Diekmann V, Scherb W, Reess J, Kornhuber HH (1990a) EEG-spectra parameters distinguish pathophysiological and pharmacological influences on the EEG in treated schizophrenics. Arch Ital Biol 128:55–66

Westphal KP, Grözinger B, Diekmann V, Scherb W, Reess J, Leibing U, Kornhuber HH (1990b) Slower theta activity over the midfrontal cortex in schizophrenic patients. Acta Psychiatr Scand 81:132–138

Westphal KP, Grözinger B, Reess J, Leibing U, Kornhuber AW, Diekmann V, Kornhuber HH (1992) Anticholinergic influences of biperidene on the EEG effects of haloperidol. Clin Physiol and Biochem 9:26–34

Wickler A (1952) Pharmacologic dissociation on behavior and EEG sleep patterns in dogs: morphine, N-allylnormorphine and atropine. Proc Soc Exp Biol Med 79:261–265

Wieneke GH, Verhoeven WMA, Westenberg HGM, de Wilde H, Lopes da Silva FH, van Praag HM, Storm van Leeuwen (1981) The effects of haloperidol on the EEG spectrum. Psychopharmacology 74:33–34

Williamson P, Mamelak M (1987) Frontal spectral EEG findings in acutely ill schizophrenics. Biol Psychiatry 22:1021–1024

Multimodal Application

Simultaneous Electroencephalographic and Cerebral Metabolic Rate Measurement

M.S. Buchsbaum[1], L. Abel, A. Mucci, S. Guich, and C. Tang

Introduction

With alertness and mental activity, the slower rhythms of the electroencephalogram (EEG), θ and δ, are usually replaced by faster activity. Since local functional activity of the brain is closely tied to the use of glucose, the major energy source of the brain (Sokoloff 1977), we expected a relationship between EEG activity and local cerebral glucose use as assessed by positron emission tomography (PET).

We are currently examining our data base of 50 off-medication patients with schizophrenia and 26 normal controls on whom we have simultaneous EEG and PET information. Based on the reports of our group and others of: (a) relatively reduced metabolic rates and cerebral blood flow in the frontal lobes of patients with schizophrenia relative to the occipital lobe (Buchsbaum 1990) and (b) increased frontal δ activity (Guich et al. 1990), we are interested in examining the detailed distribution of δ in the frontal lobe and its regional metabolic correlates. The relationship of glucose metabolic rate to occipital α would also provide information on hypofrontality. In a preliminary analysis of EEG epochs screened for eye activity, we have found that frontal δ during the activating Continuous Performance Task (CPT) is associated with increased metabolic rate while temporal, especially right temporal δ, is associated with reduced activity (Guich et al. 1990). A frontal δ increase with motor activity has also been observed by Guenther et al. (1988), who found a regionally different relationship between δ and blood flow. These differential regional and task interpretations of the traditional EEG rhythms are important to the understanding of the functional significance of scalp recorded EEG.

[1] Department of Psychiatry, Mt. Sinai School of Medicine, One Gustave L. Levy Place, New York, NY 10079, USA.

Imaging of the Brain in Psychiatry
and Related Fields
Edited by K. Maurer

Methods

Patient Sample

The patient group consisted of 25 never-medicated patients with schizophrenia (24 men, 1 woman; mean age 32.4 years, SD 8.4 years). These patients were recruited from clinical and research programs at the University of California at Irvine, Los Angeles, and San Diego. There is no overlap with earlier samples from an NIMH study (Buchsbaum et al. 1982a; Buchsbaum and Haier 1987). Of the 25 patients, 23 were right-handed and 2 left-handed. Patients were screened based on their medical history and laboratory tests including a day of scan urine drug screen. Patients with a history of seizure disorder, major head trauma, or substance abuse were excluded. All patients received an expanded version of the Brief Psychiatric Rating Scale (BPRS) (Overall and Gorham 1962; Lukoff et al. 1986). The mean BPRS score (sum of the first 18 items) was 44.3 (SD = 13). The control group for this analysis consisted of 13 right-handed volunteers (10 men, 3 women, mean 34.0 years, SD 6.9 years). There was no significant difference in age between the two groups (t = 1.57, ns). The control subjects were in good health as assessed by physical examination, medical history, and laboratory examination. Normals had the same exclusion criteria except that we required no history of psychiatric disorder in self or first-degree relatives.

Computerized Electroencephalographic Topography

For EEG recording, a set of 32 Grass gold disc electrodes were placed on subjects' scalps using 19 standard international 10–20 system leads, linked ears reference, and 3 additional midline leads (FF and FC at 10% steps and OZ), 2 additional temporal leads (TT1, 2) between T3–T5 and T4–T6 at 5% steps, and 8 additional leads (FTC1, 2; CP1, 2; TCP1, 2; and PO1, 2) at the centers of squares formed by other electrodes.

The EEG was recorded, digitized on-line (with a PDP-11/34) at 200 buffer points per second, and low frequency subharmonics removed by an autoregressive filter (Coppola 1979). The amplifiers were calibrated by recording a 10 Hz, 100 μv sine wave through all channels and determining the calibration factor for each channel; each channel was then proportionally adjusted before analysis. A standard fast Fourier transform was applied to the 2.56 s epochs, and the power spectrum estimates computed at 0.39 Hz steps (see Guich et al. 1990 for details). For smoothing, four adjacent estimates were summed to yield 1.56 Hz resolution, with the final estimates expressed as magnitude values in microvolts (square root of power). The activity estimated for the following bands was computed by summing adjacent values: δ, 0.78–4.30 cps; θ, 4.34–7.80 cps; α, 8.20–12.90 cps; and $\beta 1$, 13.30–19.90 cps.

Each 2.56 s epoch was visually inspected without information on diagnostic group for artifacts and any epoch containing artifacts was eliminated. Pilot data collected before our 1982 study (Buchsbaum et al. 1982a) indicated that leads FP1 and FP2 detected horizontal eye movements of 2° or greater and were quite sensitive to blinks. This was determined by having subjects make eye movements between targets at 1°, 2°, 3°, and 6° apart. The power spectral values for the artifact-free 2.56 s epochs (8–12 epochs/person/condition) were then averaged to yield one representative 2.56 s epoch of power spectral values for each subject in each condition.

Topographic maps were computed by linear interpolation from the four nearest electrodes (Buchsbaum et al. 1982b).

We have measured the average positions of the standard electrode positions using magnetic resonance imaging (MRI) as a method to express these locations in the coordinate system we use for PET cortical surface measurement. Each PET slice has an axial level, expressed by visual comparison to the Matsui and Hirano (1978) axial slice atlas to correct for individual differences in head height and brain proportions. Each cortical location within a slice is expressed as a proportion of the distance along the circumference of the slice from front to back. This corrects for individual differences in slice size.

Seven subjects selected as sequential cases (3 normals, 3 affective, 1 schizophrenic) were scanned. The electrode positions were marked with vaseline-filled 5 mm tubes and the canthomeatal (CM) line marked with a vaseline-filled 8 cm tube. They received axial, sagittal, and coronal MRI (TR = 2800, TE = 30, echo 1/4) parallel to the CM line. The CM line was assessed on a sagittal series by examining the position of the horizontal tube. Each MR image was matched to the corresponding level above the CM line in the Matsui and Hirano atlas. The position of each lateral electrode and midline FF and OZ was measured as a percent of the distance along the circumference from the anterior midline to the posterior midline. The average percentage and the average Matsui and Hirano level were computed for the group. For the highest midline electrodes (FZ, FC, CZ, PZ) the location on the midsagittal plane was projected down onto the highest axial slice.

For the lateral electrodes, slice levels above and below the average value were chosen. A weight, corresponding to the contribution from each slice, was also given; weights summed to 1.00.

Task and Procedure

Subjects arrived in the laboratory and were briefed on the procedure. Before the PET scan, an individually molded, thermosetting, plastic head holder was made for each subject to minimize head movement. Next, two IV lines were inserted, one in each arm for the administration of fluorodeoxyglucose (FDG) and withdrawal of blood samples. Subjects were then seated in a comfortable chair in a darkened acoustically attenuated isolation room. Subjects were requested to rest with their eyes closed while the EEG was recorded. Next, they were instructed about the procedure and the CPT to be performed. A 5 min practice session was given; the EEG was then recorded during performance. Next, a dark curtain was drawn around the subject, with the subject's left arm protruding through an opening to allow blood sampling. The left arm was wrapped in a hot pack for arterialization of venous blood. The CPT was started and an injection of 4.0–5.2 mCi FDG administered.

The CPT has been widely used in studies of schizophrenia and in studies of individuals with relatives with schizophrenia (Cornblatt et al. 1988, 1989). In the version of the CPT used here (Nuechterlein et al. 1983), single digits (0–9) were presented for 40 ms at a rate of 1 every 2 s. Subjects were told to respond with a button press using their right hand each time that they detected the digit 0 and that it was equally important to respond to zeros and not respond to non-zeros. Targets were presented irregularly with a probability of occurrence of 0.25. Stimuli were presented silently by rear projection and blurred to a degree that makes digits barely recognizable (such that a 2.8 diopter correction is required to refocus clearly). The subject's eyes were 1.2 m from the rear projection screen. Subjects were not spoken to during uptake, and all remained quiet and cooperative. Subjects were continuously observed to insure that they were following instructions. Small low-level penlights were kept on for blood sampling behind the curtain. Subjects received 4–5.2 mCi of FDG. After 30–35 min of FDG uptake, the right arm IV was removed, the subject was allowed to void, and the subject was then transferred to the adjacent scanning room.

Positron Emission Tomography

Nine planes (CTI NeuroECAT) at 10 mm increments and parallel to the CM line were acquired 45–100 min after FDG injection in a configuration with measured in-plane resolution of 7.6 mm and 10.9 mm resolution in the Z-dimension (axial). A calculated attenuation correction and a smoothing filter were used. The scanner was calibrated each scan day with a cylindrical phantom and compared to well counter data.

Scan Slice Processing and Selection

Scans were transformed to glucose metabolic rate as described elsewhere (Buchsbaum et al. 1984a,b, 1989). Each slice was then neuroanatomically matched to a standard atlas (Matsui and Hirano 1978) by an observer without reference to diagnostic group. We then outlined the cortex and

Table 1. Midline electrode position and circumferential position electrode

Midline electrodes	MH level	On midline (%)	Size of box	Weight
FZ	2	8.7	25	1.00
FC	2	25.2	25	1.00
CZ	2	44.2	25	1.00
PZ	2	86.4	25	1.00
FF	4	15.0	25	0.50
	5	15.0	25	0.50
OZ	4	96.1	25	0.33
	5	94.3	25	0.33
	6	96.3	25	0.33

averaged metabolic rates in a strip along the slice perimeter as described elsewhere (Buchsbaum et al. 1989). A weighted average of these strip segments was then calculated across slices to obtain estimates of metabolic rate in the major gyri of the brain as indicated in Table 1. Values were expressed as relative metabolic rate; for the cortex, as metabolic rate/whole brain metabolic rate.

Statistical Analysis

All analyses were performed on ratio data: EEG amplitude is calculated as the ratio of the individual lead at a given frequency to the mean of the respective frequency for all 32 leads for eyes closed and task conditions separately. Attention scores were calculated by subtracting CPT condition from resting EEG. We used a three-way analysis of variance (ANOVA) (BMDP 4V; Dixon 1988) with one grouping factor: cohort (controls, never-medicated schizophrenics) and two within factors (anterior-posterior position by lateral position) (see Table 2). Correlation coefficients were calculated with a BMDP 8D program (Dixon 1988).

Results

Differences in EEG Response Between Normals and Schizophrenics

Controls had less θ during CPT than when resting with their eyes closed for frontal leads (positive attention scores) and showed more θ posteriorly (negative scores). Schizophrenics yielded negative attention scores in frontal leads while exhibiting positive ones posteriorly (Table 3). A different

Table 2. Lateral electrodes

Electrode	Mean MH level	Exact circumference (%)	ML level	Boundaries on MH level (%)	Weight
FP1	8.6	11.4	8	8–20	0.46
			9	9–23	0.54
FP2	8.6	11.4	8	8–20	0.46
			9	9–23	0.54
F3	3.6	22.0	3	18–27	0.53
			4	17–25	0.47
F4	3.6	22.0	3	17–27	0.52
			4	17–26	0.48
F7	10.6	34.9	10	29–38	0.48
			11	31–41	0.52
F8	10.6	34.9	10	30–39	0.43
			11	27–39	0.57
FTC1	5.5	38.9	5	34–42	0.47
			6	34–43	0.53
FTC2	5.5	38.9	5	34–42	0.47
			6	34–43	0.53
C3	3.5	43.1	3	37–45	0.50
			4	38–46	0.50
C4	3.5	43.1	3	36–45	0.50
			4	37–46	0.50
T3	9.1	54.1	8	34–43	0.29
			9	24–38	0.43
			10	47–56	0.29
T4	9.1	54.1	8	34–43	0.29
			9	24–38	0.43
			10	49–58	0.29
TCP1	4.5	62.1	4	54–62	0.50
			5	57–65	0.50
TCP2	4.5	62.1	4	54–63	0.56
			5	58–65	0.44
TT1	7.2	60.7	6	54–63	0.33
			7	54–63	0.33
			8	44–53	0.33
TT2	7.2	60.7	6	54–63	0.36
			7	54–63	0.36
			8	44–51	0.29
CP1	2.0	53.3	2	49–59	0.52
			3	46–55	0.48
CP2	2.0	53.3	2	51–61	0.50
			3	46–56	0.50
T5	7.0	70.0	6	64–72	0.28
			7	64–73	0.31
			8	54–66	0.41
T6	7.0	70.0	6	64–72	0.28
			7	65–74	0.31
			8	52–64	0.41

Table 2. Continued

Electrode	Mean MH level	Exact circumference (%)	ML level	Boundaries on MH level (%)	Weight
P3	1.5	67.7	2	61–71	1.00
P4	1.5	67.7	2	63–73	1.00
PO1	2.3	91.0	2	84–94	0.52
			3	81–90	0.48
PO2	2.3	91.0	2	84–94	0.50
			3	84–94	0.50
O1	5.0	87.6	4	79–87	0.32
			5	81–89	0.32
			6	79–88	0.36
O2	5.0	87.6	4	79–88	0.34
			5	82–90	0.31
			6	79–88	0.34

MH, slice level in atlas (Matsui and Hirano, 1978).

anterior-posterior pattern in θ attention scores between controls and schizophrenics was confirmed by multivariate analysis with the anterior-posterior by group interaction ($F = 6.04$, $df = 1.5, 54.4$, $p < 0.01$, Huynh-Feldt corrected). Attention effects for δ exhibited a trend towards significance in the complex interaction of group by anterior-posterior direction by lead ($F = 1.78$, $df = 8.3, 300$, $p = 0.077$).

Correlation of EEG Change During Task with Glucose Metabolic Rate

Controls showed a negative correlation between θ change scores and glucose metabolic rate underlying the EEG lead in 19 of 32 leads, reaching significance for frontal FC (−0.618, $p < 0.02$, one-tailed), and in midline PZ (−0.510, $p < 0.05$, one-tailed). No positive correlation reached a two-tailed significance, the highest correlation was at P4 (0.522). Schizophrenics exhibited the highest positive correlation (18 of 32 positive correlations) at FP1 (0.38). Fisher's t test on correlation coefficients confirmed a significant difference at leads PZ ($F = -2.02$, $p < 0.05$), and FP2 ($F = 2{:}21$, $p < 0.05$).

Controls correlated negatively for δ change score with glucose in areas underlying the leads in 19 of 32 leads, reaching significance at FC (−0.544, $p < 0.025$, one-tailed) and C4 (−0.594, $p < 0.025$, one-tailed). Only one correlation was observed positive at TT2 (0.81). Schizophrenics showed negative correlations in 19 of 32 leads, with correlations at FC (−0.342, $p < 0.05$, one-tailed), TT1 (−0.39, $p < 0.05$, one-tailed), and F4 (−0.373, $p < 0.05$, one-tailed) reaching significance. In addition, they exhibited

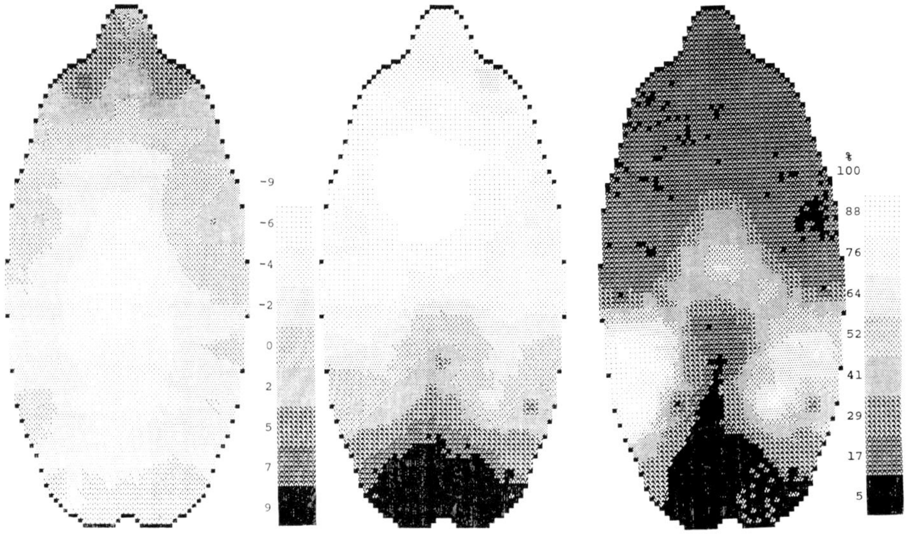

Fig. 1. Comparison of attention scores in controls (*left*), schizophrenics (*middle*), and *t* test (*right*) demonstrating the difference in the pattern of attention between the two groups. *Scale bar* between normals and schizophrenics is difference score (resting EEG − EEG during continuous performance task) ×100 calculated from ratio data (lead/lead average for each frequency). Thus *black* (*9*) indicates less θ (0.09 or 9%) during the continuous performance task. Probability bar (*right*) indicates *p* level for two-tailed *t* tests comparing difference scores in normals and schizophrenics. Note that either normals > schizophrenics or schizophrenics > normals is *black* (0.05). Note common scale for control and schizophrenic attention scores; *black* in the *t* tests picture indicates significance

Table 3. Anteroposterior θ attention scores (resting minus CPT)

	Controls	Schizophrenics
F7-F3-FZ-F4-F8	0.018	−0.049
T3-C3-FC-C4-T4	−0.018	−0.054
TT1-TCP1-CZ-TCP2-TT2	−0.017	−0.016
T5-P3-PZ-P4-T6	−0.008	0.040
O1-PO1-OZ-PO2-O2	0.002	0.109

Values represent θ activity expressed as ratio for each lead to total of all 32 leads. A positive score indicates a decrease in θ with attentional performance on the continuous performance task (CPT). Since mean θ activity is in the range of 50 μV, a change of 0.05 is roughly equivalent to 2.5 μV. The θ attention scores were also significantly different across the two groups in a 2-way ANOVA (groups × 32 leads; interaction of lead by group, $F = 3.25$, $df = 4.8, 171.6$, $p < 0.001$).

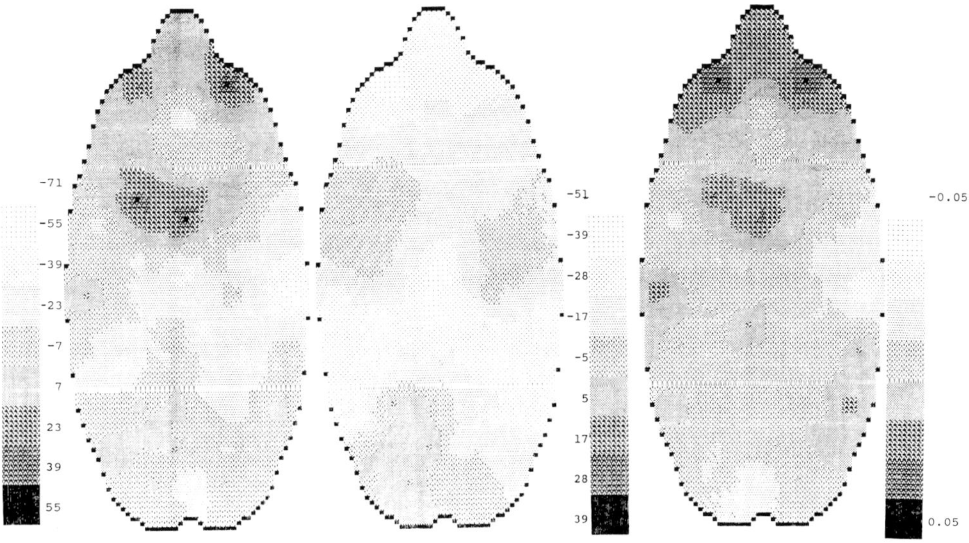

Fig. 2. Correlation coefficients between EEG θ during continuous performance task (CPT) and glucose metabolic rate in controls (*left*), schizophrenics (*middle*), and Fisher's *t* test (*right*) for differences in correlation coefficients between the two groups portrayed to the *left*. These maps describe the correlation of EEG with glucose metabolic rate in regions immediately underlying the scalp areas from which the EEG has been recorded. *Scale bars* for normals and schizophrenics indicate the correlation coefficients (*asterisk* = 0.01) with both the *white* (negative) and *black* (positive) areas indicating significant correlation coefficients. Note individual scales for the correlation maps, reflecting the different group sizes (controls exhibit significance at $r < -0.55$ and $r > 0.55$; schizophrenics are significant at $r < -0.39$ and $r > 0.39$). Probability bar (*right*) indicates p level for two-tailed Fisher's t test for correlation coefficients with both white (*negative*) and black (*positive*) showing leads of significantly different t tests for correlation coefficients

positive correlations at FP1 (0.342), C3 (0.529), P3 (0.399), and T4 (0.466). Fisher's t test on correlation coefficients confirmed significant differences between groups at leads C3 ($F = -2.11$, $p < 0.05$, two-tailed) and TT2 ($F = 2.84$, $p < 0.01$, two-tailed).

Correlation of EEG During CPT with Glucose Metabolic Rate

We next examined correlations between glucose metabolic rate and EEG during the CPT task. Controls showed negative correlations between θ and glucose metabolic rate underlying leads in 17 of 32 leads, reaching significance at T4 (−0.618, $p < 0.025$, one-tailed), while they exhibited positive correlations at F3 (0.577, $p < 0.05$, two-tailed), FP2 (0.584, $p < 0.025$, two-tailed), and FC (0.557, $p < 0.025$, two-tailed). Schizophrenics showed negative correlations in 24 of 32 leads, with correlation coefficients at FP1 (−0.386, $p < 0.05$, one-tailed), and CZ (−0.365, $p < 0.05$, one-tailed) reaching significance. Fisher's t test on correlation coefficients characterized FP1 ($F = 2.22$, $p < 0.05$) and FP2 ($F = 2.34$, $p < 0.05$) as leads in which the correlation coefficients are significantly different between groups.

Correlations between δ and glucose metabolic rate showed a positive correlation at FC (0.567, $p < 0.025$, one-tailed), and a negative correlation at T4 (−0.866, $p < 0.005$, one-tailed) for controls. Schizophrenics were negatively correlated at FP1 (−0.514, $p < 0.01$, one-tailed), and TCP1 (−0.530, $p < 0.01$, one-tailed), while they exhibited a positive correlation at O1 (0.421, $p < 0.025$, one-tailed). Fisher's t test on correlation coefficients confirmed a significant difference at FP1 ($F = 2.37$, $p < 0.05$) and T4 ($F = -3.13$, $p < 0.01$).

Discussion

In this study we found that controls and never-medicated schizophrenics differ in the slower wave rhythms of EEG, especially θ, in the anterior-posterior pattern they show during attentional tasks. Controls activate their frontal regions during CPT, decreasing their slow wave activity. Schizophrenics, on the contrary, show increased slow wave activity over the frontal regions during CPT while decreasing their slow wave activity over the occipital regions. The increased slow wave activity over the frontal lobes in schizophrenics is associated with decreased glucose metabolic rate as indicated by the negative correlations of δ and θ during CPT with glucose metabolic rate at FP1. These findings are not dissimilar to those of Westphal et al. (1990) who found slower frequency θ increased in an anteroposterior gradient in schizophrenics.

Controls showed a different association of θ during CPT with glucose metabolic rate at the frontal lobes as they correlated positively at FP2, F3, and FC and negatively for attention score with glucose metabolic rate at FC. The direction of these correlations (lower glucose metabolic rate with less θ) could indicate efficiency.

The observed difference in attention scores mainly in θ and with only a trend towards significance in δ might be due to the majority of the effect stemming from the higher range of δ to the lower range of θ as suggested by the data of Westphal et al. (1990). Further analysis needs to be done to determine the exact range of the effect.

The finding of a correlation of increased slow wave rhythms with decreased glucose metabolism at FP1 in never-medicated schizophrenics is a partial replication of our previous study (Guich et al. 1990). The current study allowed us to directly match areas of the scalp from which electrical activity is recorded to glucose metabolic rate in immediately underlying brain. We have previously suggested that the relationship of excess slow wave activity and hypofrontality in schizophrenics is congruent (Buchsbaum and Haier 1987; Guich et al. 1990), as separate EEG and PET studies have reported both increases in slow wave rhythms in schizophrenics and hypofrontality in schizophrenics (for review see Buchsbaum 1990). In this study we have been able to confirm the congruency of this relationship using simultaneous measurements of EEG and PET linked together through MRI derived templates.

References

Buchsbaum MS (1990) The frontal lobes, basal ganglia and temporal lobes as sites for schizophrenia. Schizophr Bull 16:379–390

Buchsbaum MS, Haier RJ (1987) Functional and anatomical brain imaging: impact on schizophrenia research. Schizophr Bull 13:115–132

Buchsbaum MS, Ingvar DH, Kessler R, Waters RN, Cappelletti J, van Kammen DP, King AC, Johnson JJ, Manning RG, Flynn RM, Mann LS, Bunney WE Jr, Sokoloff L (1982a) Cerebral glucography with positron tomography in normals and in patients with schizophrenia. Arch Gen Psychiatry 39:251–259

Buchsbaum MS, Rigal R, Coppola R, Cappelletti J, King C, Johnson J (1982b) A new system for gray-level surface distribution maps of electrical activity. Electroencephalogr Clin Neurophysiol 53:237–242

Buchsbaum MS, DeLisi LE, Holcomb HH, Cappelletti J, King AC, Johnson J, Hazlett E, Dowling-Zimmerman S, Post RM, Morihisa J, Carpenter W, Cohen R, Pickar D, Weinberger DR, Margolin R, Kessler RM (1984a) Anteroposterior gradients in cerebral glucose use in schizophrenia and affective disorders. Arch Gen Psychiatry 41:1159–1166

Buchsbaum MS, Mirsky AF, DeLisi LE, Morihisa J, Karson CN, Mendelson WB, King AC, Johnson J, Kessler R (1984b) The Genain quadruplets: electrophysiological, positron emission, and X-ray tomographic studies. Psychiatry Res 13:95–108

Buchsbaum MS, Gillin JC, Wu J, Hazlett E, Sicotte N, DuPont RM (1989) Regional cerebral glucose metabolic rate in human sleep assessed by positron emission tomography. Life Sci 45:1349–1356

Coppola R (1979) Isolating low frequency activity in EEG spectrum analysis. Electroencephalogr Clin Neurophysiol 46:224–226

Cornblatt BA, Risch NJ, Faris G, Friedman D, Erlenmeyer-Kimling L (1988) The continuous performance test, identical pairs version (CPT-IP): new findings about sustained attention in normal families. Psychiatry Res 26:223–238

Cornblatt BA, Lenzenweger MF, Erlenmeyer-Kimling L (1989) The continuous performance test, identical pairs version (CPT-IP). II. Contrasting attentional profiles in schizophrenic and depressed patients. Psychiatry Res 29:65–85

Dixon WJ (1988) BMDP statistical software. University of California Press, Berkeley

Guenther W, Davous P, Godet J-L, Guillibert E, Breitling D, Rondot P (1988) Bilateral brain dysfunction during motor activation in type II schizophrenia measured by EEG mapping. Biol Psychiatry 23:295–311

Guich SM, Buchsbaum MS, Burgwald L, Wu J, Haier R, Asarnow R, Nuechterlein K, Potkin S (1989) Effect of attention on frontal distribution of delta activity and cerebral metabolic rate in schizophrenia, Schiz Res 2:439–448

Lukoff D, Nuechterlein KH, Ventura J (1986) Manual for expanded brief psychiatric rating scale (BPRS). Schizophr Bull 12:594–602

Matsui T, Hirano A (1978) An atlas of the human brain for computerized tomography. Igaku-Shoin, Tokyo

Nuechterlein KH, Parasuraman R, Jiang Q (1983) Visual sustained attention: image degradation produces rapid decrement over time. Science 220:327–329

Overall JE, Gorham DR (1962) The brief psychiatric rating scale. Psychol Rep 10:799–812

Sokoloff L (1977) Relation between physiological function and energy metabolism in the central nervous system. J Neurochem 29:13–26

Westphal KP, Grözinger B, Diekmann V, Scherb W, Reess J, Kornhuber HH (1990) EEG spectra parameters distinguish pathophysiological influences on the EEG in treated schizophrenics. Arch Italiennes de Biologie 128:55–66

Simultaneous Electroencephalogram Mapping and Positron Emission Tomography in Chronic Schizophrenia: Preliminary Results in Neuroleptic Treated Patients*

W. Wünther, K. Alper, E. Bartlett, F. Barouche, A.P. Wolf, S.L. Dewey, F. Henn, R. Riedel, U. Klages, J.D. Brodie, and R. John

Introduction

Neuroimaging methods have provided an important contribution to the search for pathophysiologic correlates of schizophrenia, as outlined in this volume and emphasized by Buchsbaum and Haler (1987). Information on results of positron emission tomography (PET) is provided, e.g., by Brodie (this volume); information on findings obtained with computerized electroencephalogram (EEG) and mapping are reviewed by Duffy (this volume). Here, we report on preliminary results obtained utilizing the simultaneous application of PET and computerized EEG mapping.

Volkow et al. (1987) reported a PET study in 18 DSM III chronic schizophrenics using [^{11}C]deoxyglucose. They studied resting condition and a challenge paradigm (eye tracking) and gave special consideration to the psychopathology of the patients in regard to the positive-negative dimension. For this purpose, they calculated correlations between glucose uptake in various parts of the brain and the amount of positive/negative symptomatology during baseline and task conditions. They found for these patients (all treated with neuroleptic and anticholinergic medication) signs of relative hypofrontality and nonreactivity for the task conditions (i.e., no significant changes as compared to baseline). Interestingly, these researchers reported a consistent trend towards positive correlations between the absolute regional glucose metabolism and the number of positive symptoms and negative correlations between metabolism and the number of negative symptoms.

We attempted to adopt the resting/activation paradigm of Volkow and colleagues with similar PET methodology and to monitor carefully for the positive/negative dimension, initially investigating markedly "negative" DSM III chronic patients. Additionally, however, we engaged in extending their correlational approach to brain function variables using PET and EEG

* Supported in part by National Institute of Mental Health grant MH-42647, National Institute of Health grant NS-15368, NATO grant 0700/87, Deutsche Forschungsgemeinschaft Sachbeihilfen Gu 207/2-1, 4-1, 5-1.
[1] Abt. für Psychiatrie, Universität München, Nussbaumstr. 7, W-8000 München 2, FRG.

Imaging of the Brain in Psychiatry
and Related Fields
Edited by K. Maurer

in the same schizophrenic subjects, taking into account the following experimental evidence. Previous EEG mapping and single photon emission computerized tomography (SPECT) findings of the Munich working group of this conjoint project suggested during simple motor activity of the dominant right hand possible uncoupling of bioelectrical and circulatory parameters in subgroups of schizophrenic patients (Günther et al. 1986, 1988). Additionally, there was a pathological activation pattern to manumotor stimulation, as shown both by SPECT and EEG results.

Thus, the purpose of this ongoing PET/EEG study is: (1) To check on our previous SPECT findings (Gunther et al. 1986) of an inability to raise focal brain activity during a motor stimulation challenge in chronic schizophrenics (DSM III diagnosis; Scale for Assessment of Negative Symptoms, SANS, total score above 25 as a cutoff value). This finding was indeed replicated by PET: nonreactivity on a complex finger movement task was found in DSM III-R chronic schizophrenics (average SANS total score 30, SD 21), which will be reported in detail by E.J. Bartlett et al. (in preparation). (2) To investigate the relationship of some quantitative EEG parameters (namely, absolute power frequency analyzed in conventional EEG bands) to glucose consumption (relative to whole brain) in various brain regions of patients and check on possible differences of this coupling as compared to normal persons.

For the second objective, 21-channel EEG mapping was performed simultaneously with the PET investigation in five schizophrenics. For technical reasons, however, we were not able to study more patients with EEG mapping and PET truly simultaneously since the laboratories were at distant locations with no permanent EEG mapping system installed at the PET site. Therefore, this EEG/PET project was continued in a synchronous manner, i.e., EEG and PET investigations were performed within 24 h, at the same time of two consecutive days). This seems acceptable given the high test-retest reliability coefficients, which were reported for resting conditions for EEG mapping (Günther et al. 1989), and PET parameters, as used in our study (Bartlett et al. 1988). Accordingly, relations between EEG and PET data shall be reported for this condition only (and not for motor activation).

In this ongoing study all but one of the patients were treated exclusively with haloperidol. Thus, this preliminary report refers to neuroleptic treated patients only; enlargement of both untreated and neuroleptic treated patient subgroups, along with the investigation of controls, is in progress.

For preliminary comparisons, the control group of the EEG/PET study of Buchsbaum and coworkers (1984) will be utilized. This comparison was enabled by the adjustment of our methodology for calculating EEG/PET correlations to the methodology used by that group.

Subjects and Methods

A total of 14 normal control persons and 13 schizophrenic patients took part in the PET study on motor dysfunction, reported in detail by E.J. Bartlett et al. (in preparation). Of the schizophrenic patients, nine were examined by both PET and EEG mapping methods. These patients can be described as follows: DSM III-R criteria for chronic schizophrenia yielding the following diagnoses: 295.1 (disorganized/hebephrenic subtype), $n = 2$; 295.3 (paranoid subtype) $n = 4$; 295.9 (undifferentiated subtype), $n = 3$. Haloperidol plasma levels ranged from 5.3 to 21.8 ng/ml.

The mean age was 32.0 (SD 6.0) years, the mean duration of disease 15.6 years (SD 6.1). Psychopathology was assessed as follows: Brief Psychiatric Rating Scale (BPRS) total score 19–54 (mean 32, SD 10); Scale for Assessment of Positive Symptoms (SAPS) total score 27–59 (mean 42, SD 12); SANS total score 6–67 (mean 30, SD 21), i.e., comparable to type II/negative patients of our previous EEG and SPECT studies.

PETT VI measurements using 11-2-deoxyglucose as tracer were obtained in 16 cortical regions of interest (ROIs). Details as to the boundary finding procedure and the reliability measures are provided in Bartlett et al. (1988; in preparation) along with full details of the PET methodology. Patients were examined during resting/eyes closed conditions (the two motor tasks are not reported here).

In addition to the PET data, 21-channel EEG mapping recordings during resting/eyes closed condition were obtained in nine schizophrenic patients. Linked ear reference leads were used after automatic artifact rejection confirmed by visual analysis, providing the basis for further analysis. Fast Fourier transform was applied yielding (among other parameters not used for further analysis) absolute power values for each individual. They were transformed into normally distributed z-scores, i.e., normalized to a data base of reference subjects. We used the four frequency bands δ 1.5–3.5, θ 3.5–7.5, α 7.5–12.5, and β 12.5–25.0. Further details as to this neurometric methodology are reported in several publications (e.g., John et al. 1988).

Following the procedures proposed by Buchsbaum and his group (1984) EEG/PET correlations were established as follows: The 16 nearest 10–20 positions to the predefined cortical PET ROIs were selected. The placements of these electrodes are given in both Table 1 and Fig. 1; the exact location of PET/ROIs must be obtained from E.J. Bartlett et al. (in preparation).

Normalized data sets have been used for further analysis (as required for calculating product-moment correlations), as outlined for the EEG data before. For PET data, rates of glucose consumption in each particular ROI were related to the overall cerebral metabolism in order to control for spontaneous fluctuations (Bartlett et al. 1988).

Table 1. Product-moment correlation coefficients between absolute EEG power and regional cerebral metabolic rate of glucose

Region of interest	Electrode position	δ 1.5–3.5 cps	θ 3.5–7.5 cps	α 7.5–12.5 cps	β 12.5–25 cps	Total 1.5–25 cps
MF	Fz	0.011	−0.297	−0.354	−0.355	−0.299
LPF	F3	−0.11	−0.385	−0.478	−0.537	−0.432
LPM	F3	0.412	0.15	0.016	−0.167	0.138
LSM	C3	0.034	0.175	0.128	0.063	0.158
RPF	F4	0.415	0.153	−0.037	−0.447	0.079
RPM	F4	0.655	0.777	0.741	0.509	0.765
RSM	C4	−0.101	−0.079	−0.437	−0.048	−0.189
LMF	Fp1	−0.015	−0.292	−0.052	−0.218	−0.707
LIMF	F7	0.691	0.707	0.7	0.464	0.326
RMF	Fp2	0.338	0.221	0.371	0.147	0.192
RIMF	F8	−0.101	0.071	0.157	0.26	0.317
LP	P3	0.197	0.194	0.347	0.321	0.168
LT	T3	0.366	0.212	0.249	−0.065	0.462
RP	P4	0.338	0.332	0.534	0.244	0.549
RT	T4	−0.353	−0.523	−0.54	−0.499	−0.461
OCC	O1/2	−0.354	−0.484	−0.428	−0.549	−0.461

MF, mesiofrontal; LPF, left prefrontal; LPM, left promotor; LSM; left sensorimotor; RPF, right prefrontal; RPM, right premotor; RSM, right sensorimotor; LMF, left midfrontal; LIMF, left inferior midfrontal; RMF, right midfrontal; RIMF, right inferior midfrontal; LP, left parietal; LT, left temporal; RP, right parietal; RT, right temporal; OCC, occipital.

EEG absolute power values in four frequency bands (and the total power) were then related to glucose consumption in 16 PET/EEG ROIs yielding 80 product-moment correlation coefficients, which are displayed in Table 1. These coefficients have been z-transformed and multiplied by 100 for display in a color and gray scale, a procedure identical to that used by Buchsbaum and coworkers in 1984 (Fig. 1). Since Buchsbaum provides the coefficients only for δ and α frequency bands, we restrict the coefficients reported in Fig. 1 to these bands also.

Results

Table 1 shows the correlation coefficients EEG/PET, obtained in haloperidol treated schizophrenic patients in resting/eyes closed condition.

As can be seen in this table and (more easily) in Fig. 1, the most striking finding is that in chronic schizophrenics total energy and power values are coupled very similarly to glucose consumption across all frequency bands.

The relative lack of influence of EEG bandwidth on the relationship of EEG to glucose consumption appears to be also present in the left hemisphere of normals, as reported by Buchsbaum and coworkers (1984).

The topography of points of maximal and minimal correlation between EEG and PET appear to differ somewhat in the two groups. Due to the similarity of the relationship of EEG and PET across frequency bands, and, as mentioned above, because Buchsbaum et al. (1984) confined their study of normal individuals to the α and δ bands, we will limit our discussion to these bands only.

The δ coefficents range from −0.354 in occipital and −0.353 in right temporooccipital regions to 0.691 in left inferior frontal and right premotor areas.

Since significance in correlations is an ambiguous measure (if variances are low, meaninglessly small coefficients may become significant and vice versa), we prefer to use ranges of absolute values for further discussion.

If we consider coefficients between −0.300 and +0.300 as no correlation (only 9% common variance), seven coefficients for δ are in this category, and the same number yield positive correlations. Only two negative correlations are found in our schizophrenics. This seems to be different, at least in some brain regions, to the correlations in healthy control persons reported by Buchsbaum et al. (1984; displayed in Fig. 1).

In left frontal and temporal regions, normals have positive and chronic schizophrenics no correlations, whereas in other brain regions of the left hemisphere schizophrenics and normals are alike. Thus, there is possible evidence of maximal uncoupling in left frontotemporal regions for chronic schizophrenic patients as compared to normal controls (Fig. 1).

Unfortunately, until we have examined our own controls, no comparisons between schizophrenic and healthy persons are available for the right hemisphere (since this is not reported by Buchsbaum et al. 1984).

The α coefficients in chronic schizophrenic patients (Table 1, Fig. 1) range from −0.540 in occipital and −0.478 in left prefrontal regions to +0.741 in right prefrontal (note the extreme hemispheric differences for prefrontal regions) and +0.700 in left inferior frontal regions.

Five coefficients are negative (in bilateral posterior and left midfrontal regions), five are positive (in right frontal and biparietal areas), and six indicate no correlation.

If we compare these coefficients to those reported by Buchsbaum (Fig. 1), maximal differences appear to exist, as already in the δ frequency band, in left inferior frontal and temporal areas. Whereas there are negative correlations in normals in these regions, either markedly positive correlations (+0.700; left inferior frontal) or no correlations (left temporal area) are found in chronic schizophrenic patients. However, again, nothing can be said about the right hemisphere until our own control data are available.

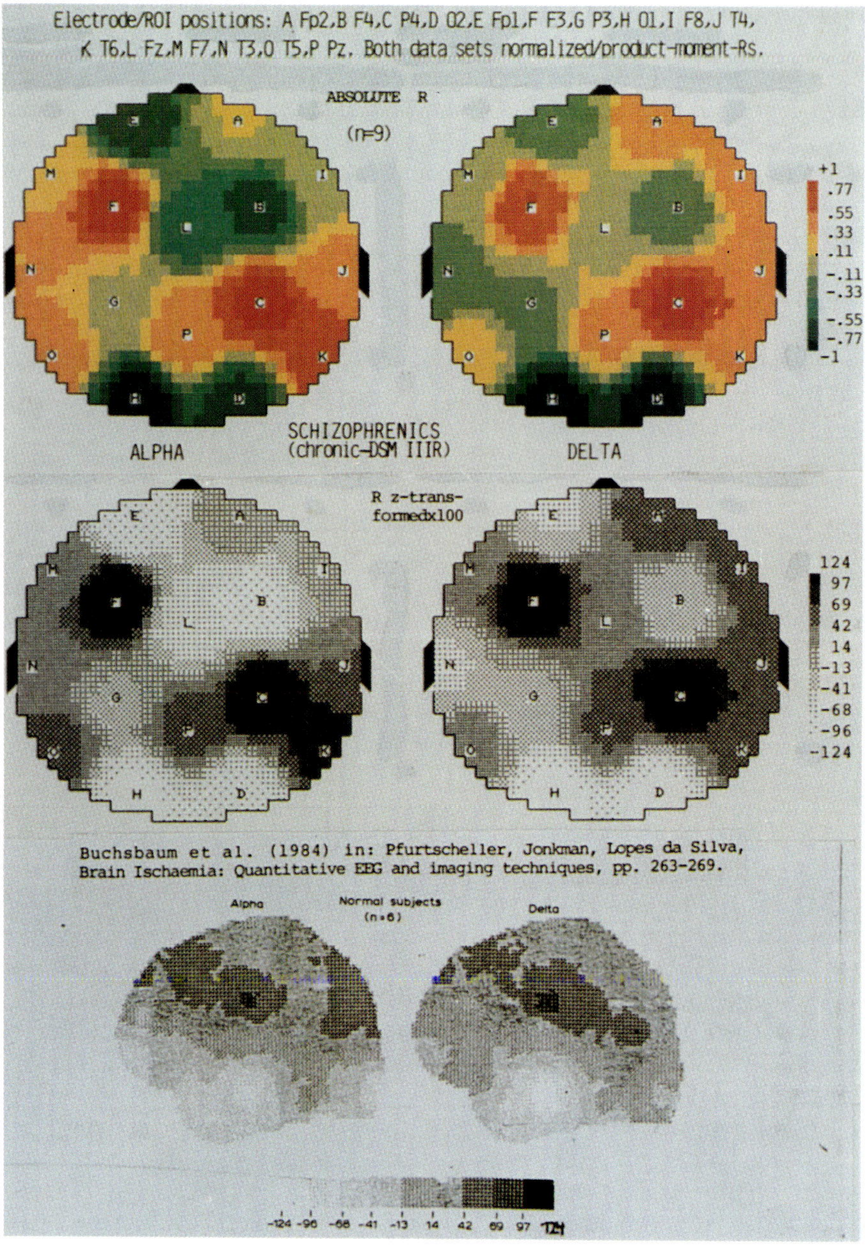

a

Fig. 1a,b. Product-moment correlation coefficients between metabolic rate of glucose and absolute EEG power (see Table 1) displayed in absolute values (color scale) and z-transformed ×100 (gray scale) in haloperidol treated DSM III-R chronic schizophrenics. EEG electrode positions as shown; PET regions of interest (ROIs) as shown in Table 1; further EEG/PET methodology see text. **a** Coefficients in α (7.5–12.5 cps) and δ (1.5–3.5 cps). *Upper row*, absolute *R*s; *middle row*, z-transformed *R*s; *lower row*, normal values of the left hemisphere, as reported by Buchsbaum and colleagues (1984). Identical gray scales used. Note similiar coupling patterns in most brain regions except the left temporal regions, where normals show negative coefficients in both bands and schizophrenics zero to maximal positive ones

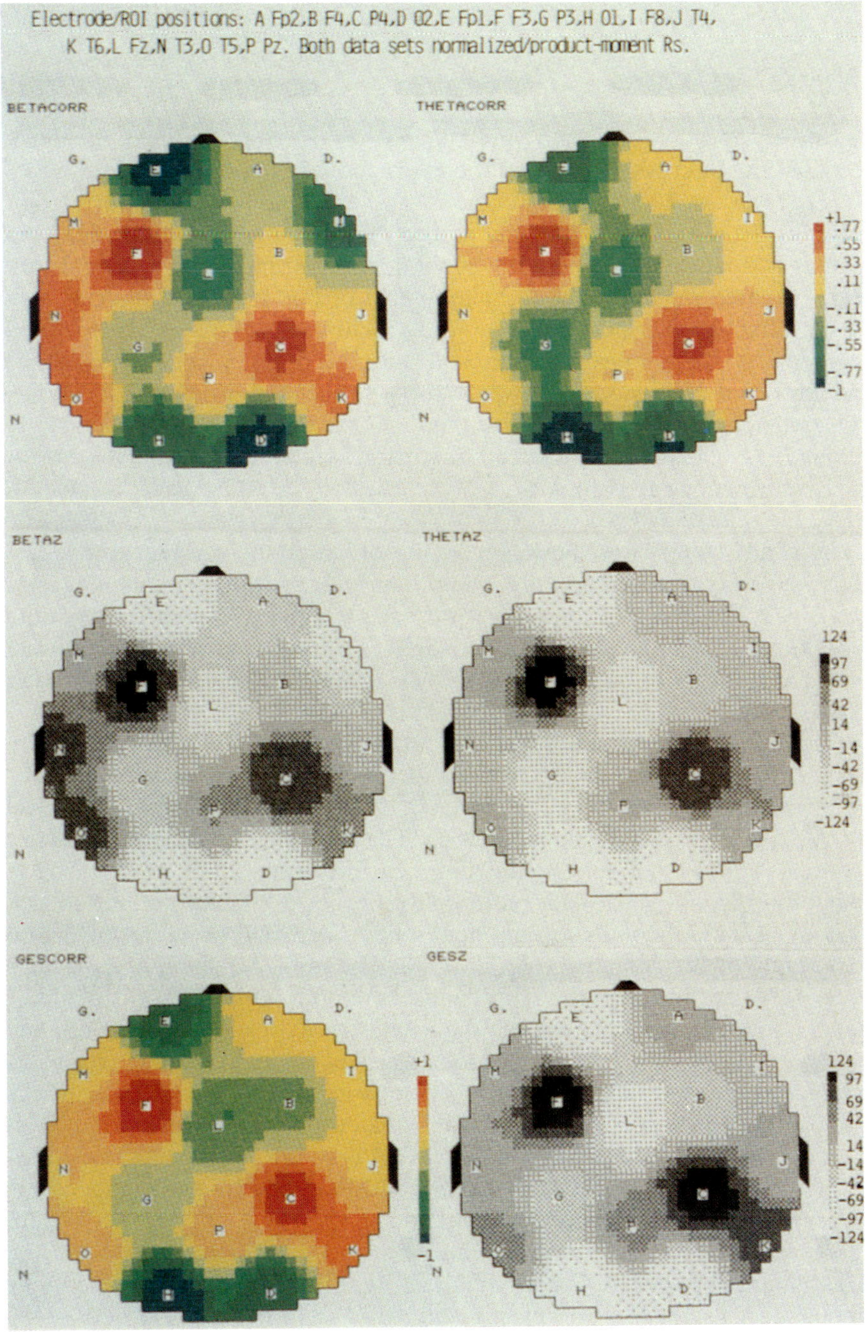

b

b Coefficients for θ (3.5–7.5 cps), β (12.5–25.0 cps), and total power (1.5–25.0 cps) in absolute values (color scale) and z-transformed ×100 (gray scales). (GESCORR/GESZ = coefficients in absolute values/z-transformed for total energy/power). Note the striking similarity between glucose consumption and EEG power in schizophrenics in all frequency bands. There are major hemispheric differences of coupling distributions. Both findings seem unexpected; however, since no controls have been examined (ongoing), no further speculations can be made

Discussion

Since we consider our data preliminary, for reasons outlined in above sections, the discussion here shall be restricted to a few speculative issues.

First, no exact anatomical relations can be established by our correlation methods. However, we follow the procedure of the pioneers in the field. As long as it is not known where the generators of various EEG potentials are really situated in the brain, the major goal of our type of study can only be to establish constant topographical relations of PET ROIs (defined according to anatomical structures as displayed by magnetic resonance imaging) and the nearest EEG ROI (with defined electrode location). Following the widely accepted assumption that the EEG is predominantly (though not exclusively) produced in cortical brain layers in the absence of gross morphological pathology, only cortical PET ROIs were related to EEG variables.

Second, comparison between results of different working groups are always to be considered tentative, until data with the same methodology are available. With this precaution we present preliminary evidence suggesting differences of coupling of EEG and PET in chronic schizophrenics during resting conditions as compared to normals investigated by Buchsbaum et al. (1984).

Two findings may be consistent with the literature: left hemisphere dysfunction in subgroups of right-handed schizophrenics is supported by both functional (review, e.g., Flor-Henry 1987; Gaebel 1988) and anatomical data (e.g., Jakob and Beckmann 1986). This may have speculative relations to areas of maximal uncoupling between EEG and PET in left fronto-temporal regions. Since data on normals are not available, nothing can be said about the nondominant right hemisphere. A recent simultaneous EEG/PET study of Buchbaums group in DSM III chronic schizophrenics (Guich et al. 1989) has included the right hemisphere both in their 15 schizophrenic and 9 healthy persons. However, their data report relations between δ and glucose consumption in unmedicated (washout at least 30 days, mean 30 weeks) patients during continous performance task which appear hardly comparable to our data in haloperidol treated patients during resting/eyes closed conditions and shall not be discussed here further for that reason.

Finally, Nagata et al. (1989) performed EEG and PET simultaneously in patients with unilateral cerebral infarction at various stages of illness. Since there was no group of normal controls included in their study, again no information on the EEG/PET relations in the right hemisphere can be obtained. This renders the examination of our own control group, along with the examination of an unmedicated sample of chronic and acute schizophrenics, an essential part of our ongoing EEG/PET study.

References

Bartlett EJ, Brodie JD, Wolf AP, Christman DR, Laska E, Meissner M (1988) Reproducibility of cerebral glucose metabolic measurements in resting human subjects. J Cereb Blood Flow Metab 8:502–512

Buchsbaum MS, Haler RJ (1987) Functional and anatomical brain imaging: impact on schizophrenia research. Schizophr Bull 30:115–132

Buchsbaum MS, Kessler R, King A, Johnson J, Cappelletti J (1984) Simultaneous cerebral glucography with PET and topographic EEG. In: Pfurtscheller G, Jonkman EJ, Lopes da Silva FH (eds) Brain ischaemia: quantitative EEG and imaging techniques. Elsevier, Amsterdam, pp 263–269 (Progress in brain research, vol 62)

Flor-Henry P (1987) Cerebral dynamics, laterality and psychopathology: a commentary. In: Takahashi R, Flor-Henry P, Gruzelier J, Niwa S (eds) Cerebral dynamics, laterality and psychopathology. Elsevier, Amsterdam, pp 3–21

Gaebel W (1988) Hemisphärenfunktion und psychische Erkrankungen. Nervenarzt 59:437–448

Guich SM, Buchsbaum MS, Burgwald L, Wu J, Haier R, Asarnow R, Nuechterlein K, Potkin S (1989) Effect of frontal distribution of delta activity and cerebral metabolic rate in schizophrenia. Schizophr Res 2:439–448

Günther W, Moser E, Mueller-Spahn F, Voefele K, Buell U, Hippius H (1986) Pathological cerebral blood flow during motor function in schizophrenic and endogenous depressed patients. Biol Psychiatry 21:889–899

Günther W, Davous P, Godet JL, Guillibert E, Breitling D, Rondot P (1988) Bilateral brain dysfunction during motor activation in type II schizophrenia measured by EEG mapping. Biol Psychiatry 23:295–311

Günther W, Streck P, Steinberg R, Guenther R, Raith L, Backmund M (1989) Psychomotor disturbances in psychiatric patients as a possible basis for new attempts at differential diagnosis and therapy. IV. Brain dysfunction during motor activation measured by EEG mapping. Eur Arch Psychiatry Neurol Sci 239:194–209

Jakob H, Beckmann H (1986) Prenatal developmental disturbances in the limbic allocortex in schizophrenics. J Neural Transm 65:303–326

John ER, Prichep LS, Fridman J, Easton P (1988) Neurometrics: computer-assisted differential diagnosis of brain dysfunctions. Science 239:162–169

Nagata K, Tagawa K, Hiroi S, Shishido F, Uemara K (1989) Electroencephalographic correlates of blood flow and oxygen metabolism provided by positron emission tomography in patients with cerebral infarction. Electroencephalogr Clin Neurophysiol 72:16–30

Volkow ND, Wolf AP, van Gelder P, Brodie JD, Overall JE, Cancro R, Gomez-Mont F (1987) Phenomenological correlates of metabolic activity in 18 patients with chronic schizophrenia. Am J Psychiatry 187:151–158

Adenosine Receptors and Second Messengers in Rat Hippocampus After Unilateral Entorhinal Cortex Lesion: An Autoradiographic Study

J. DECKERT[1] and M.B. JORGENSEN

Introduction

The entorhinal cortex is the source of the major afferent input into the hippocampus, making up the perforant path. Some 85% of the synaptic input to the outer two-thirds of the molecular layer of the ipsilateral dentate gyrus is provided by entorhinal cortex neurons. Morphologically, pathological changes in the entorhinal cortex have been demonstrated in several brain disorders with cognitive impairment, such as schizophrenia (Jakob and Beckmann 1986), Alzheimer's disease, and Parkinson's disease (Braak and Braak 1990). The major inhibitory neuromodulator of entorhinal cortex neurons is the nuleoside adenosine. We therefore decided to investigate the effect of unilateral surgical removal of the entorhinal cortex on, among others, adenosine A1 receptors and adenylate cyclase using radioactive ligand probes in a quantitative autoradiographic study.

Material and Methods

Ten male Wistar rats weighing between 300 and 400 g were used in this study. The right entorhinal cortex of five animals was removed surgically (Jorgensen et al. 1987). On the fourth postoperative day operated and control animals were anesthetized with halothane, perfused with 50 ml isotonic NaCl, and decapitated. The brains were processed and 20 μm thick cryostat sections were obtained, as previously described (Deckert et al. 1988).

Binding of 2.5 n*M* [^{3}H]cyclohexyladenosine (A1) and 10 n*M* [^{3}H]forskolin (adenylate cyclase) was performed according to published protocols (Deckert et al. 1988; Gehlert et al. 1985). Comparable sections through the rostrodorsal hippocampus of all animals were processed in parallel. The slide-mounted sections and Amersham ^{3}H microscales, kindly provided and equilibrated by J. Unnerstall, were then exposed to LKB ultrafilm. The films were processed as described (Deckert et al. 1988). Quantitative

[1] Psychiatrische Klinik und Poliklinik, Universitäts-Nervenklinik Würzburg, Füchsleinstr. 15, W-8700 Würzburg, FRG.

Imaging of the Brain in Psychiatry and Related Fields
Edited by K. Maurer

Table 1. [^{3}H]cyclohexyladenosine and [^{3}H]forskolin binding in rat brain after surgical removal of the right entorhinal cortex

	[^{3}H]CHA		[^{3}H]FOR	
	Right	Left	Right	Left
Parietal motor cortex	88 ± 18	87 ± 21	71 ± 4	73 ± 5
Radiatum (CA1)	138 ± 25	145 ± 23	35 ± 4	37 ± 3
Oriens (CA1)	119 ± 25	122 ± 30		
Upper blade of molecular layer (DG)	85 ± 16[a]	136 ± 16	76 ± 5[b]	101 ± 6
Lower blade of molecular layer (DG)	80 ± 18[a]	133 ± 18	83 ± 4[b]	104 ± 6

Values of fmol/mg dry tissue represent the mean ± S.E.M. (n = 5). The value for each of the five animals is based on three measurements.
[^{3}H]CHA, [^{3}H]cyclohexyladenosine; [^{3}H]FOR, [^{3}H]forskolin.
[a] Significant at $p < 0.01$ level (ANOVA and Scheffe F test).
[b] Significant at $p < 0.05$ level (ANOVA and Scheffe F test).

analysis was performed using the image analysis system first described by Goochee et al. (1980). Brain microregions and the lesion efficacy were determined on adjacent thionin and Fink-Heimer stained sections.

Results

[^{3}H]cyclohexyladenosine and [^{3}H]forskolin binding were reduced by 40% and 25%, respectively, in the molecular layer of the right dentate gyrus when compared to the molecular layer of the left dentate gyrus in the lesioned animals or the molecular layer of the ipsi- and contralateral side of the control animals. No differences between the lesioned and the non-lesioned side of the lesioned animals or the lesioned side of the lesioned animals and either side of the control animals were observed in any of the other brain microregions investigated (Table 1 and Fig. 1).

Discussion

Of several components of a putative adenosinergic neuromodulatory system in human hippocampus, A1 receptors and adenylate cyclase will probably be the most affected by loss of human entorhinal cortex neurons.

Disturbances of adenosinergic neuromodulation in hippocampus have therefore to be expected as a consequence of pathological changes in the human entorhinal cortex.

Correction of disturbed adenosinergic neuromodulation by pharmacological intervention may thus be of therapeutic value in human diseases with

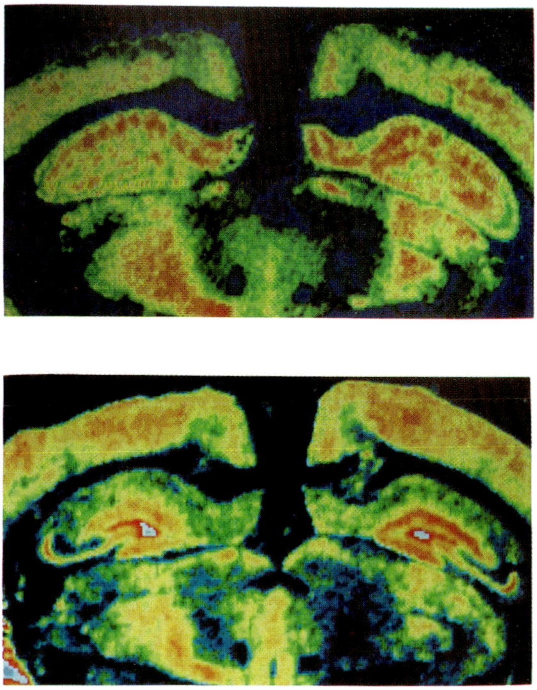

Fig. 1. [^{3}H]cyclohexyladenosine (*top*) and [^{3}H]forskolin (*bottom*) binding on adjacent sections through the rostrodorsal hippocampus of a rat after surgical removal of the right entorhinal cortex. Note the decrease in labeling in the outer two-thirds of the molecular layer of the right dentate gyrus as compared to the left dentate gyrus. Density of labeling decreases from *red* over *yellow*, *green* and *blue* to *black*

cognitive impairment as different as schizophrenia, Alzheimer's and Parkinson's disease.

References

Braak H, Braak E (1990) Cognitive impairment in Parkinson's disease: amyloid plaques, neurofibrillary tangles and neuropil threads in the cerebral cortex. J Neurotransm (PD) 2:45–58

Deckert J, Bisserbe JC, Klein E, Marangos PJ (1988) Adenosine uptake sites in brain: regional distribution of putative subtypes in relationship to adenosine A1 receptors. J Neurosci 8:2338–2349

Gehlert D, Dawson TW, Yamamura HJ, Wamsley JK (1985) Localization of [^{3}H]forskolin binding sites in the rat brain using quantitative autoradiography. Eur J Pharmacol 106:223–225

Goochee C, Rasband W, Sokoloff L (1980) Computerized densitometry and colour coding of [^{14}C]deoxyglucose autoradiographs. Ann Neurol 7:359–370

Jakob H, Beckmann H (1986) Prenatal developmental disturbances in the limbic allocortex in schizophrenics. J Neurotransm 65:303–326

Jorgensen MB, Johansen FF, Diemer NH (1987) Removal of the entorhinal cortex protects hippocampal CA1 neurons from ischemic damage. Acta Neuropathol 73:189–194

Imaging of Cat Cerebellar Cortex Responses*

F.P. Kolb[1], R. Lerch, and G. Arnold

Introduction

Purkinje cells (PCs) are the only output from the cerebellar cortex. They are activated via the climbing fiber (CF) and mossy fiber (MF) systems. With respect to the CF system both anatomical (Voogd 1969) and electrophysiological (Oscarsson 1969) studies leave no doubt that it is parasagittally organized. Thus, PCs oriented within a parasagittal strip are activated via CFs originating from the same group of cells in the inferior olive.

With respect to the MF system debate continues concerning the orientation of the spread of excitation. Based on anatomical findings the MF system was assumed to activate PCs primarily in a beam-like fashion, i.e., along the parallel fibers (Braitenberg and Atwood 1958; Ekerot and Larson 1983; Andersson and Garwicz 1988). However, recent results have been reported describing a patch-like activation of PCs, and thus indicating a more vertical organization in the granule cell – PC relationship (Shambes et al. 1978; Bower and Woolston 1983).

The present study examines this question using a method developed in our laboratory which allows display of the momentary state of the spatial excitation, expressed by the two-dimensional distribution of the cerebellar potentials. The results of the study confirm the latter of the above hypotheses.

Methods

Experiments were carried out on α-chloralose anesthetized, paralyzed adult cats. Cerebellar field potentials were evoked by peripheral and central stimuli. The peripheral stimulus consisted of passive movements around the wrist joint and of electrical activation of different nerves of both forelimbs. In order to simulate a central command, the right sensory motor cortex was intracortically stimulated with constant current pulses (200 μs, 200–

* Supported by the Deutsche Forschungsgemeinschaft SFB 220, D9.
[1] Physiologisches Institut, Universität München, Pettenkoferstr. 12, W-8000 München 2, FRG.

Imaging of the Brain in Psychiatry
and Related Fields
Edited by K. Maurer

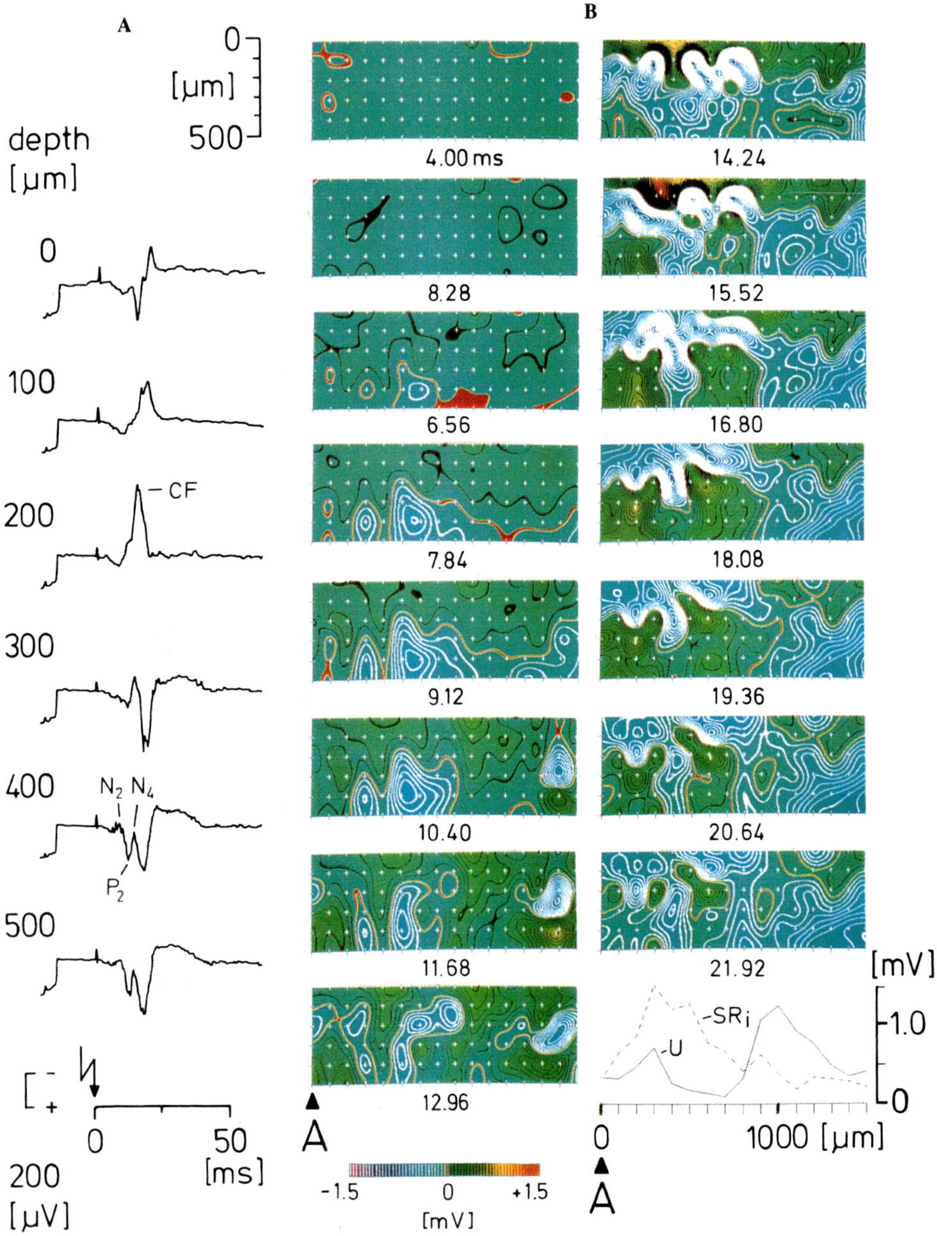
A
B
depth
[μm]
0
[μm]
500
0
100
200
— CF
300
400
N2 N4
P2
500
0
50
[ms]
200
[μV]
4.00 ms
8.28
6.56
7.84
9.12
10.40
11.68
12.96
14.24
15.52
16.80
18.08
19.36
20.64
21.92
A
-1.5
0
+1.5
[mV]
-SRi
-U
[mV]
1.0
0
0
1000 [μm]
A

500 μA). These various stimuli were applied sequentially. Averaged field potentials were recorded by a single glass micropipette within a frontal plane of lobule Vc of the left intermediate cerebellar cortex. By repetitive penetrations of the electrode an equidistant grid of recording points was achieved. In order to obtain a continuous distribution of the field potentials, the values between the recording points were interpolated using the cubic spline algorithm. This results in the so-called intracortical potential image (ICPI).

Results

The responses in Fig. 1 were obtained within the sensory representation area (lobule Vc) of the cat cerebellar cortex. They result from electrical stimulation of the corresponding superficial radial nerve (SRi). Figure 1A shows averaged field potentials displayed as conventional plots recorded from different depths of a single track. According to a terminology described elsewhere (e.g., Eccles et al. 1967), all the distinct components observed in different depths can be undoubtedly attributed to the activation via the CF and MF system (CF, N_2, N_4, P_2). Figure 1B depicts a temporal sequence of images constructed from 16 recording tracks. Each of these ICPI represents the momentary spatial (i.e., two-dimensional) activity profile. Within the area of interest, covering the c1 and c2 zones (Voogd 1969; Oscarsson 1969), and during the period covering the arrival of the short latency MF responses, a clear patch-like or columnar activation was observed in the ICPIs. Multiple columnar activated centers, approximately equidistant and about 250 μm apart, were found (see Fig. 1B, e.g., 10.40 ms panel). They arose from the granule cell layer waxing towards the surface

←

Fig. 1A,B. Cerebellar responses to electrical stimulation of the superficial radial nerve (SRi). **A** Conventional presentation of field potentials obtained from different depths (N_2, N_4, P_2) indicate the relative polarities and components of the mossy fiber input. The climbing fiber (CF) input is also shown. **B** A sequence of intracortical potential images (ICPIs) is constructed from 16 electrode tracks covering a cortical area of 500 μm (depth) ×1500 μm (mediolateral direction) with a regular grid distance of 100 μm in each direction. The letter *A* and the *arrowhead* mark the track from which field potentials in Fig. 1A are recorded. The *background colors* represent amplitudes. Isopotential lines are drawn with a distance of $\Delta U = 50\,\mu V$. The zero line is shown in *red*, lines of negative values in *white*, and those of positive values *black*. The 15 ICPIs represent a time sequence ranging from 4.00 ms to 21.92 ms (time increment $\Delta t = 1.28$ ms). The *bottom right* diagram shows two amplitude profiles obtained from the surface recordings, related to the CF input. The *broken line* represents the values for the CF input following SRi stimulation and the *solid line* those following ulnar stimulation

which, however, was not reached. This was true for the different nerves stimulated. With respect to latencies, amplitudes, spatial representation, and the size of activated areas, significant differences were found.

With respect to the CF system, responses also showed focal activation at a depth based on of approximately 200 μm. In contrast to the MF responses, the CF activation was localized negative potentials within the molecular layer. Corresponding reversed potentials were found above and below. Covering the period of 15.52–19.36 ms, the foci merged to form a superficial band which, however, was restricted to the left half of these SRi evoked ICPIs. This can also be derived from the bottom right portion of Fig. 1, displaying the distribution of the maximal CF amplitudes observed during the above mentioned period. Furthermore, it can be clearly seen that the maximal CF amplitudes resulting from ulnar (U) stimulation showed a completely different spatial distribution.

Following the central sensory motor cortex stimulation, an activation closer to the PC somata was observed, indicating more pronounced information processing in favor of central inputs. This holds for both MF and CF systems.

Discussion

The present study reports a method allowing visualization of the generally complex responses of the cerebellar cortex generated by the activation of different cerebellar afferents. Based on a detailed field potential analysis and calculating the spatial distribution of potentials it was possible to achieve some insight into the physiological organization of the cerebellar cortex. With respect to the MF system the present study confirms the electrophysiological findings of Shambes et al. (1978) and Bower and Woolston (1983), which indicated a patch-like rather than a beam-like activation of PCs. In contrast to the majority of anatomical data favoring beam-like activation there are also histological data which are not inconsistent with our present findings (Scheibel 1977; Heckroth and Eisenman 1988).

The CF responses in this study also agree well with those reported elsewhere, e.g., by Trott and Armstrong (1987). The different foci observed (Fig. 1B, 14.24 ms ICPI) spaced approximately 200 μm apart may result from differentially activated zones. Ekerot and Larson (1982) and Campbell and Armstrong (1985) were able to demonstrate that the medial and lateral halves of the c1 zone receive inputs from quite distinct regions in the inferior olive.

The present state of research does not allow us to reject the concept of the propagation of specific information along the parallel fibers. Further experiments in which larger areas are analyzed must be undertaken to establish the functional significance of the observed information processing as well as to confirm the hypothesis of patch-like activation.

References

Andersson G, Garwicz M (1988) Parallel fiber mediated field potentials in the cat cerebellum evoked by peripheral stimulation. Eur J Neurosci (abstract)

Bower JM, Woolston DC (1983) Congruence of spatial organization of tactile projections to granule cell and Purkinje cell layers of cerebellar hemispheres of the albino rat: vertical organization of cerebellar cortex. J Neurophysiol 49:745–766

Braitenberg V, Atwood RP (1958) Morphological observations on the cerebellar cortex. J Comp Neurol 109:1–33

Campbell NC, Armstrong DM (1985) Origin in the medial accessory olive of climbing fibres to the x and lateral c_1 zones of the cat cerebellum: a combined electrophysiological/WGA-HRP investigation. Exp Brain Res 58:520–531

Eccles JC, Ito M, Szentágothai J (1967) The cerebellum as a neuronal machine. Springer, Berlin Heidelberg New York

Ekerot CF, Larson B (1980) Termination in overlapping sagittal zones in cerebellar anterior lobe of mossy and climbing fiber paths activated from dorsal funiculus. Exp Brain Res 38:163–172

Ekerot CF, Larson B (1982) Branching of olivary axons to innervate pairs of sagittal zones in the cerebellar anterior lobe of the cat. Exp Brain Res 48:185–198

Heckroth JA, Eisenman LM (1988) Parasagittal organization of mossy fiber collaterals in the cerebellum of the mouse. J Comp Neurol 270:385–394

Oscarsson O (1969) The sagittal organization of the cerebellar anterior lobe as revealed by the projection patterns of the climbing fiber system. In: Llinás R (ed) Neurobiology of cerebellar evolution and development. American Medical Association, Chicago, pp 525–537

Scheibel AB (1977) Sagittal organization of mossy fiber terminal systems in the cerebellum of the rat: a Golgi study. Exp Neurol 57:1067–1070

Shambes GM, Beermann DH, Welker W (1978) Multiple tactile areas in cerebellar cortex: another patchy cutaneous projection to granule cell columns in rats. Brain Res 157:123–128

Trott JR, Armstrong DM (1987) The cerebellar corticonuclear projection from lobule Vb/c of the cat anterior lobe: a combined electrophysiological and autoradiographic study. Exp Brain Res 66:318–338

Voogd J (1969) The importance of fiber connections in the comparative anatomy of the mammalian cerebellum. In: Llinás R (ed) Neurobiology of cerebellar evolution and development. American Medical Association, Chicago, pp 493–514

Topographic Mapping of Biochemical Data

P. RIEDERER[1] and W. GSELL

Numerous chemical and biochemical data from postmortem analyses of human brain are available and cover almost all psychiatric and neurologic diseases of the central nervous system (CNS). Most data give a static representation of the human brain, i.e., they represent the results of an endpoint measurement. These data concern differences between: (a) groups of patients and healthy controls and (b) regions of the brain with respect to numerous parameters, such as enzyme activities, neurotransmitter and metabolite concentrations, and receptor densities and affinities, and are of a one-dimensional format. Dynamic or two-dimensional data are less well represented within the literature of postmortem brain analyses. They mainly include data from enzymatic or receptor analysis (Michaelis-Menten equation, Lineweaver-Burke plots, Scatchard analysis) and/or regression analysis of the dependency or independency of parameters on postmortem analysis-specific variables, e.g., age, postmortem delay, storage time of tissue, and gender. These latter approaches for estimating the quality of one's data are often poorly carried out.

Data are normally presented by plotting a curve for two-dimensional data or by plotting bars; for one-dimensional data, tables are given. However, clearness of results is often darkened by both the amount and our limited ability for abstract thinking. Both can be overcome by converting data from absolute to relative modes, i.e., from a dimensional to a dimensionless status, when possible. In this way the number of data is easily reduced by half and a reference point for easier abstraction is created.

When abstraction, i.e., reduction in attributes, is finished, determination, or addition of attributes, for computer handling and presentation can start. This means that frames both for form and content must be created. The form is given by the anatomical structure of the brain. The frame is then built up by digitalizing the shapes of specified regions by convenient methods such as scanning or using a digitalizing table. We have chosen a low-cost possibility easily reproduced by all labs owning an IBM-compatible computer. We used a simple IBM MS-DOS compatible "mouse" (Genius

[1] Abt. für Psychiatrie, Universitäts-Nervenklinik Würzburg, Füchsleinstr. 15, W-8700 Würzburg, FRG.

Imaging of the Brain in Psychiatry
and Related Fields
Edited by K. Maurer

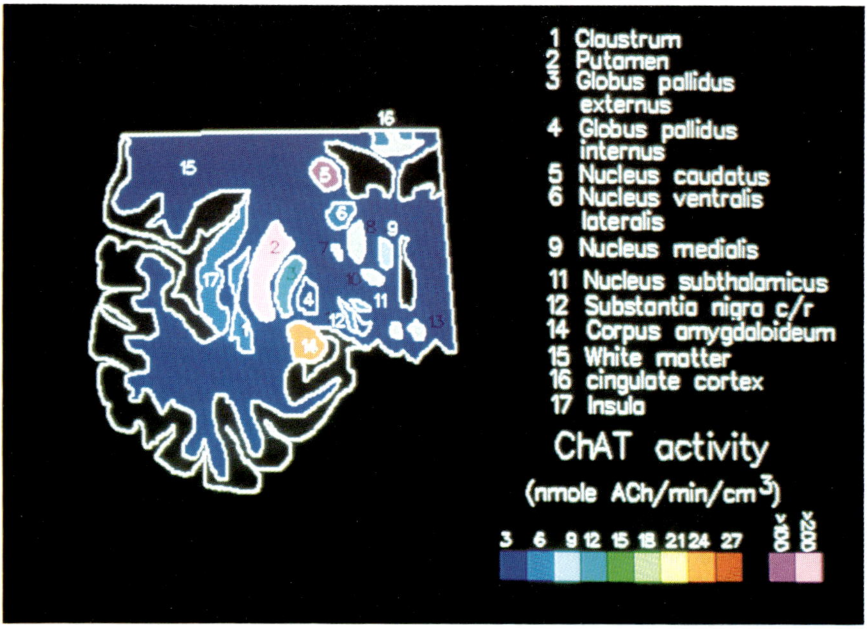

1

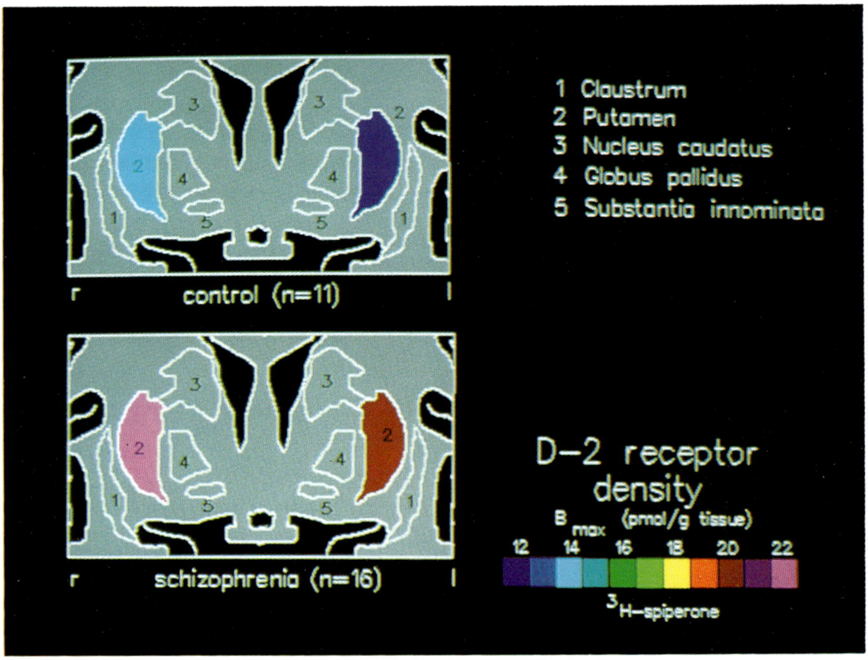

2

Fig. 1. Full view of a slice of a coronal section. Regions were drawn out of an anatomy book and digitalized as described in the text. ChAT, choline acetyltransferase. (Data were taken from the work of Aquilonius (1980))

Fig. 2. One half slice of a coronal section was copied once and mirrored then fixed to the original slice to mimic a coronal section through both halves of the brain. The slice was then copied again. (Data were taken from Reynolds et al. (1987))

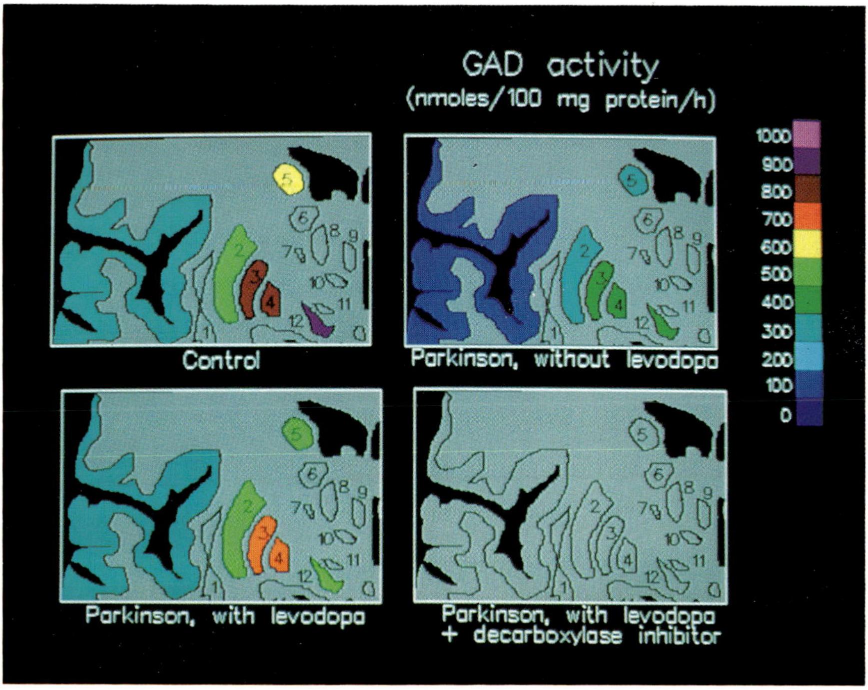

Fig. 3. Multiple copies of one slice of a coronal section were drawn and placed beside each other to allow comparison of a parameter within different groups within the same regions of the brain. GAD, glutamic acid decarboxylase; data were taken from Rinne et al. (1979)

Dyna Mouse GM-6000) with an easy to learn painting program. Different hard copies of coronal sections of human brain were drawn out of an anatomy book (Nieuwenhuys et al. 1987) on a transparency which then was fixed in front of the monitor. The mouse pointer was then turned to full brightness and contrast and the shapes of the regions were drawn by mouse. The frame to bring content into the form was made by a color bar. The 12 colors which represented specific values of the parameters were chosen from the 16 colors of the painting program.

The following examples demonstrate the abstraction of attributes (use of relative mode) and the determination of form and content (Fig. 1). The once digitalized form is easy to handle. One can cut out specific regions of interest, rotate/mirror a slice (Fig. 2), or make multiple copies for comparisons of different groups of patients or time series (Fig. 3).

Other advantages of this method are that regions which were of minor interest and appeared as white spots in the past are now high lighted. Crude preparations of regions can be readily improved by more skilled techniques.

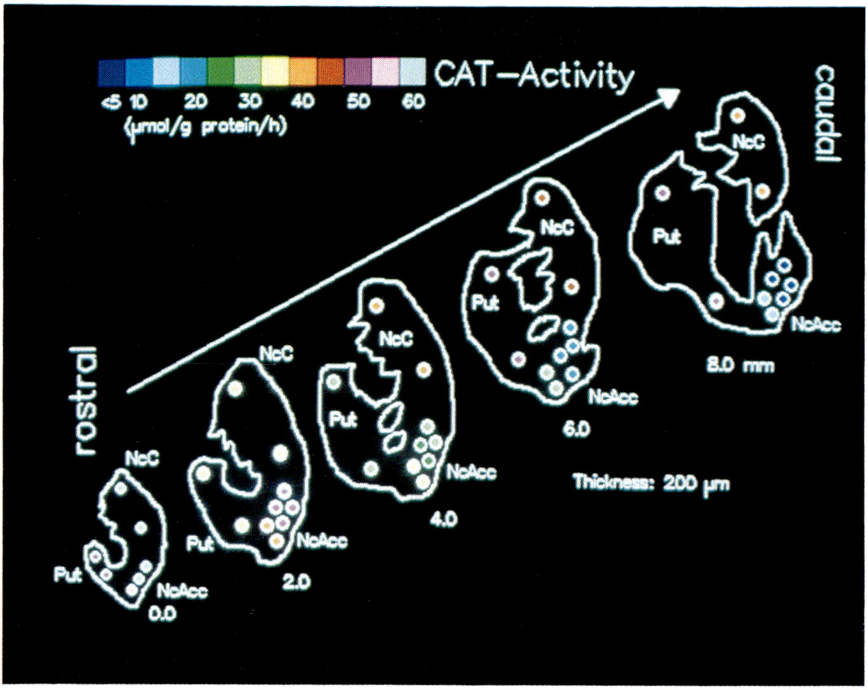

Fig. 4. Caudal-rostral distribution of choline acetyltransferase (CAT) activity in the striatum; slices of 200 µm thickness; assays for CAT activity were performed using a punch technique according to Kanazawa (1982)

For example, punch techniques, using serial slices, can be easily performed with this technique (Fig. 4).

Chemical and biochemical data from postmortem brain analyses will increase as long as new methods and their easy use succeed. We hope and believe that clearness in data presentation will help in a better understanding of the ever growing amount of data in complex systems like the brain.

References

Aquilonius S-M (1980) Cholinergic mechanisms in the CNS related to Parkinson's disease. In: Rinne UK, Klingler M, Stamm G (eds) Parkinson's disease – current progress, problems and management. Elsevier/North-Holland, Amsterdam

Kanazawa I (1982) The rostral-caudal distribution of choline acetyltransferase, glutamic acid decardoxylase and substance P in the human accumbens area. In: Pope A (ed) Human brain dissection. 3rd Human brain dissection meeting, Hall

Nieuwenhuys R, Voogd J, van Huijzen C (1987) The human central nervous system. A synopsis and atlas. Springer, Berlin Heidelberg New York

Reynolds GP, Czudek C, Bzowej N, Seeman P (1987) Dopamine receptor asymmetry in schizophrenia. Lancet 979

Rinne UK, Sonninen V, Laaksonen H (1979) Responses of brain neurochemistry to levodopa treatment in Parkinson's disease. Adv Neurol 24:259–274

Behavioral Imaging: The Neuropsychological Assessment*

R.C. Gur[1], A.J. Saykin, and R.E. Gur

Neuropsychological assessment is becoming an integral part of the workup of neurological disorders affecting the central nervous system and is used increasingly in psychiatry as well. This presents some potential benefits but there is also a danger in its indiscriminate use and overinterpretation. Here we will describe our attempts to integrate measures derived from neuropsychological assessment with measures of regional brain function using neuroimaging.

Neuropsychological Assessment: Linkage of Regional Brain Function to Behavioral Dimensions

Psychological testing is already incorporated in the process of psychiatric evaluation, including measurement of intellectual functioning, such as tests intelligence; personality assessment, such as the Minnesota Multiphasic Personality Inventory (MMPI) and Thematic Apperception Test (TAT), and evaluation of intrapsychic conflicts, such as the Rorschach and other projective techniques. Neuropsychological assessment will include many of the same measurements. For example, a battery of neuropsychological tests will usually include several subscales from the standard intelligence tests and may overlap several other tools used for personality assessment and other behavioral functions.

The defining characteristic of neuropsychological assessment is that each behavioral measure derived from the testing is linked to brain function. Thus, when a subscale of an intelligence test is given, the purpose is not to assess an individual's intellectual endowment but because performance on this subscale has been linked to regional brain function. For example, performance on the Block Design subscale of the Wechsler Adult Intelligence Test (WAIS) is impaired in patients with right hemispheric lesions, particularly in posterior regions of the brain (e.g., Goodglass and Kaplan 1983).

* This investigation was supported by NIMH grants MH-43880, MH-42191, and MH-00586.

[1] Department of Psychiatry, 10th floor Gates Building, University of Pennsylvania, PA, USA

Imaging of the Brain in Psychiatry and Related Fields
Edited by K. Maurer

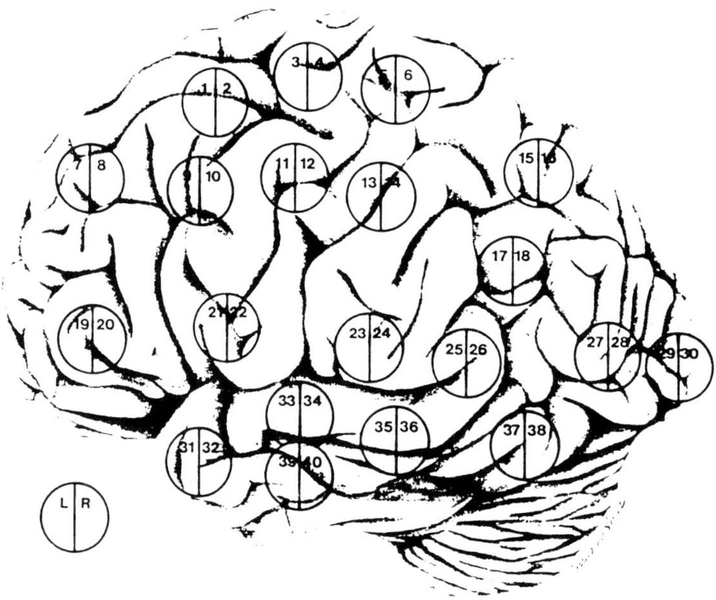

Fig. 1. The brain template used by the experts indicating location of regions of interest (ROIs). (From Gur et al. 1990a)

It is important to note that by this definition of neuropsychological tests some tests not currently linked to brain function could become so in the future. Indeed, most personality and psychodynamic tests are not considered neuropsychological because there is meager knowledge on how the brain regulates intrapsychic conflicts. Nonetheless, since the neuropsychological perspective views behavior as a product of brain processes, all behavioral measures can ultimately, in principle, be used in the neuropsychological assessment process.

The Behavioral Imaging Method

We will focus on a method proposed for topographic display of neuropsychological test scores so that the display reflects the integrity or impairment of brain regions as suggested by the pattern of performance. The method, which we called behavioral imaging (BI) (Gur et al. 1988a,b, 1990a; Trivedi and Gur 1987, 1989), uses an algorithm which joins observed scores with a weight table to produce values in a set of regions of interest (ROIs). The values reflect the probability that the observed pattern of deficits is associated with a lesion in that ROI. These values are determined by expert weightings indicating, for each performance measure, the sensitivity of each ROI to this measure. The following formula is used to calculate pixel intensity (Gur et al. 1988a):

$$Bj = \frac{\Sigma\ W(i,j)Si}{\Sigma\ W(i,j)}$$

where Bj is the index of behavioral functioning for a given region; $W(i,j)$ is the weight assigned to the jth brain region for the ith behavioral score; and Si is the test score.

The weights currently used were supplied by expert neuropsychologists (Drs. Arthur Benton, University of Iowa; Edith Kaplan, Boston University; Harvey Levin, University of Texas; and Andrew J. Saykin, University of Pennsylvania). These weights were obtained for each of 40 ROIs (20 homotopic regions in the two hemispheres, see Fig. 1), and from each expert twice, at 8–14 month intervals. The battery of tests and scores that were rated is shown in Table 1.

Reliability of Expert Weightings

There was substantial interexpert agreement and intraexpert reliability (Gur et al. 1990a). For interexpert agreement, the correlations of the 1720 theoretical weights (43 test scores × 20 ROIs × 2 hemispheres) were calculated between all pairs of experts (Table 2). Intraclass correlations (ICCs) were inappropriate because the "objects" being rated (brain-behavior relationships) are not independent of one another and so the ICC model does not describe these data. The highest correlation for both initial and 1 year ratings were between raters AJS and EK, while AB showed the lowest agreement with the other experts.

Inspection of the distribution of weights indicated that AB applied a trichotomous rating scheme (1, 5, or 10) while others used the entire range (from 1 to 10). This attenuated his estimate of agreement based on a product-moment correlation. Applying Sheppard's (1887) correction for grouping to the correlations between AB and the other experts improved the correlations somewhat. Furthermore, difference scores (AJS − EK, AJS − AB, etc.) indicated a modal difference of 0 (perfect agreement) for all experts (Fig. 2).

Intraexpert reliability correlations between the two sets of ratings were 0.64 (0.81 with Sheppard's correction), 0.79, 0.65, and 0.82 for AB, EK, HL, and AJS, respectively. These can be considered acceptable, particularly given the nature of the task and the time interval. Again, distribution of the difference scores (rating 1–rating 2) indicated a modal score of 0 for all experts (Fig. 3).

Table 1. Behavioral image core neuropsychological battery by function and score. (From Gur et al. 1990a)

Test	Scores obtained	Reference
Abstraction		
Wisconsin Card Sorting Test	Total perseverations Categories obtained	1
Modified Card Sort Test	Total perseverations Categories obtained	2
Verbal		
WAIS-R		
Information	Scaled score	3
Vocabulary		3
Spatial		
WAIS-R		
Block design	Scaled score	3
Judgment of line orientation	Total correct	4
Design fluency free condition	Total acceptable figures	5
Semantic memory		
Wechsler Memory Story Recall		6, 7
Immediate 30 min delay	Raw total	
Visual memory		
Wechsler Memory Design Reproduction		6
Immediate recall 30 min delay	Raw total	
Recognition of unfamiliar faces		8
Immediate 30 min delay	Number correct	
Verbal learning		
California Verbal Learning Test	Sum trials 1–5 Sum perseverations trials 1–5	9
Language		
First Name Fluency	Total output in 60 s	10
Animal Naming (Semantic Fluency)	Total output in 60 s	11
Controlled Oral Word Association (CFL)	Total output in 180 s	12
Sentence Repetition	Number correct	12
Boston Naming Test	Total correct	13
Verbal Comprehension		
Complex ideational material	Number correct	11
Token test	Total correct	12
Visual motor		
Trail making A	Time in seconds	14
Trail making B	Time in seconds	14
WAIS-R		
digit symbol	Scaled score	3

Table 1. Continued

Test	Scores obtained	Reference
Attention		
Continuous Performance Task		
Vigilance	Total correct	
Distractibility	Total correct	
WAIS-R		
Digit span	Scaled score	3
Levin 2–5 Auditory vigilance task	Total correct	16
Motor		
Fine Motor Speed		
Finger tapping (right and left hands)	Mean of 5 trials	14
Fine Motor Sequencing		
Thumb-finger sequential touch (right and left hands)	Total in 10 s	17
Sensory		
Graphesthesia (Right and left hands)	Total errors	14
Double simultaneous stimulation		
Tactile (right and left sides) Auditory (right and left ears) Visual (right and left sides)	Total suppressions	14

References: 1, Heaton (1981); 2, Nelson (1976); 3, Wechsler (1981); 4, Benton et al. (1983); 5, Jones-Gotman and Milner (1977); 6, Wechsler (1945); 7, Russell (1975); 8, Saykin (1982); 9, Delis et al. (1983); 10, Kaplan (1987); 11, Goodglass and Kaplan (1983); 12, Benton and Hamsher (1978); 13, Kaplan et al. (1978); 14, Reitan (1979); 15, Gordon (1988); 16, Levin (1987); 17, Christensen (1975)
WAIS-R, Wechsler Adult Intelligence Test, revised.

Table 2. Correlations – interexpert agreement. (From Gur et al. 1990a)

	Rating A			Rating B		
	Kaplan	Levin	Saykin	Kaplan	Levin	Saykin
Benton	0.33 (0.37)	0.36 (0.40)	0.34 (0.38)	0.39 (0.44)	0.34 (0.38)	0.31 (0.35)
Kaplan		0.55	0.64		0.47	0.74
Levin			0.62			0.53

Sheppard's correction for grouping in parentheses. All $p < 0.0001$.

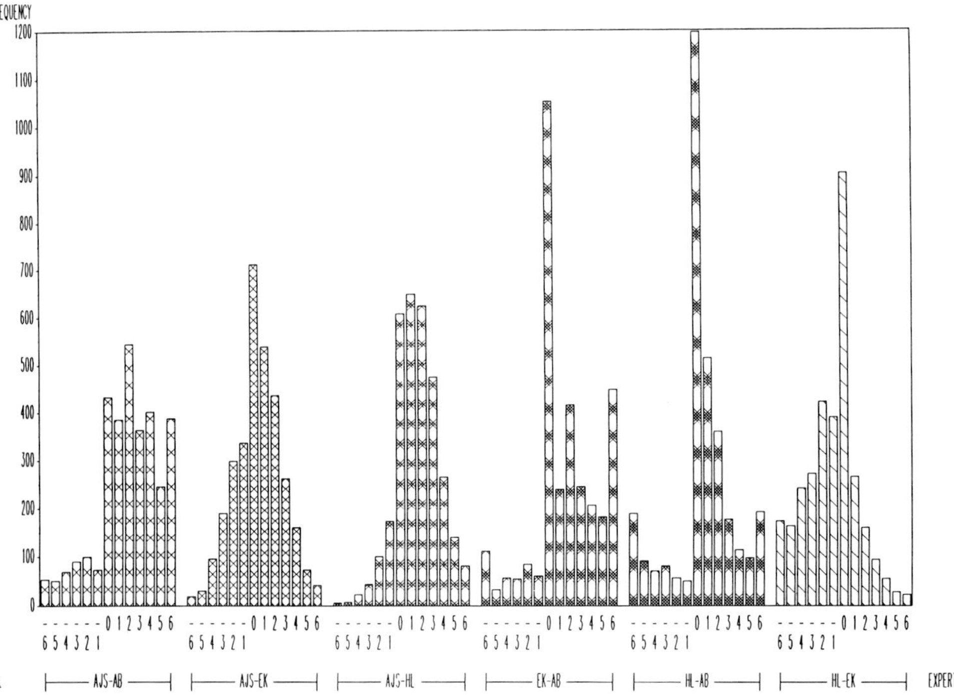
FREQUENCY
1200
1100
1000
900
800
700
600
500
400
300
200
100
0
- - - - - - 0 1 2 3 4 5 6
6 5 4 3 2 1
AJS-AB
AJS-EK
AJS-HL
EK-AB
HL-AB
HL-EK
EXPERT

A

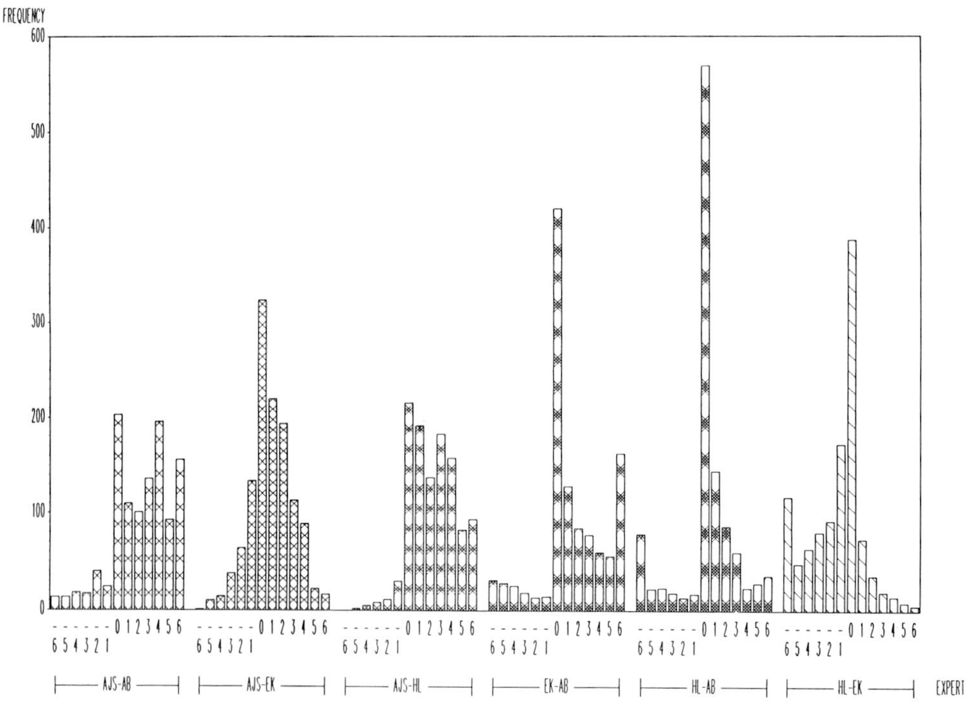
FREQUENCY
600
500
400
300
200
100
0
- - - - - - 0 1 2 3 4 5 6
6 5 4 3 2 1
AJS-AB
AJS-EK
AJS-HL
EK-AB
HL-AB
HL-EK
EXPERT

B

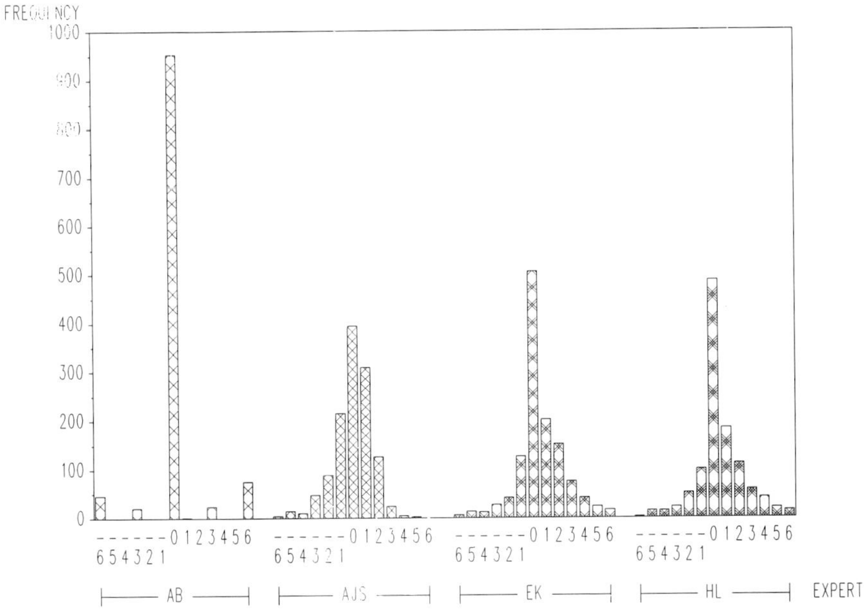

Fig. 3. Intraexpert reliability of ratings between initial (Time 1) and 1 year (Time 2) sessions. The *abscissa* shows the difference score between the two ratings for each expert (Time 1 − Time 2). As in Fig. 2, *0* reflects identical scores, *negative values* indicate higher ratings in Time 2 than Time 1, and *positive values* the opposite. The *ordinate* shows frequency of each difference score. (From Gur et al. 1990a)

Initial Validation Studies

Initial testing of the algorithm in clinical cases and populations was encouraging (Gur et al. 1988a,b). There was consistency between the behavioral images and the location of lesions in patients with unilateral cerebral infarcts (Fig. 4). The topographic displays showed correspondence with clinical, CT, and metabolic data and were congruent with the clinical interpretation of the neuropsychological assessment. Patients with focal ischemic lesions have been a major source of information on the validity of neurobehavioral theories. This is because of the circumscribed nature of

←

Fig. 2A,B. Interexpert agreement for the initial (**A**) and 1 year ratings (**B**). The *abscissa* shows the difference score for each pair of experts (EK-AB, EK's ratings minus AB's ratings, etc.), with *0* reflecting perfect agreement, *negative values* indicating that, e.g., EK's ratings are higher than AB's, and *positive values* reflecting the opposite for each expert pair. The *ordinate* shows frequency of each difference score. (From Gur et al. 1990a)

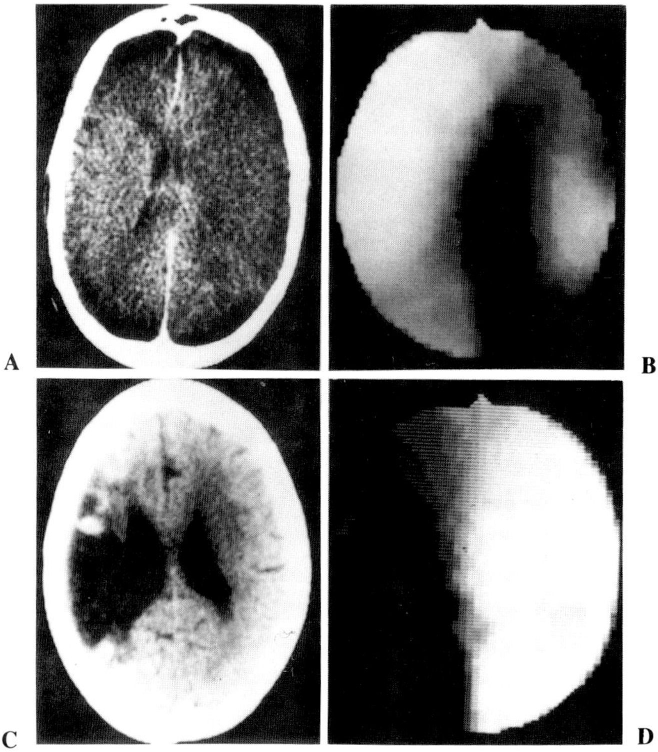

Fig. 4A–D. Computerized tomography (CT) scans and corresponding behavioral images of two patients with cerebral infarcts, one in the right hemisphere (**A** and **B** for CT and behavioral image, respectively) and one in the left (**C** and **D**). The CT scans show the left hemisphere is to the viewer's left. (From Gur et al. 1988a)

many infarcts and the tendency of such lesions to occur in adult, neurally mature, brains.

The potential of the algorithm was also evaluated in a sample of patients with hemiparkinsonism (Blonder et al. 1989; Gur et al. 1988b). The hypothesis of greater neurobehavioral deficits associated with the hemisphere ipsilateral to the side of striatal deficiency was evaluated quantitatively using this algorithm for averaged ROIs which were grouped into larger regions. As can be seen in Fig. 5, this hypothesis was supported.

We are currently evaluating the algorithm in other clinical populations with focal and diffuse brain disorders. Such data can help us to apply BI cautiously in psychiatric populations, in whom the location of regional brain dysfunction is not well circumscribed.

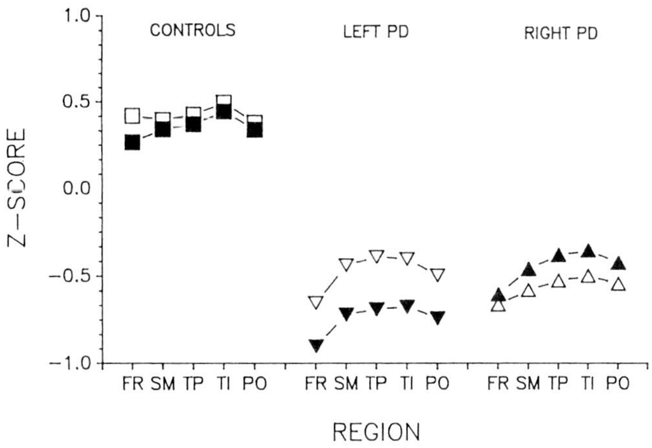

Fig. 5. Lobar neuropsychological values for hemiparkinson patients and controls produced by the behavioral imaging algorithm. Regions are frontal (*FR*), sensorimotor (*SM*), temporoparietal (*TP*), inferior temporal (*TI*), and parietooccipital (*PO*). Left hemisphere scores are *open symbols*; right hemisphere scores are *filled symbols*. (From Gur et al. 1988b)

Future Directions

The BI method has just passed the initial steps of verification and testing. Although we believe the specific criticisms of it by Yeo et al. (1990) are invalid (Gur et al. 1990b), alternative algorithms should be considered and developed. Other steps we are planning to improve the generalizability and utility of BI are:

1. Expand the range of experts to include experts in specific behavioral domains, such as memory and attention, who could provide more detailed specification of ROIs in the network of regions involved in regulating these functions. This may also result in revision of the neuropsychological core battery to contain tests that more specifically target components of behavioral functions.
2. Develop a three-dimensional version of weights.
3. Compare BI to results of other neuroimaging studies using anatomic measures or resting physiologic measures of regional brain function. The correspondence between BI and neuroanatomic measures will provide a first stage for testing the neurobehavioral hypotheses embedded in the theoretical weightings. Differences could be due to suppressed metabolic activity in the penumbra or remote regions (e.g., Kuhl et al. 1975). Residual differences will necessitate an additional revision of neuro-

psychological theory, and this can be done quantitatively by adjusting the weightings.

4. The correlation of BI with anatomic measures and resting physiologic measures will only give a limited power to testing hypotheses on brain behavior relationships. A more powerful tool is to use "neurobehavioral probes" (Gur et al., 1992) in conjunction with the physiologic measures; these results can be directly contrasted with BI. However, the available "library" of suitable neurobehavioral probes is extremely limited at present and much more work is needed in this area.
5. Finally, aside from its potential as a heuristic tool for hypothesis testing, BI may have clinical and didactic applications. Clinically it can convey in a simple and readily interpretable form results of complex integration of test scores with theoretical considerations. This can help both in an interdisciplinary context and compared to other neuroimaging data for diagnostic considerations. In this context BI can also help clarify regional distribution of dysfunction. In a didactic situation, students can be asked to generate interpretations of test scores and compare them to the results of BI. Alternatively, it would be a valuable educational experience to produce theoretical weights and test their adequacy against our experts and, most importantly, real data.

Acknowledgements. We thank Drs. Arthur Benton, Edith Kaplan, and Harvey Levin for their collaboration on the behavioral imaging project and D. Brian Kester, M.S. and Margaret Taleff, M.S. for their assistance.

References

Benton AL, Hamsher KdeS (1978) Multilingual aphasia examination. (Manual, revised). University of Iowa, Iowa City

Benton AL, Hamsher KdeS, Varney NR, Spreen O (1983) Contributions to neuropsychological assessment. Oxford University Press, New York

Blonder LX, Gur RE, Gur RC, Saykin AJ, Hurtig HI (1989) Neuropsychological functioning in hemiparkinsonism. Brain Cogn 9:177–190

Christensen A (1975) Luria's neuropsychological investigation. Spectrum, New York

Delis DC, Kramer JH, Kaplan EF, Ober BA (1983) California verbal learning test. Jovanovich, New York

Goodglass H, Kaplan E (1983) The assessment of aphasia and related disorders, 2nd edn. Lea and Febiger, Philadelphia

Gordon M (1988) The Gordon diagnostic system (Manual). Gordon, Dewitt

Gur RC, Trivedi SS, Saykin AJ, Gur RE (1988a) "Behavioral imaging" – a procedure for analysis and display of neuropsychological test scores: I. Construction of algorithm and initial clinical application. Neuropsychiatr Neuropsychol Behav Neurol 1:53–60

Gur RC, Saykin AJ, Blonder LX, Gur RE (1988b) "Behavioral imaging": II. Application of the quantitative algorithm to hypothesis testing in a population of hemiparkinsonian patients. Neuropsychiatr Neuropsychol Behav Neurol 1:87–96

Gur RC, Saykin AJ, Benton A, Kaplan E, Levin H, Kester DB, Gur RE (1990a) "Behavioral imaging": III. Inter-rater agreement and reliability of weightings. Neuropsychiatr Neuropsychol Behav Neurol 3:113–124

Gur RC, Saykin AJ, Muenz LR, Trivedi S, Gur RE (1990b) Response to Yeo et al.'s critique of behavioral imaging. Neuropsychiatr Neuropsychol Behav Neurol 3:304–312

Gur RC, Erwin RJ, Gur RE (1992) Neurobehavioral probes for physiologic neuroimaging studies. Arch Gen Psychiatry

Heaton RK (1981) Wisconsin card sorting test (Manual). Psychological Assessment Resources, Odessa

Jones-Gotman M, Milner B (1977) Design fluency: the invention of nonsense drawings after focal cortical lesions. Neuropsychologia 15:305–324

Kaplan EF (1987) First name fluency task. Unpublished test.

Kaplan EF, Goodglass H, Weintraub S (1978) The Boston naming test. Lea and Febiger, Philadelphia

Kuhl DE, Reivich M, Alavi A et al. (1975) Local cerebral blood volume determined by three-dimensional reconstruction of radionuclide scan data. Circ Res 36: 610–619

Levin H (1987) Auditory search task. Unpublished test.

Nelson HE (1976) A modified card sorting test sensitive to frontal lobe deficits. Cortex 12:313–324

Reitan R (1979) Manual for administration of neuropsychological test batteries for adults and children. Neuropsychological Laboratory, Tucson

Russell EW (1975) A multiple scoring method for assessment of complex memory functions. J Consult Clin Psychol 43:800–809

Saykin AJ (1982) Facial memory test. Unpublished test.

Sheppard WF (1887) A correction for grouping. Proc Lond Math Soc 29:353–380

Trivedi SS, Gur RC (1987) Computer graphics for neuropsychological data. Proc Natl Comput Graph Assoc 3:22–32

Trivedi SS, Gur RC (1989) Topographic mapping of cerebral blood flow and behavior. Comput Biol Med 19:219–229

Wechsler D (1945) A standardized memory scale for clinical use. J Psychol 19:87–95

Wechsler D (1981) Wechsler Adult Intelligence Scale–Revised (Manual). Harcourt Brace Jovanovich, New York

Yeo RA, Turkheimer E, Bigler ED (1990) Neuropsychological methods of localizing brain dysfunction: clinical versus empirical approaches. Neuropsychiatr Neuropsychol Behav Neurol 3:290–303

Topographical Variation of Equivalent EEG Generators During Cognitive Decline in Patients with Dementia of Alzheimer Type

T. Dierks[1], K. Maurer, L. Frölich, and R. Ihl

Introduction

Since Berger described the human EEG in 1929 (Berger 1929) clinicians as well as researchers have attempted to conceptualize electrical activity of the brain as a reflection of mental processes. Due to recent advances in computer software and hardware it is now possible to sample more electrical information from the brain and make the concept of the EEG as an electrical brain mirror tangible. However, the increasing amount of data make a sensible interpretation of the data difficult. One way to reduce data in a reasonable way is to calculate equivalent dipoles, which describe the electrical activity of the brain as one or more dipoles generating the electrical field over the surface of the scalp. The calculation of dipoles have mostly been accomplished in the time domain, for example, epileptic discharges or evoked potentials. For the investigation of psychiatric diseases, however, the analysis of frequency bands is of higher interest than an analysis of the time domain.

In 1989 Lehmann and Michel presented the FFT approximation as a simple and elegant method to calculate equivalent dipoles of frequency components of EEG. The FFT approximation allows an estimation of the intracranial representation of mental processes of the brain which generate the electrical fields measured upon the scalp. These equivalent dipoles are independent of the choice of reference. In the conventional reports of FFT power, variation of the reference will alter results (Lehmann and Michel 1989).

Whereas a number of studies have investigated the alterations of peak frequency and activity in different frequency bands in dementia of Alzheimer type (DAT), reports regarding topographical EEG alterations in patients with DAT are relatively sparse. The aim of the present study was, hence, to investigate by a confirmative statistical analysis whether topographical changes occur in various stages of cognitive decline in patients suffering from DAT.

[1] Abt. für Psychiatrie, Universitäts-Nervenklinik Würzburg, Füchsleinstr. 15, W-8700 Würzburg, FRG.

Imaging of the Brain in Psychiatry
and Related Fields
Edited by K. Maurer

Methods

We studied 35 patients suffering from probable DAT (19 women, 16 men, mean age ± standard deviation, 69 ± 11 years, age range from 42 to 83 years) in various stages of mental deterioration. All patients were right handed and only those who were not taking drugs influencing cerebral functions were included in the study. All patients fulfilled the criteria for probable DAT (McKhann et al. 1984). They were hospitalized for a period of 2–3 weeks for diagnostic evaluation. Diagnostic assessment included history, physical and neurological examination and routine laboratory tests (including thyroid hormone levels and vitamin B_{12} and folic acid). The modified Hachinski ischemic score (score < 4) (Rosen et al. 1984) was used to exclude multi-infarct dementia. Further selection was based on computed tomography (CT) scans in all patients who showed only cerebral atrophy, ventricular dilatation, and no more than one lacunar infarction, if abnormal. In no case were there territorial infarctions. In most patients, single photon emission computed tomography with ^{99m}Tc hexamethylpropylene-amine-oxime (HMPAO-SPECT) was performed and did not reveal signs of multi-focal flow deficits. Typically, temporoparietal and/or frontal flow deficits were found (Froelich et al. 1989). All patients were investigated with a battery of neuropsychological tests for cognitive function, language, apraxia, agnosia, visospatial abilities, mood, and behavioral changes. The stage of mental impairment was assessed by means of Mini Mental Status Examination (MMS; Folstein et al. 1975), the Brief Cognitive Rating Scale (BCRS; Reisberg et al. 1983), the Short Syndrome Test (SKT; Erzigkeit 1986), and the Alzheimer Disease Assessment Scale (ADAS; Mohs and Cohen 1988). The patients were divided into three groups of severity on the basis of their BCRS scores: (1) slight degree of dementia; BCRS < 29 ($n = 11$), (2) moderate degree of dementia; BCRS 29–39 ($n = 14$), and (3) severe degree of dementia; BCRS > 39 ($n = 10$).

Electrodes were applied to the scalp according to the international 10–20 system. The EEGs were recorded using a channel Bio-Logic Brain Atlas III Plus with linked mastoids as reference. The EEG was sampled with a rate of 128 Hz per channel and stored onto magnetic disks for further analysis off-line; however, before AD conversion the EEG was filtered analogous with a band pass of 1–30 Hz. Overall amplification was 20 000 times. Care was taken to keep the subjects in a stable state of vigilance. For data analysis the first ten successive artifact-free 2-s epochs, 20-s after eyes were closed, were selected from the off-line stored EEG.

Data Processing

Fast Fourier analysis were done on each 2-s epoch, multiplied with a Hamming window. The resulting sine and cosine coefficients for each

Table 1. Correlations between psychometric scales and dipole-strength in frequencybands, fronto-occipital localization of the equivalent dipole, and the peak frequency

	Delta	Theta	Alpha	Beta1
Dipole strength				
BCRS	0.15	0.26	−0.36*	−0.23
SKT	0.34*	0.47**	−0.19	−0.10
MMS	−0.27	−0.26	0.37*	0.19
ADAS	0.35*	0.47**	−0.24	−0.17
Tronto-occipital localization for equivalent dipole				
BCRS	0.03	0.01	0.24	0.31*
SKT	0.01	−0.09	0.28	0.47**
MMS	−0.04	0.08	−0.21	0.46**
ADAS	0.05	−0.09	0.33*	0.43**
Peak frequency				
BCRS	−0.41**			
SKT	−0.42**			
MMS	0.38*			
ADAS	−0.29			

BCRS, Brief Cognitive Rating Scale; SKT, Short Syndrome Test; MMS, Mini Mental Status Examination; ADAS, Alzheimer Disease Assessment Scale.

electrode and each frequency point (0.5 Hz resolution) were placed into a sine–cosine diagram (Norcia et al. 1985). Through the FFT constellation a best-fit straight line is placed, onto which the entries are orthogonally projected. The projections on the line describes a map of potential distribution which is used for single source dipole estimation (Lehmann and Michel 1989, 1990). For each frequency point in the FFT approximation a localization was calculated with three resulting parameters: 1, right–left (x = transversal) localization; 2, frontal–occipital (y = saggital) localization; 3, depth of the source (z).

For statistical purposes, the data was reduced into frequency bands. A mean localization of the equivalent dipole was calculated for delta (1–3.5 Hz), theta (4–7.5 Hz), alpha (8–11.5 Hz), betal (12–15.5 Hz), beta2 (16–19.5 Hz), and beta3 (20–23.5 Hz). For statistical evaluation an analysis of variance was used. Furthermore, linear correlations between localization of the frequency bands and degree of cognitive deterioration (by the various psychometric tests) was calculated.

Results

For each subject the frequency was calculated where the equivalent dipole reached its maximum (peak frequency). There was a clear correlation

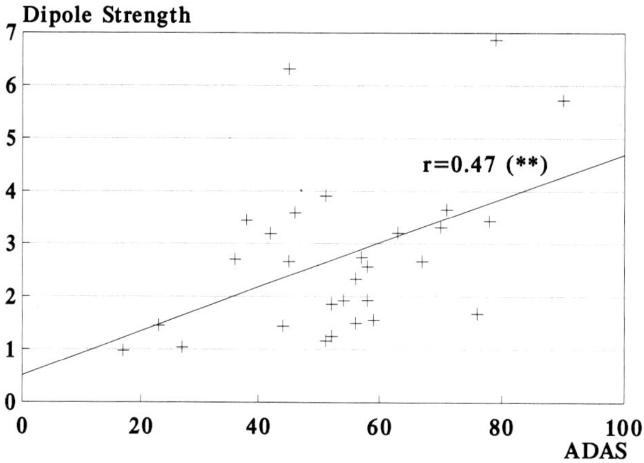

Fig. 1. Theta band (4–7.5 Hz). Plot of the association between strength of dipole (y, μV) and cognitive decline (x, score) measured by the Alzheimer Disease Assessment Scale (*ADAS*)

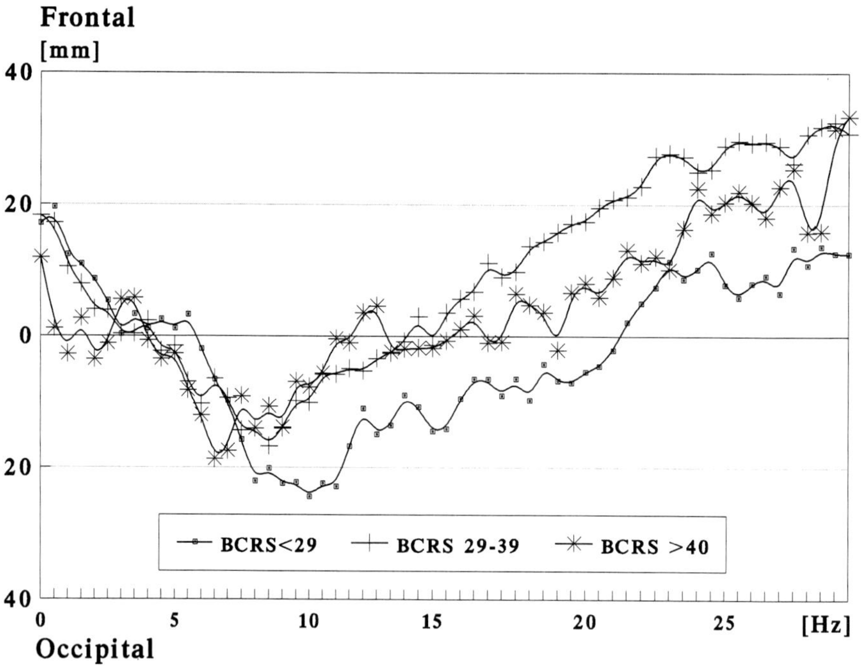

Fig. 2. Mean localization in the three subgroups of demented patients in 0.5-Hz steps in fronto-occipital direction of the calculated single equivalent dipole

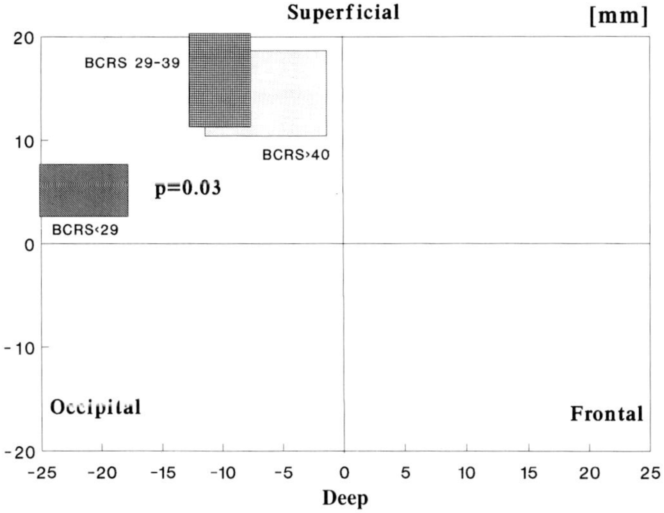

Fig. 3. Alpha band (8–11.5 Hz). Mean localization (± standard error) of alpha activity in two dimensions (frontal-occipital and superficial-deep direction) for the three subgroups. *BCRS*, Brief Cognitive Rating Scale

between peak frequency and cognitive decline (e.g., with BCRS; $r = -0.41$; $p < 0.01$; Table 1). With regard to left–right localization, no correlation to psychometric tests could be found. The strength of the theta band exhibited a positive correlation with increasing cognitive decline (e.g., with ADAS; $r = 0.47$; $p < 0.01$; Fig. 1, Table 1). An adverse effect could be seen regarding the alpha-strength, where an increasing cognitive impairment correlated with a decrease of strength (e.g., with MMS; $r = 0.37$; $p < 0.05$; Table 1). In fronto-occipital direction neither the delta band nor the theta band showed a significant correlation with any psychometric scale. On the other hand, the alpha and the beta bands demonstrated a positive correlation between severity of cognitive decline and frontal localization of the equivalent dipole (Table 1). Concerning the superficial direction only the beta bands showed a significant correlation, in the sense that decreased cognitive capability correlated with a more superficially localized equivalent source. With respect to localization in fronto-occipital direction, the slightly demented showed the maximal occipitally localized equivalent dipole at 10.0 Hz, the moderately demented group at 8.5 Hz, and the severely demented group at 6.5 Hz (Fig. 2). Concerning the localization in two dimensions (fronto-occipital and superficial) for the alpha band, in the slightly demented patients they were significantly more occipital and deeply localized compared to the moderately and severely demented group ($p <$ 0.05; Fig. 3). The two latter-mentioned groups did not show a significant difference in localization of the equivalent dipole in the two dimensions.

Discussion

Summarizing our investigation, we showed (a) a decrease of dipole strength, (b) a move of the equivalent dipole of alpha and beta activity towards frontal regions, and (c) a slowing of the EEG with increasing cognitive deterioration.

Our results regarding the strength of a dipole may be compared to studies which have investigated the activity of frequency bands with the help of conventional FFT results. A number of investigations have described increased slow wave activity with increasing cognitive deterioration (Coben et al. 1983; Penttilä et al. 1985; Brenner et al. 1986). This is analogous to our finding of a positive correlation between equivalent dipole strength in the theta band and mental deterioration. Similar holds true for the alpha band where several authors have described decreased activity with increasing cognitive decline, comparable to our finding of reduced dipole strength in the alpha band with increasing mental deterioration (Letemendia and Pampligione 1958; Gordon and Sim 1967).

Studies investigating topographical changes of electrical activity in relation to severity of cognitive deterioration are few. Breslau et al. (1989) reported a change towards increased beta activity over central regions in aged normals compared to younger ones, but did not comment on findings in their DAT population with cognitive impairment. Ihl et al. (1988) found a stage-dependent decrease of beta activity in temporo-parietal regions. In our own study where we investigated the topography of the peak frequency, we found a clear anteriorization of the peak frequency in demented patients; however, no correlation was found between anteriorizing of peak frequency and degree of dementia (Dierks et al. 1991). Our finding of anteriorization of the beta dipole may be interpreted as an increased vulnerability of parieto-temporal and occipital regions, with normal beta activity maintained in frontal regions for a longer duration. Significant correlations between the localization of the equivalent dipole of the alpha band in frontal direction and neuropsychological testing, also reported for conventional alpha activity in occipital region with MMS by Primavera et al. (1990), supports this hypothesis.

The strength in the FFT approximation lies in its ability to reduce multichannel data into few parameters, which allows a comfirmative conservative statistical evaluation of topographical differences between groups. On the other hand, one should not be led to believe that the resulting single equivalent dipoles shows the exact localization of anatomical structures which are generating the surface potential. It should be considered as the sum of all neuronal processes which are simultaneously active and are generating the potential measured upon the scalp. Nevertheless, the statistical difference between groups in localization of the calculated single equivalent dipole allows the conclusion that different localized neuronal structures have been active in the various groups.

The clinical advantages of the present method are, as for the EEG, obvious: noninvasiveness, ease of measurement, possibility of follow-up, and low cost. Thus, a tool for a sensible objective quantification of cognitive impairment in patients with Alzheimer disease may be available.

References

Berger H (1929) On the electroencephalogram of man. Arch Psychiatr Nervenkr 87:527–570

Brenner RP, Ulrich RF, Spiker DG et al. (1986) Computerized EEG spectral analysis in elderly normal, demented and depressed subjects. Electroencephalogr Clin Neurophysiol 64:483–492

Breslau J, Starr A, Sicotte N, Higa J, Buchsbaum MS (1989) Topographic EEG changes with normal aging and SDAT. Electroencephalogr Clin Neurophysiol 72:281–289

Coben LA, Danziger WL, Berg L (1983) Frequency analysis of the resting awake EEG in mild senile dementia of Alzheimer type. Electroencephalogr Clin Neurophysiol 55:372–380

Dierks T, Perisic I, Frölich L, Ihl R, Maurer K (1991) Topography of the quantitative electroencephalogram in dementia of the Alzheimer type: Relation to severity of dementia. Psychiatry Res 40:181–194

Erzigkeit H (1986) Manual zum SKT Formen A-E (Ein Kurztest zur Erfassung von Aufmerksamkeits- und Gedächnisstörungen). Vless, Ebersberg

Folstein MF, Folstein SE, McHugh PR (1975) "Mini-mental state", a practical method for grading the cognitive state of patients for the clinician. J Psychiatr Res 12:189–198

Froelich L, Eilles C, Ihl R, Maurer K, Lanczik M (1989) Stage-dependent reductions of regional blood flow measured by HMPAO-SPECT in dementia of Alzheimer type. Psychiatry Res 29:347–350

Gordon EB, Sim M (1967) The EEG in presenile dementia. J Neurol Neurosurg Psychiatry 30:285–291

Ihl R, Froelich L, Maurer K, Dierks T, Perisic I (1988) Electrical activity and degree of cognitive impairment in dementia of alzheimer-type. Brain Topogr 1/2:146 (abstr)

Lehmann D, Michel CM (1989) Intracerebral dipole sources of EEG FFT power maps. Brain Topogr 2:155–164

Lehmann D, Michel CM (1990) Intracerebral dipole source localization for FFT power maps. Electroencephalogr Clin Neurophysiol 76:271–276

Letemendia F, Pampligione G (1958) Clinical and electroencephalographic observations in Alzheimer's disease. J Neurol Neurosurg Psychiatry 21:167–172.

McKhann G, Drachman D, Folstein M, Katzman R, Price D, Stadlan EM (1984) Clinical diagnosis of Alzheimer's disease: report of NINCDS-ADRDA work group under the auspices of department of health and human services task force on Alzheimer's disease. Neurology 34:939–944

Mohs RC, Cohen L (1988) Alzheimer's disease assessment scale (ADAS). Psychopharmacol Bull 24/4:627–628

Norcia AM, Sutter EE, Tyler CW (1985) Electrophysiological evidence for the existence of coarse and fine disparity mechanism in human. Vision Res 25: 1603–1611

Penttilä M, Partanen JV, Soininen H, Riekkinen PJ (1985) Quantitative analysis of occipital EEG in different stages of Alzheimer's disease. Electroencephalogr Clin Neurophysiol 60:1–6

Primavera A, Novello P, Finocchi C, Canevari E, Corsello L (1990) Correlation between mini-mental state examination and quantitative electroencephalography in senile dementia of Alzheimer type. Neuropsychobiology 23:74–78
Reisberg B, London E, Ferris SH, Borenstein BA, Scheler L, de Leon MJ (1983) The brief cognitive rating scale: language, motoric, and mood concomitans in primary degenerative dementia. Psychopharmacol Bull 19/4:702–708
Rosen WG, Mohs RC, Davies KL (1984) A new rating scale for Alzheimer's disease. Am J Psychiatry 14:1356–1364

Subject Index